REFERENCE EDITION

Pediatric ESAP™ 2025-2026

Endocrine Society's
Pediatric Endocrine Self-Assessment Program
Questions, Answers, and Discussions

Liuska M. Pesce, MD, Co-Chair
Clinical Professor
Pediatric Thyroid Clinic Director
Stead Family Children's Hospital
Division of Pediatric Endocrinology and Diabetes
University of Iowa Carver College of Medicine

Ryan S. Miller, MD, Co-Chair
Clinical Associate Professor
George Washington School of Medicine
and Health Sciences

Sasigarn A. Bowden, MD
Professor of Pediatrics
Nationwide Children's Hospital
The Ohio State University

Li Chan, MD
Reader in Molecular Endocrinology
and Metabolism
Honorary Consultant in
Paediatric Endocrinology
Centre for Endocrinology
William Harvey Research Institute

Andrew Dauber, MD, MMSc
Professor of Pediatrics
George Washington University
School of Medicine and Health Sciences
Chief of Endocrinology,
Children's National Hospital

Cem S. Demirci, MD
Director, Type 1 Diabetes Program
Connecticut Children's Medical Center

Evgenia A. Gourgari, MD
Associate Professor of Pediatrics
Georgetown University

Colin P. Hawkes, MB BCh BAO, MD, PhD
Associate Professor of Pediatrics
University College Cork
Perelman School of Medicine
University of Pennsylvania

Shana McCormack, MD
Assistant Professor of Pediatrics
Children's Hospital of Philadelphia

Siobhan Pittock, MB, BAO, BCH
Pediatric Endocrinologist
Mayo Clinic

Sripriya Raman, MD
Pediatric Endocrinologist
K S Pediatrics

Kyriakie Sarafoglou, MD
Professor
Department of Pediatrics-Divisions of
Endocrinology and Genetics & Metabolism
Department of Experimental
& Clinical Pharmacology
University of Minnesota
Director, Center for Congenital
Adrenal Hyperplasia
MHealth Masonic Children's Hospital

Christine Trapp, MD
Pediatric Endocrinology,
Connecticut Children's Medical Center
Associate Fellowship Director,
Pediatric Endocrinology
Assistant Professor of Pediatrics,
University of Connecticut
School of Medicine

Halley Wasserman, MD
Associate Professor
Cincinnati Children's Hospital
Medical Center

Ari Wassner, MD
Medical Director, Thyroid Center
Director, Endocrinology
Fellowship Training Program
Associate Professor of Pediatrics
Boston Children's Hospital
Harvard Medical School

Abbie L. Young, MS, CGC, ELS(D)
Medical Editor

Endocrine Society
2055 L Street NW, Suite 600, Washington, DC 20036
1-888-ENDOCRINE • www.endocrine.org

ENDOCRINE SOCIETY
Hormone Science to Health

ENDOCRINE SOCIETY
Hormone Science to Health

The Endocrine Society is the world's largest, oldest, and most active organization working to advance the clinical practice of endocrinology and hormone research. Founded in 1916, the Society now has more than 18,000 global members across a range of disciplines. The Society has earned an international reputation for excellence in the quality of its peer-reviewed journals, educational resources, meetings, and programs that improve public health through the practice and science of endocrinology.

For between-edition updates, visit us at:
endocrine.org/education-and-training/book-updates

Other publications:
endocrine.org/publications

ISBN: 978-1-936704-64-4

OVERVIEW

The Pediatric Endocrine Self-Assessment Program (Pediatric ESAP™) is a self-study curriculum specifically designed for endocrinologists seeking initial certification or recertification in pediatric endocrinology, program directors interested in a training instrument, and clinicians seeking a self-assessment and a broad review of pediatric endocrinology. Pediatric ESAP consists of 100 multiple-choice questions in all areas of pediatric endocrinology, diabetes, growth, and metabolism. There is extensive discussion of each correct answer and references.

Pediatric ESAP is composed of two key components: the online interactive module and the printed book. Upon purchase, learners initially receive access to the online module. To use Pediatric ESAP as a true self-assessment tool, learners are strongly encouraged to complete the online interactive self-assessment module first before continuing self-study with the printed book; the online module may be accessed at education.endocrine.org.

LEARNING OBJECTIVES

Pediatric ESAP 2025-2026 allows learners to assess their knowledge of all aspects of pediatric endocrinology. Upon completion of this educational activity, participants will be able to:

- Recognize clinical manifestations of pediatric endocrine, growth, and metabolic disorders and select among current options for diagnosis, management, and therapy.
- Identify risk factors for endocrine and metabolic disorders in pediatric patients and develop strategies for prevention.
- Evaluate pediatric endocrine and metabolic manifestations of systemic disorders.
- Use current, evidence-based clinical guidelines and treatment recommendations to guide diagnosis and treatment of pediatric endocrine and metabolic disorders.

TARGET AUDIENCE

Pediatric ESAP is a self-study curriculum aimed at physicians seeking initial certification or recertification in endocrinology, program directors interested in a testing and training instrument, and clinicians simply wanting a self-assessment and broad review of endocrinology.

STATEMENT OF INDEPENDENCE

The Endocrine Society has a policy of ensuring that the content and quality of this educational activity are balanced, independent, objective, and scientifically rigorous. The scientific content of this activity was developed under the supervision of the Endocrine Society's Pediatric ESAP Faculty Working Group.

DISCLOSURE POLICY

The faculty, committee members, and staff who are in position to control the content of this activity are required to disclose to the Endocrine Society and to learners any relevant financial relationship(s) of the individual or spouse/partner that have occurred within the last 12 months with any commercial interest(s) whose products or services are related to the content. Financial relationships are defined by remuneration in any amount from the commercial interest(s) in the form of grants; research support; consulting fees; salary; ownership interest (eg, stocks, stock options, or ownership interest excluding diversified mutual funds); honoraria or other payments for participation in speakers' bureaus, advisory boards, or boards of directors; or other financial benefits. The intent of this disclosure is not to prevent planners with relevant financial relationships from planning or delivering content, but rather to provide learners with information that allows them to make their own judgments of whether these financial relationships may have influenced the educational activity with regard to exposition or conclusion. The Endocrine Society has reviewed all disclosures and resolved or managed all identified conflicts of interest, as applicable.

The following faculty reported relevant financial relationship(s): **Sasigarn Bowden, MD**, is an advisory board member of Alexion. **Li Chan, MD**, is an advisory board member of OMass Therapeutics and Great Ormond Street Hospital Children's Charity Research. **Andrew Dauber, MD**, is an advisory board member of Ascendis, BioMarin, BridgeBio, Novo Nordisk, and Pfizer. He serves as a consultant for Novo Nordisk and Tyra Pharmaceuticals. He is also a grant recipient from BioMarin and Pfizer. **Shana McCormack, MD**, is an NIH grantee and grant reviewer. She is a grantee of the Doris Duke Charitable Foundation and the Friedreich Ataxia Research Alliance. She is a consultant for Rhythm Pharmaceuticals and Reata Pharmaceuticals. She is also a principal investigator for Rhythm Pharmaceuticals and Aegerion. **Ryan S. Miller, MD**, is an NIH grantee and a consultant for Novo Nordisk. **Kyriakie Sarafoglou, MD**, receives research support from the Office of Orphan Products Development of the Food and Drug Administration, National Institutes of Health, Neurocrine Biosciences, Spruce Biosciences, Crinetics Pharmaceuticals, Adrenas Therapeutics (BridgeBio), Alexion Pharmaceuticals, and BioMarin Pharmaceutical. She serves as a consultant for Novo Nordisk, Eton Pharmaceuticals, Neurocrine Biosciences, Spruce Biosciences, and Crinetics Pharmaceuticals on behalf of the University of Minnesota but does not receive personal income for these activities. **Christine Trapp, MD**, is an advisory panel member for Rhythm Pharmaceuticals. **Ari Wassner, MD**, is a topic peer reviewer for UpToDate (thyroid).

The following faculty reported no relevant financial relationships: **Cem S. Demirci, MD**; **Evgenia Gourgari, MD**; **Colin Hawkes, MB BCh BAO, MD, PhD**; **Liuska M. Pesce, MD**; **Siobhan Pittock, MB, BAO, BCH**; **Sripriya Raman, MD**; and **Halley Wasserman, MD**.

The medical editor for this program, **Abbie L. Young, MS, CGC, ELS(D)**, reported no relevant financial relationships.

The Endocrine Society staff associated with the development of this program reported no relevant financial relationships.

DISCLAIMERS

The information presented in this activity represents the opinion of the faculty and is not necessarily the official position of the Endocrine Society.

USE OF PROFESSIONAL JUDGMENT:

The educational content in this self-assessment test relates to basic principles of diagnosis and therapy and does not substitute for individual patient assessment based on the health care provider's examination of the patient and consideration of laboratory data and other factors unique to the patient. Standards in medicine change as new data become available.

DRUGS AND DOSAGES:

When prescribing medications, the physician is advised to check the product information sheet accompanying each drug to verify conditions of use and to identify any changes in drug dosage schedule or contraindications.

POLICY ON UNLABELED/OFF-LABEL USE

The Endocrine Society has determined that disclosure of unlabeled/off-label or investigational use of commercial product(s) is informative for audiences and therefore requires this information to be disclosed to the learners at the beginning of the presentation. Uses of specific therapeutic agents, devices, and other products discussed in this educational activity may not be the same as those indicated in product labeling approved by the Food and Drug Administration (FDA). The Endocrine Society requires that any discussions of such "off-label" use be based on scientific research that conforms to generally accepted standards of experimental design, data collection, and data analysis. Before recommending or prescribing any therapeutic agent or device, learners should review the complete prescribing information, including indications, contraindications, warnings, precautions, and adverse events.

ACKNOWLEDGMENT OF COMMERCIAL SUPPORT

This activity is not supported by educational grant(s) or other funds from any commercial supporter.

PUBLICATION DATE: March 2025

Common Abbreviations Used in Pediatric ESAP

ACTH ---------- corticotropin
ACE inhibitor ---------- angiotensin-converting enzyme inhibitor
ALT ---------- alanine aminotransferase
AST ---------- aspartate aminotransferase
BMI ---------- body mass index
CNS ---------- central nervous system
CT ---------- computed tomography
DHEA ---------- dehydroepiandrosterone
DHEA-S ---------- dehydroepiandrosterone sulfate
DNA ---------- deoxyribonucleic acid
DPP-4 inhibitor ---------- dipeptidyl-peptidase 4 inhibitor
DXA ---------- dual-energy x-ray absorptiometry
FDA ---------- Food and Drug Administration
FGF-23 ---------- fibroblast growth factor 23
FNA ---------- fine-needle aspiration
FSH ---------- follicle-stimulating hormone
GH ---------- growth hormone
GHRH ---------- growth hormone–releasing hormone
GLP-1 receptor agonist ---------- glucagonlike peptide 1 receptor agonist
GnRH ---------- gonadotropin-releasing hormone
hCG ---------- human chorionic gonadotropin
HDL ---------- high-density lipoprotein
HIV ---------- human immunodeficiency virus
HMG-CoA reductase inhibitor ---------- 3-hydroxy-3-methylglutaryl coenzyme A reductase inhibitor
IGF-1 ---------- insulinlike growth factor 1
LDL ---------- low-density lipoprotein
LH ---------- luteinizing hormone
MCV ---------- mean corpuscular volume
MIBG ---------- *meta*-iodobenzylguanidine
MRI ---------- magnetic resonance imaging
NPH insulin ---------- neutral protamine Hagedorn insulin
PCSK9 inhibitor ---------- proprotein convertase subtilisin/kexin 9 inhibitor
PET ---------- positron emission tomography
PSA ---------- prostate-specific antigen
PTH ---------- parathyroid hormone
PTHrP ---------- parathyroid hormone–related protein
SGLT-2 inhibitor ---------- sodium-glucose cotransporter 2 inhibitor
SHBG ---------- sex hormone–binding globulin
T_3 ---------- triiodothyronine
T_4 ---------- thyroxine
TPO antibodies ---------- thyroperoxidase antibodies
TRH ---------- thyrotropin-releasing hormone
TRAb ---------- TSH-receptor antibodies
TSH ---------- thyrotropin
VLDL ---------- very low-density lipoprotein

QUESTIONS

PEDIATRIC ENDOCRINE SELF-ASSESSMENT PROGRAM 2025-2026

Part I

1 A 9-year-old boy born to consanguineous parents presents with poor oral intake and vomiting for 3 days. He was born via a normal vaginal delivery at term, with a birth weight of 7 lb, 11.5 oz (3500 g). There were no complications during pregnancy. His brother has a diagnosis of autoimmune Addison disease diagnosed at age 5 years (detectable antiadrenal antibodies).

On physical examination, he has enamel dysplasia and hyperpigmentation. His height and weight are between the 10th and 25th percentiles.

Laboratory test results:

Sodium = 133.0 mEq/L (135.0-145.0 mEq/L) (SI: 133 mmol/L [135.0-145.0 mmol/L])
Potassium = 4.7 mEq/L (3.5-5.5 mEq/L) (SI: 4.7 mmol/L [3.5-5.5 mmol/L])
Calcium = 9.6 mg/dL (8.8-10.8 mg/dL) (SI: 2.4 mmol/L [2.2-2.7 mmol/L])
Phosphate = 5.5 mg/dL (3.9-5.8 mg/dL) (SI: 1.8 mmol/L [1.3-1.9 mmol/L])
PTH = 61.7 pg/mL (15-65 pg/mL) (SI: 6.5 pmol/L [1.6-6.9 pmol/L])
Glucose = 95 mg/dL (70-110 mg/dL) (SI: 5.3 mmol/L [3.9-6.1 mmol/L])
TSH = 1.67 mIU/L (0.35-4.94 mIU/L)
Total T_3 = 121 ng/dL (58-159 ng/dL) (SI: 1.86 nmol/L [0.89-2.45 nmol/L])
Free T_4 = 1.10 ng/dL (0.70-1.48 ng/dL) (SI: 14.2 pmol/L [9.0-19.0 pmol/L])
ACTH = 1182.0 pg/mL (7.2-63.3 pg/mL) (SI: 260.0 pmol/L [1.6-13.9 pmol/L])
Cortisol = <0.4 μg/dL (6.7-22.6 μg/dL) (SI: 11.0 nmol/L [184.8-623.5 nmol/L])
Renin = 2.9 ng/mL per h (0.5-3.3 ng/mL per h)
Aldosterone = 7.5 ng/dL (4.0-48.0 ng/dL) (SI: 208.1 pmol/L [111.0-1331.5 pmol/L])
17-Hydroxyprogesterone = 6 ng/dL (11-108 ng/dL) (SI: 0.18 nmol/L [0.33-3.27 nmol/L])

Which of the following conditions most likely explains this patient's adrenal insufficiency?

A. Autoimmune polyglandular syndrome type 1
B. Autoimmune polyglandular syndrome type 2
C. IPEX syndrome (immune dysregulation, polyendocrinopathy, enteropathy, X-linked)
D. Sphingosine phosphate lyase insufficiency syndrome
E. X-linked adrenoleukodystrophy

2 An 11-year-old girl is referred for evaluation of short stature. Her growth chart shows her height following the 10th percentile through 4 years of age, but her height is now well below the 1st percentile. She has a history of mild developmental delays and attention-deficit/hyperactivity disorder that has been treated with a stimulant medication for the past 3 years. She wears glasses for distance vision and has follow-up care with a neurologist for chronic headaches. Midparental height is 63.5 in (161.3 cm) (40th percentile).

Physical examination findings are normal. She is prepubertal and has no notable neurological findings and no cardiac murmurs. Her height is 47.4 in (120.4 cm) (<1st percentile), and BMI is normal.

Laboratory test results:

Complete blood cell count, normal
Complete metabolic panel, normal
IGF-1 = 158 ng/mL (91-610 ng/mL) (SI: 20.7 nmol/L [11.9-79.9 nmol/L])
TSH = 3.43 mIU/L (0.45-4.5 mIU/L)
Free T_4 = 1.41 ng/dL (0.93-1.60 ng/dL) (SI: 18.1 pmol/L [12.0-20.6 pmol/L])

On karyotype analysis, 4 metaphases show a 45,X karyotype and 16 metaphases show 1 normal X and a ring chromosome.

Which of the following is needed to determine the next step in this patient's care?

A. Cardiac MRI
B. Chromosomal microarray
C. DXA
D. Pelvic ultrasonography
E. *SRY* fluorescence in situ hybridization

3 A 4-year-old boy with an older sibling with type 1 diabetes has laboratory evidence of detectable antibody levels for zinc transporter 8, glutamic acid decarboxylase 65, and islet-cell. Insulin autoantibodies are undetectable. He has no symptoms of hyperglycemia and no polyuria, polydipsia, nocturia, or weight loss. The family reports that they have used his sibling's glucose meter to measure his blood glucose values, which they say have been "normal" (although values are not available for review). His point-of-care hemoglobin A_{1c} measurement during the office visit is 5.6% (38 mmol/mol), and his random blood glucose concentration is 105 mg/dL (5.8 mmol/L). Urinalysis shows undetectable glucose and ketones.

Which of the following is the best next step in assessing this patient's risk of developing type 1 diabetes?

A. Measure fasting C-peptide
B. Perform oral glucose tolerance testing every 6 months
C. Perform testing for HLA-DR3-DQ2/DR4-DQ8
D. Start low-dosage basal insulin therapy at 0.05 to 0.1 unit/kg daily
E. Start nasal insulin therapy

4 A 6-year-old boy who was recently diagnosed with isolated GH deficiency presents for the first follow-up visit 4 months after starting once-weekly GH therapy with lonapegsomatropin. His parents state that they have not missed a single dose of the weekly injection despite his history of needle phobia. He received his most recent dose of the medication 2 days before the current appointment. He has had no headaches, hip pain, knee pain, or other symptoms.

His pretreatment height was −2.9 SDS, and pretreatment growth velocity was 4 cm/y with a baseline IGF-1 value that was −2 SD. His annualized growth velocity since starting treatment is 13 cm/y, and his height is now −2.4 SDS. His IGF-1 concentration measured immediately after the clinic visit is +2.3 SD.

Which of the following is the best next step in the treatment of this patient's GH deficiency?

A. Continue the current treatment plan
B. Decrease the dosage by 10% to 20%
C. Discontinue GH therapy until IGF-1 normalizes and restart lonapegsomatropin at 50% of the initial dosage
D. Remeasure IGF-1 on day 6 postinjection
E. Switch to daily GH therapy

5 A 5-week-old male infant is being evaluated for thyroid dysfunction. He was born at term with a birth weight of 7 lb, 1 oz (3200 g) and was diagnosed with hypoplastic left heart syndrome. He had a normal result on newborn screening for congenital hypothyroidism (TSH-based). He underwent cardiac catheterization and cardiac surgery 3 weeks ago. His postoperative course has been complicated by sepsis and a wound infection, and his chest has remained open postoperatively. He was placed on extracorporeal membrane oxygenation (ECMO) 4 days ago.

On physical examination, his weight is 9 lb, 4 oz (4200 g) (25th percentile) and length is 22.4 in (57 cm) (75th percentile). His chest wound is covered but open.

Laboratory test results:

TSH = 34.0 mIU/L (0.7-11.0 mIU/L)
Free T_4 = 0.9 ng/dL (0.9-2.2 ng/dL) (SI: 11.6 pmol/L [11.6-28.3 pmol/L])

Which of the following is the best next step in this infant's management?

A. Initiate intravenous levothyroxine
B. Measure free T_4 by equilibrium dialysis
C. Measure reverse T_3
D. Measure urinary iodine excretion
E. Repeat thyroid testing in 2 weeks

6 A 3-day-old male newborn is diagnosed with congenital hypothyroidism on the basis of low T_4 concentrations on newborn screening. No complications occurred during the pregnancy. Subsequent test results are consistent with central hypothyroidism. Brain MRI shows a small anterior pituitary, an ectopic posterior pituitary, and a thin and interrupted pituitary stalk. At 6 weeks of life, a low random cortisol concentration prompts initiation of hydrocortisone. Intramuscular testosterone is also initiated for microphallus. Linear growth is initially reassuring in the 25th percentile, but it declines to the 3rd percentile by age 18 months. Growth factors are low despite adequate nutrition, and recombinant GH is started with good response. Physical examination findings are normal, and neurodevelopment has been typical. His parents would like to understand why the child's condition developed. The family is counseled that it is not possible to identify the cause for most children, but testing can provide an answer in some cases.

Which of the following assessments is most likely to yield a definitive cause of this patient's underlying condition?

A. Microarray
B. Review of maternal history for exposures (eg, alcohol) during pregnancy
C. Sanger sequencing of the *GH1* gene
D. Skeletal survey
E. Whole-exome sequencing

7 A 10-year-old boy presents for a new patient visit. His parents report that due to weight gain, his pediatrician ordered bloodwork, and they were told he has a "cholesterol problem" that may require treatment. There is a family history of dyslipidemia in older relatives, but his parents do not know details. No family members have early-onset cardiovascular disease.

On physical examination, his height is 51.2 in (130 cm) (8.69th percentile), weight is 136.7 lb (62 kg) (99.45th percentile), and BMI is 29 kg/m^2 (>99th percentile).

Laboratory test results (sample drawn nonfasting):

Total cholesterol = 175 mg/dL (acceptable <170 mg/dL) (SI: 4.53 mmol/L [<4.40 mmol/L])
HDL cholesterol = 39 mg/dL (acceptable >45 mg/dL) (SI: 1.01 mmol/L [>1.17 mmol/L])
Triglycerides = 400 mg/dL (acceptable <90 mg/dL) (SI: 4.52 mmol/L [<1.02 mmol/L])
LDL cholesterol = 96 mg/dL (acceptable <110 mg/dL) (SI: 2.49 mmol/L [<2.85 mmol/L])
Non–HDL cholesterol = 136 mg/dL (acceptable <120 mg/dL) (SI: 3.52 mmol/L [<3.11 mmol/L])

His parents have made no recent changes to his eating patterns; he is a picky eater who does not like vegetables and fruits. He has physical education class twice weekly at school and sometimes plays basketball with friends. However, he has no other structured physical activity during the week.

Which of the following is the most appropriate recommendation for this child?

A. Adopt a low-fat, carbohydrate-appropriate diet
B. Order another lipid panel (sample drawn while fasting)
C. Restrict dietary fat to less than 10% to 15% of daily caloric intake (<20 g daily)
D. Start a statin
E. Start over-the-counter omega-3 fatty acid supplementation

8 A full-term male baby was born 2 days ago to a woman (G1, P1) with Graves disease. The mother was treated with methimazole, 7.5 mg daily, during the third trimester of pregnancy and is still on this regimen. The pregnancy and delivery were uncomplicated, and findings on fetal ultrasonography were normal. The infant has been asymptomatic since birth and is breastfeeding normally. Laboratory testing for TRAb in the newborn's cord blood has been sent and results are pending.

Mother's laboratory test results:

	Time point		
Measurement	**20 weeks' gestation**	**1 week prior to delivery**	**Reference range**
TRAb	3.6 IU/L	...	<1.75 IU/L
TSH	...	0.42 mIU/L	0.5-5.0 mIU/L
Free T_4	...	1.9 ng/dL (SI: 25.45 pmol/L)	0.8-1.8 ng/dL (SI: 10.30-23.17 pmol/L)

Which pattern of thyroid function is most likely to be observed in this neonate?

A. Central hypothyroidism
B. Euthyroidism
C. Hyperthyroidism
D. Primary hypothyroidism
E. Primary hypothyroidism followed by hyperthyroidism

9 A 7-year-old boy is referred to pediatric endocrinology with pubic and axillary hair development. He was born full term and has no notable medical history. He is an only child, and there is no family history of consanguinity.

On physical examination, pubertal development is Tanner stage 1 for genitalia and stage 2 for pubic hair, and he has 3-cc testes bilaterally. He has axillary hair. Height and weight are at the 90th percentile.

Bone age is advanced by 3 years.

Laboratory test results:

ACTH = 20 pg/mL (<50 pg/mL) (SI: 4.4 pmol/L [<11.0 pmol/L])
DHEA-S = 221.4 µg/dL (0-14.8 µg/dL) (SI: 6.0 µmol/L [0-0.4 µmol/L])
Androstenedione = 25.7 ng/dL (0-20.1 ng/dL) (SI: 0.9 nmol/L [0-0.7 nmol/L])
Random cortisol = 7.3 µg/dL (4.3-9.4 µg/dL) (SI: 201 nmol/L [119-259 nmol/L])
17-Hydroxyprogesterone = 49.5 ng/dL (11-108 ng/dL) (SI: 1.5 nmol/L [0.33-3.27 nmol/L])
Testosterone = 28.8 ng/dL (<14.4 ng/dL) (SI: 1.0 nmol/L [<0.5 nmol/L])

Urinary steroid profile:

Glucocorticoid metabolites:

Tetrahydrocortisol = 362 mg/24 h (94-720 mg/24 h)
5α-Tetrahydrocortisol = 54 mg/24 h (152-820 mg/24 h)
α-Cortol = 15 mg/24 h (11-87 mg/24 h)
β-Cortol = 54 mg/24 h (40-302 mg/24 h)
Tetrahydrocortisone = 7329 mg/24 h (235-1781 mg/24 h)
α-Cortolone = 812 mg/24 h (61-530 mg/24 h)
β-Cortolone = 1449 mg/24 h (64-475 mg/24 h)
Sum of glucocorticoid metabolites = 10,075 mg/24 h (832-4312 mg/24 h)

Diagnostic ratios:

5α-Tetrahydrocortisol + tetrahydrocortisol-to-tetrahydrocortisone = 0.06 (0.7-1.3)
Cortols/cortolones = 0.03 (0.26-0.50)

Androgen metabolites:

Androsterone = 295 μg/24 h (2-254 μg/24 h)
Etiocholanolone = 198 μg/24 h (1-184 μg/24 h)
DHEA = 79 μg/24 h (0.5-31 μg/24 h)
Sum of androgen metabolites = 572 μg/24 h (5-455 μg/24 h)

Pathogenic variants in which of the following genes are the most likely cause of this patient's condition?

A. *CYP11B1* (cytochrome P450 family 11 subfamily B member 1)
B. *CYP17A1* (cytochrome P450 family 17 subfamily A member 1)
C. *HSD11B1* (hydroxysteroid 11-beta dehydrogenase 1)
D. *HSD3B1* (hydroxy-delta-5-steroid dehydrogenase)
E. *HSD3B2* (hydroxy-delta-5-steroid dehydrogenase, 3 beta- and steroid delta-isomerase 2)

10 A 4-year-old girl presents for initial evaluation for short stature. Her parents state that she has always been on the small side, and she has struggled with weight gain since infancy. Pregnancy was uncomplicated except that she measured small for dates throughout. She was born at 38 weeks' gestation with a birth weight of 4 lb, 13.6 oz (2200 g) (−2.2 SD), length of 16.5 in (42 cm) (−3.1 SD), and head circumference of 13.4 in (34 cm) (0 SD). Her neonatal course was otherwise uneventful. She did not have neonatal hypoglycemia.

At age 1 year, failure to thrive and gastroesophageal reflux were diagnosed. She was referred for feeding therapy and nutrition and was eventually placed on cyproheptadine to assist with appetite stimulation. She has mild speech delay and receives speech therapy.

On physical examination, her height is currently −3.3 SD and weight is −3.5 SD. She has a triangular-shaped face, and her right leg is slightly longer (~1 cm) than her left leg. She has bilateral clinodactyly of the fifth finger.

Which of the following is most likely to identify this patient's underlying diagnosis?

A. Chromosomal microarray
B. Karyotype analysis
C. Methylation testing of chromosome 11p15
D. *PTPN11* sequencing
E. Whole-exome sequencing

11 An 11-year-old girl and her 4-year-old brother both have osteogenesis imperfecta and are transferring care to a multidisciplinary metabolic bone clinic. Neither child has indwelling hardware. DXA will be performed to assess the children's bone density.

Which of the following sets of DXA scans best aligns with guidance offered by the 2019 International Society of Clinical Densitometry Pediatric Position statement and available reference ranges?

Answer	11-year-old	4-year-old
A.	• Total body less head • Lumbar spine	• Total body less head • Lumbar spine
B.	• Total body less head • Lumbar spine • Proximal femur	• Total body less head • Lumbar spine
C.	• Total body less head • Lumbar spine • Distal radius	• Total body less head • Lumbar spine • Distal radius
D.	• Total body less head • Lumbar spine	• Lumbar spine
E.	• Lumbar spine • Proximal femur	• Lumbar spine • Proximal femur

12 A 15-year-old boy is undergoing evaluation for severe headaches. MRI shows a 5.3 × 5.6 × 5.0-cm lesion (*see image*).

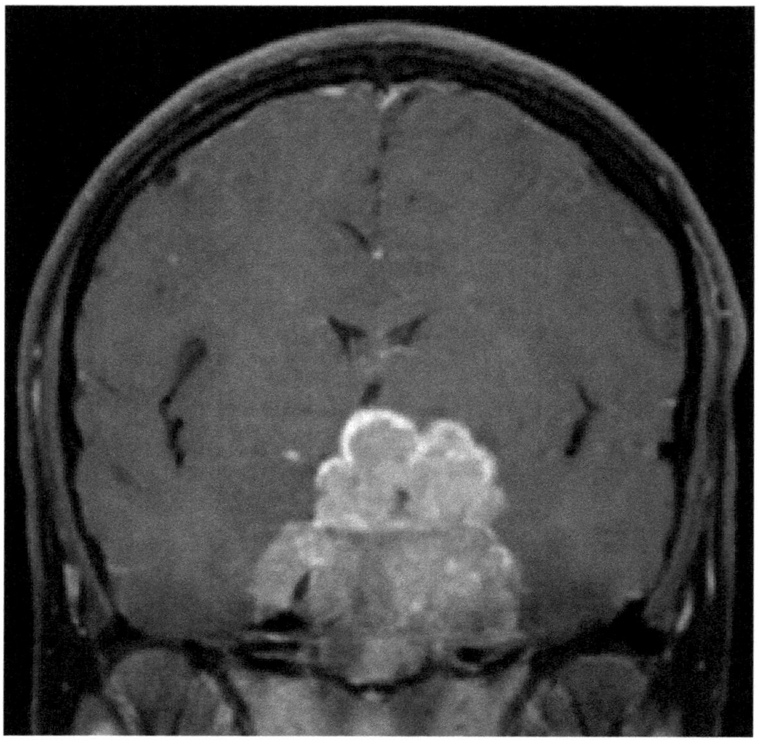

Initial MRI of the brain/pituitary; coronal section, post gadolinium, T1-weighted image.

He has substantial peripheral visual field deficits that are more pronounced on the left side (*see image*). Visual acuity is 20/500 on the left side and 20/20 on the right side.

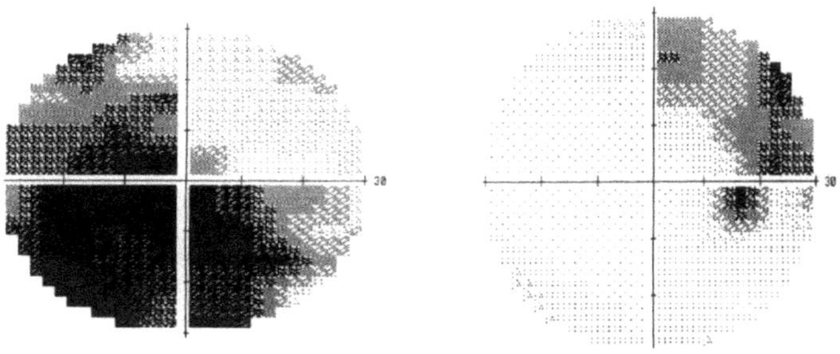

Humphrey visual fields (30-2); left (on the left side) and right (on the right side). The visual fields show the extent of an area visible to an individual during steady fixation of the eye, where white is visible and black is not visible.

His initial prolactin concentration is greater than 3259 ng/mL (>141.7 nmol/L). His IGF-1 concentration is normal. Cabergoline is started at a dosage of 0.25 mg twice weekly and is escalated. Visual symptoms rapidly improve and his prolactin concentration decreases, but the persistent visual threat leads to multiple operative resections for debulking. Eighteen months later, he develops polyuria and is found to have hyperglycemia and diabetes mellitus. IGF-1 is substantially elevated for age and Tanner stage, and GH levels are nonsuppressed on oral glucose tolerance testing. Another operative resection is pursued.

Which of the following pathologic findings on the most recent operative specimen would be most likely to reflect the cause of this patient's clinical presentation?

A. Infiltration of the anterior pituitary by inflammatory cells
B. Mixed pituitary neuroendocrine tumor with 2 discrete cellular populations
C. Monomorphous pituitary neuroendocrine tumor with a single cellular population
D. Pituitary cellular hyperplasia
E. Tumor with blastemal cells, Rathke pouch epithelium, and adenohypophyseal neuroendocrine cells

13 Each of the answer choices represents a patient who has new-onset diabetes with diabetic ketoacidosis.

Which of the following patients is at the greatest risk for cerebral edema?

Answer	Age, y	pH	Bicarbonate	Glucose	Serum urea nitrogen	Pco_2
A.	4	7.1	7.0 mEq/L (SI: 7.0 mmol/L)	623 mg/dL (SI: 34.6 mmol/L)	17 mg/dL (SI: 6.1 mmol/L)	23 mm Hg
B.	5	7.1	5.0 mEq/L (SI: 5.0 mmol/L)	233 mg/dL (SI: 12.9 mmol/L)	16 mg/dL (SI: 5.7 mmol/L)	22 mm Hg
C.	4	7.0	7.0 mEq/L (SI: 7.0 mmol/L)	425 mg/dL (SI: 23.6 mmol/L)	23 mg/dL (SI: 8.2 mmol/L)	15 mm Hg
D.	5	7.0	5.0 mEq/L (SI: 5.0 mmol/L)	280 mg/dL (SI: 15.5 mmol/L)	19 mg/dL (SI: 6.8 mmol/L)	21 mm Hg
E.	4	7.0	6.0 mEq/L (SI: 6.0 mmol/L)	560 mg/dL (SI: 31.1 mmol/L)	24 mg/dL (SI: 8.6 mmol/L)	24 mm Hg

14 A 7-day-old Hispanic baby boy has an abnormal newborn screen with a TSH value of 42.0 mIU/L (<29.0 mIU/L). He was delivered vaginally at term after an uncomplicated pregnancy. There is no family history of thyroid disease.

On physical examination, his weight is 8 lb, 7.8 oz (3850 g). He has no goiter.

Technetium scan shows no uptake.

Compared with this infant, which of the following children is at higher risk for congenital hypothyroidism?

A. African American female
B. African American male
C. American Indian male
D. Hispanic female
E. NonHispanic White male

15 A 7-year-old girl is being evaluated for accelerated growth. She was growing along the 25th percentile until 2 years ago. In the last 2 years, she has had robust growth despite a 4-lb (2.3-kg) weight loss. Her height is now at the 75th percentile, and BMI is at the 99th percentile. She is growing out of her clothes and shoes. Her midparental height is at the 75th percentile. Her mother had menarche at age 14 years, and her father continued to grow until his first year in college.

On physical examination, she has mild thyroid enlargement. Pubic hair and breast development are Tanner stage 1.

Which of the following is the mechanism of the recent growth pattern seen in this patient?

A. Enhancement of the GH/IGF-1 axis
B. Excessive caloric intake
C. Familial tall stature
D. Pulsatile secretion of GnRH
E. Slow maturation of growth plates

16 A 16-year-old natal male/affirmed female teenager presents for follow-up transgender care. She reports that she started to feel uncomfortable with her body around age 13 years; in particular, she struggled with changes related to puberty. Her history is notable for anxiety and depression, currently managed by a psychiatrist, and her psychologist who has expertise in gender-affirming therapy has confirmed a diagnosis of gender dysphoria. She also has type 1 diabetes. Her BMI is at the 47th percentile.

Recent laboratory test results:

Hemoglobin A_{1c} = 8.6% (4.0%-5.6%) (70 mmol/mol [20-38 mmol/mol])
Total cholesterol = 139 mg/dL (<170 mg/dL) (SI: 3.60 mmol/L [<4.40 mmol/L])
Triglycerides = 129 mg/dL (<90 mg/dL) (SI: 1.46 mmol/L [<1.02 mmol/L])
HDL cholesterol = 45 mg/dL (>45 mg/dL) (SI: 1.17 mmol/L [>1.17 mmol/L])
LDL cholesterol = 71 mg/dL (<110 mg/dL) (SI: 1.84 mmol/L [<2.85 mmol/L])
TSH = 2.14 mIU/L (0.45-4.5 mIU/L)
Random glucose = 219 mg/dL (SI: 12.2 mmol/L)
Urinary albumin-to-creatinine ratio, normal
25-Hydroxyvitamin D = 34 ng/mL (30-100 ng/mL) (SI: 85 nmol/L [75-250 nmol/L])

She is interested in starting ethinyl estradiol to promote a more feminine body appearance. She has been informed of the intended effects and potential adverse effects of treatment and has support from her parents to start therapy.

Which of the following is the greatest risk for this patient after starting estradiol?

A. Dyslipidemia
B. Liver dysfunction
C. Low bone density
D. Obesity
E. Venous thromboembolism

17 A 12-year-old girl presents for evaluation of abnormal thyroid function test results obtained by her neurologist. She has refractory seizures that are managed with multiple anticonvulsant medications. She reports fatigue, mild constipation, and hair thinning. She has no other symptoms and specifically has no headache, vision changes, or vomiting. Her current medications are levetiracetam, oxcarbazepine, and valproic acid, and this regimen has been stable for 1 year. She also takes a daily biotin supplement, which was held for 3 days prior to her laboratory studies.

On physical examination, she has a normal pulse rate and blood pressure. Her growth chart shows an annualized growth velocity of 4.2 cm/y. The rest of her examination findings are normal, including those of eye exam with fundoscopy and thyroid exam.

Laboratory test results:

TSH = 1.6 mIU/L (0.7-5.7 mIU/L)
Free T_4 = 0.62 ng/dL (0.8-1.8 ng/dL) (SI: 7.98 pmol/L [10.30-23.17 pmol/L])

Which of the following is the most likely cause of the thyroid function pattern observed in this patient?

A. Biotin
B. Central nervous system tumor
C. Levetiracetam
D. Oxcarbazepine
E. Valproic acid

18 A 14-year-old girl is admitted to the adolescent medicine service with a diagnosis of anorexia nervosa and malnutrition. Menarche was at age 12 years, and her periods became regular within a few months. However, her periods stopped 6 months before hospital admission, concurrent with significant weight loss. Medications include a daily multivitamin, vitamin D_3, and multiple over-the-counter nutritional supplements.

Laboratory tests are ordered to evaluate secondary amenorrhea:

Prolactin = 69 ng/mL (3-18 ng/mL) (SI: 3.00 nmol/L [0.13-0.78 nmol/L])
Cortisol (8 AM) = 12.0 μg/dL (3.7-19.4 μg/dL) (SI: 331.1 nmol/L [102.1-535.2 nmol/L])
Thyroid function, normal
Pregnancy test, negative

Findings on brain and pituitary MRI with and without contrast are normal. The decision is made to follow-up closely. After 3 months, regular menses resume with nutritional support. Prolactin is measured again (120 ng/mL [5.2 nmol/L]).

Which of the following most likely explains the patient's persistently elevated prolactin concentration?

A. Biotin supplementation
B. Hook effect
C. Pituitary stalk disruption
D. Presence of macroprolactin
E. Prolactin-secreting pituitary neuroendocrine tumor

19 A 15-year-old girl presents for a follow-up visit to monitor for adverse effects after starting pharmacotherapy for weight loss. The patient has a history of excessive weight gain and mild dyslipidemia that has not required pharmacotherapy. Despite lifestyle modifications, she has continued to gain weight. At the last clinic visit, her height was 64.5 in (163.8 cm) (61.6th percentile), and weight was 229.3 lb (104 kg) (>99th percentile for age). At that time, she and her mother wanted to consider approved pharmacotherapy options to address ongoing weight gain. After discussing different medications and potential adverse effects, she decided to start a medication, which she has now taken for 6 weeks. She thinks that her appetite has lessened, and she has been troubled by a metallic taste when she eats. She does not endorse any other adverse effects when questioned.

Which of the following medications is the most likely cause of her symptom?

A. Liraglutide
B. Metformin
C. Naltrexone/bupropion
D. Orlistat
E. Phentermine/topiramate

20 The family of a 9-year-old girl seeks a second opinion regarding her short stature. She was initially evaluated by another pediatric endocrinologist at age 8 years. At that time, her height was −2.4 SDS. Physical examination findings were unremarkable, and she was prepubertal. Laboratory evaluation was performed, which documented normal results from a complete blood cell count, complete metabolic panel, thyroid tests, celiac screen, and IGF-1 measurement. A bone age x-ray was interpreted to be 1 year delayed compared with her chronologic age. The patient was followed for 1 year and had a growth velocity of 5 cm/y. She remained prepubertal and was diagnosed with constitutional delay of growth and puberty. The family is now seeking a second opinion.

The patient's mother has a history of short stature with an adult height of 58 in (147.2 cm). During the appointment, an abnormality is noted in the mother's forearm (*see image*). The father's height is 66 in (167.6 cm). The patient is an only child.

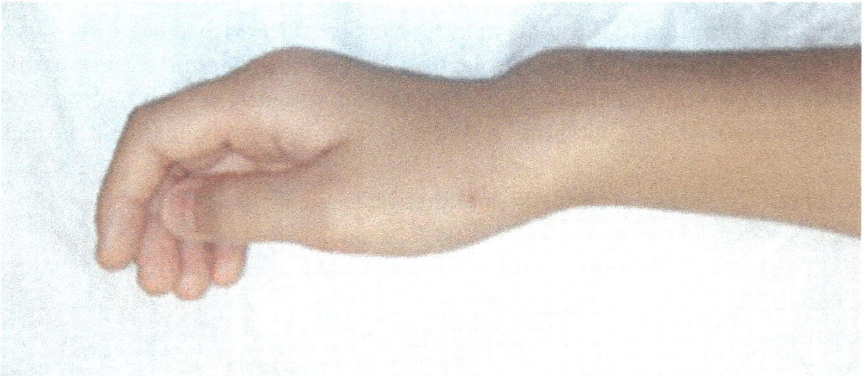

Reprinted from Toshihiko O, Daisuke I, Hiroshi S, and Kousuke I. *Clin Orthop Surg*, 2012; 4(1): 45-57.

On physical examination, the patient's height remains at –2.4 SDS. She is prepubertal. Her sitting height is measured, and her calculated sitting-height ratio is 0.55 (>97th percentile) (sitting height divided by standing height).

Which of the following is this patient's most likely diagnosis?

A. Mosaic Turner syndrome
B. Pathogenic variant in the *ACAN* (aggrecan) gene
C. Pathogenic variant in the *FGFR3* gene
D. Pathogenic variant in the *NPR2* gene
E. Pathogenic variant in the *SHOX* gene

21

An 8-year-old boy with an inoperable aneurysmal bone cyst of the cervical spine is treated with denosumab, 120 mg monthly, for 6 months. Monitoring x-rays obtained at the start of denosumab treatment and at the end of treatment are shown, depicting the development of dense metaphyseal bands (*see image*). He receives a single dose of zoledronic acid on the same day as his last denosumab injection. The oncology team asks for advice regarding ongoing monitoring of bone health in this patient.

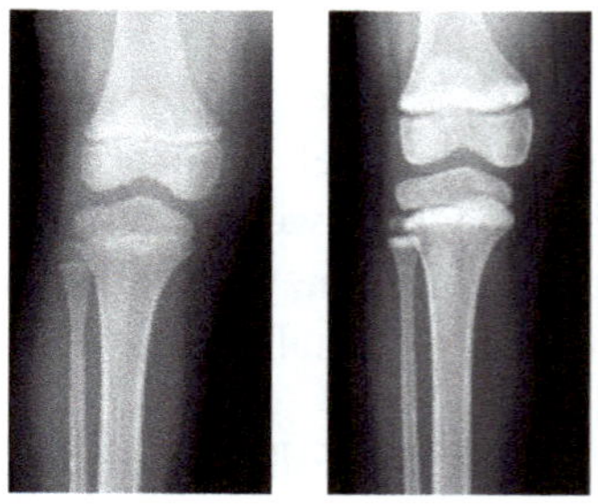

Baseline — 6 months of monthly denosumab

Which of the following is the best next step for monitoring this patient's bone health after he discontinues denosumab?

A. Administer zoledronic acid 6 months after last denosumab dose
B. Monitor serum calcium every month
C. Obtain lumbar and thoracic spine x-rays every 6 months
D. Recommend no additional monitoring
E. Repeat lower-extremity x-rays in 6 months

22 A 17-year-old girl was diagnosed with Graves disease 15 months ago. Her hyperthyroidism has been poorly controlled due to inconsistent adherence to methimazole therapy. At this visit, she states that she would like to pursue definitive therapy for hyperthyroidism with radioactive iodine ablation or thyroidectomy.

She has mild fatigue and difficulty concentrating, but no palpitations or tremor. She has Graves orbitopathy that was active and moderate in severity at her last ophthalmology visit 3 weeks ago. On social history, she reports occasional unprotected intercourse with her boyfriend and does not reliably use contraception.

Thyroid ultrasonography shows a diffusely enlarged, heterogeneous thyroid gland (thyroid volume = 52 g) with increased vascularity and multiple bilateral cysts measuring 2 to 3 mm in diameter.

Laboratory test results:

TSH = 0.07 mIU/L (0.7-5.7 mIU/L)
Free T_4 = 2.62 ng/dL (0.8-1.8 ng/dL) (SI: 33.72 pmol/L [10.30-23.17 pmol/L])
Total T_3 = 340 ng/dL (80-210 ng/dL) (SI: 5.24 nmol/L [1.23-3.23 nmol/L])
Urine pregnancy test, negative

Which of the following is the most important contraindication to radioactive iodine therapy in this patient?

A. Failure to complete at least 2 years of initial antithyroid drug treatment
B. Moderate, active thyroid eye disease
C. Presence of thyroid cysts
D. Thyroid gland volume greater than 40 mL
E. Unreliable use of contraception

23 A 13-year-old boy is referred to pediatric endocrinology for evaluation of weight gain over the past 2 years. He is the youngest of 3 children born to consanguineous parents (distant cousins). The family reports that the patient's older brother had an operation to remove a lump from one of his testes in his 20s. His height is at the 25th percentile and weight is at the 90th percentile. When reviewing and plotting his previous height and weight, there is apparent deceleration of height velocity with associated marked weight gain.

On physical examination, he has a round face, some abdominal striae, and 3 small café au-lait-spots. Pubertal development is Tanner stage 1 for genitalia and stage 2 for pubic hair, and testicular volume is 3 cc bilaterally.

Baseline laboratory test results:

Plasma ACTH (9 AM) = 0.8 pg/mL (5.0-50.0 pg/mL) (SI: 0.2 pmol/L [1.1-11.0 pmol/L])
Cortisol (9 AM) = 15.9 μg/dL (5.0-15.0 μg/dL) (SI: 438.6 nmol/L [137.9-413.8 nmol/L])
Urinary free cortisol = 445 μg/24 h (54-408 μg/24 h) (SI: 1228.2 nmol/d [149.0-1126.1 nmol/d])

Adrenal-directed MRI is performed.

Result of a low-dose (1-mg) overnight dexamethasone-suppression test:

Cortisol = 5.3 μg/dL (<1.8 μg/dL) (SI: 145 nmol/L [<50 nmol/L])

Results of the Liddle test:

Urinary free cortisol	Result	Reference range
Baseline	456 μg/24 h (SI: 1259 nmol/d)	54-408 μg/24 h (SI: 149-1126 nmol/d)
Day 2 after 0.5 mg dexamethasone administered every 6 hours for 48 hours	969 μg/24 h (SI: 2674 mol/d)	<50 μg/24 h (SI: <138 nmol/d)
Day 4 after 2 mg dexamethasone administered every 6 hours for another 48 hours	948 μg/24 h (SI: 2616 nmol/d)	<50 μg/24 h (SI: <138 nmol/d)
Day 6	912 μg/24 h (SI: 2617 nmol/d)	<50 μg/24 h (SI: <138 nmol/d)

He undergoes adrenalectomy.

Which of the following is the most likely histologic diagnosis in this patient?

A. Adrenocortical carcinoma
B. Bilateral macronodular disease
C. Isolated micronodular adrenocortical disease
D. Primary pigmented nodular adrenal disease
E. Sporadic nodular adrenocortical disease

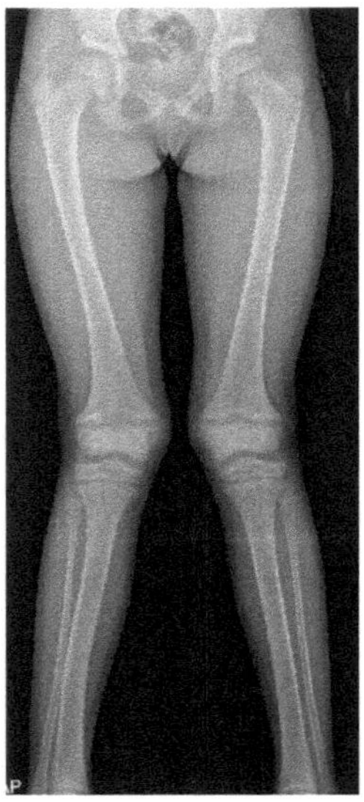

24 An 8-year-old girl is evaluated for bilateral lower-extremity pain and found to have a knock-kneed deformity with an intermalleolar distance of 11 cm. Her current height is at the 3rd percentile, and midparental height is at the 60th percentile. Examination findings are otherwise notable for dolichocephaly but no dental issues.

Treatment options are discussed, including conventional therapy with active vitamin D and multiple daily doses of phosphorus or anti–FGF-23 monoclonal antibody injections.

After initiation of therapy, which of the following options is the best next step in this patient's management?

A. GH treatment
B. Head CT
C. Kidney ultrasonography
D. Lower-extremity x-rays in 6 months
E. Orthopedics consultation

25 A 15-year-old girl is being evaluated for hypothyroidism. She has not had a visit with a pediatrician in the last 10 years. Two months ago, her mother noticed she had a neck swelling. Her mother made an appointment with a pediatrician because the swelling was progressively getting larger. In addition to the goiter, the pediatrician also noted that the girl has short stature. Her height is 57 in (145 cm) (<3rd percentile), weight is 97 lb (44 kg) (15th percentile), and BMI is 21 kg/m^2 (62nd percentile). Her midparental height is at 50th percentile. The patient has always been shorter than her peers since preschool. She had menarche at age 13 years and has spontaneous regular monthly menstrual cycles. She has no constipation, diarrhea, or abdominal pain.

Laboratory test results (sample drawn in the morning 2 weeks ago):

IGF-1 = 365 ng/mL (199-537 ng/mL) (SI: 47.8 nmol/L [26.0-70.2 nmol/L])
TSH = 10.4 mIU/L (0.5-4.8 mIU/L)
Free T_4 = 0.90 ng/dL (0.90-1.67 ng/dL) (SI: 11.6 pmol/L [11.6-21.5 pmol/L])
Basic metabolic panel, normal
Celiac disease screen, negative

Which of the following is the best next step in identifying the cause of this patient's short stature?

A. Check thyroid antibodies
B. Obtain a bone age x-ray
C. Perform GH-stimulation testing
D. Perform karyotype analysis
E. Perform upper gastrointestinal endoscopy

26 A 9-year-old girl is referred for management of precocious puberty. Her parents report that breast development started just prior to her eighth birthday and pubic hair appeared shortly thereafter. She has been growing fast over the past year. Autism was diagnosed at age 4 years and attention-deficit/hyperactivity disorder was diagnosed at 6 years. She has no history of seizures, headaches, or vision problems. Her mother reports that she underwent menarche at age 11 years, and her father reports that his pubertal timing was average.

Laboratory test results:

LH = 5.5 mIU/L (0-0.18 mIU/L) (SI: 5.5 IU/L [0-0.18 IU/L])
Estradiol = 34.6 pg/mL (0-14.9 pg/mL) (SI: 127 pmol/L [0-54.7 pmol/L])
TSH = 6.23 mIU/L (0.45-4.5 mIU/L)
Free T_4 = 1.34 ng/dL (0.90-1.67 ng/dL) (SI: 17.3 pmol/L [11.6-21.5 pmol/L])

Review of her growth chart shows that both height and weight percentiles have been increasing over the past 2 years. Her midparental height is 64.5 in (163.8 cm).

On physical examination, her height is at the 93rd percentile, weight is at the 99th percentile, and BMI is at the 98th percentile. Breast and pubic hair development are both stage 4. Examination findings are otherwise unremarkable.

Her bone age is 12 years at a chronologic age of 9 years 6 months.

Which of the following is most likely contributing to this patient's early puberty?

A. Elevated BMI
B. Family history of early menarche
C. History of autism
D. Hypothyroidism
E. Nonclassic congenital adrenal hyperplasia

27 A 13-year-old boy presents with a palpable lump in the left side of his neck. He first noticed the lump 2 weeks ago and it has not changed in size. He has had no pain, dysphagia, voice changes, tremor, temperature intolerance, palpitations, or weight changes. He has no history of recent illness or radiation exposure. There is no family history of thyroid disease, thyroid neoplasia, or other endocrine disorders. His TSH concentration is 2.7 mIU/L (0.7-5.7 mIU/L).

On physical examination, he has a normal pulse rate and blood pressure. His thyroid has a 4-cm, firm nodule palpable in the left thyroid lobe that moves with swallowing and is not fixed to surrounding tissues. He has bilateral shotty anterior cervical lymphadenopathy. The rest of his examination findings are normal.

Thyroid ultrasonography shows a nodule in the left thyroid lobe measuring 4.4 cm in maximal diameter. The nodule is mixed solid and cystic in composition, hypoechoic, and taller-than-wide in transverse view, with regular margins and no calcifications. The right thyroid lobe is normal. No abnormal lymph nodes are present. FNA of the nodule is performed, and cytology is benign.

Which of the following is the best next step in this patient's management?

A. Initiate levothyroxine treatment
B. Perform thyroid scintigraphy
C. Refer to a thyroid surgeon for consideration of hemithyroidectomy
D. Repeat FNA in 3 to 6 months
E. Repeat thyroid ultrasonography in 3 months

28 A 15-day-old female baby is admitted to the pediatric intensive care unit for tachycardia and tachypnea. She was born at 40 weeks' gestation to a 30-year-old woman (G2, P2). Her parents are nonconsanguineous. Apgar score is 5 at 1 minute and 7 at 5 minutes. Birth weight is 3 lb, 13.7 oz (1750 g). She is cushingoid in appearance with hypertrichosis and a large birth mark.

Initial laboratory test results:

TSH = <0.05 mIU/L (0.32-5.00 mIU/L)

Free T_4 = 2.98 ng/dL (0.71-1.85 ng/dL) (SI: 38.4 ng/dL [9.1-23.8 pmol/L])

ACTH (random value) = 3 pg/mL (9-54 pg/mL) (SI: 0.66 pmol/L [1.98-11.88 pmol/L])

Cortisol (8 AM) = 72.0 μg/dL (5.0-25.0 μg/dL) (SI: 1986.3 nmol/L [137.9-689.7 nmol/L])

Cortisol (8 AM) after 0.5 mg dexamethasone at midnight = 49.3 μg/dL (<5.0 μg/dL) (SI: 1360.1 nmol/L [<137.9 nmol/L])

Cortisol (8 AM) after 2.0 mg dexamethasone at midnight = 49.0 μg/dL (<5.0 μg/dL) (SI: 1351.8 nmol/L [<137.9 nmol/L])

Pathogenic variant(s) in which of the following genes is/are most likely in this patient?

A. *AIP*
B. *DICER1*
C. *GNAS*
D. *PRKAR1A*
E. *TP53*

29 A 6-month-old boy is referred for possible new-onset diabetes. His mother reports that in the last month, he has been more irritable, feeding more frequently, and having heavier wet diapers. He has not been sleeping well. He has not lost any weight, and his mother thinks he has become chubbier in the last month. His growth has slowed in the last 2 months. He was born via spontaneous normal vaginal delivery at full-term. He has been very healthy except for a persistent diaper rash for the last 6 weeks for which he saw a dermatologist and started clobetasol propionate ointment, applied to the diaper area with occlusive dressing twice daily. They have a follow-up appointment with the dermatologist next week.

On physical examination, he is irritable, has excess weight, and has a diaper rash. His blood pressure is elevated for age and sex.

His fingerstick blood glucose concentration is 180 mg/dL (10.0 mmol/L), and fingerstick hemoglobin A_{1c} value is 6.0% (42 mmol/mol).

Which of the following is the best next step in this patient's management?

A. Admit to the hospital for new-onset diabetes mellitus
B. Assess for type 1 diabetes antibodies
C. Order genetic testing for neonatal diabetes
D. Perform brain MRI
E. Start oral hydrocortisone and stop using diaper rash cream

30 A 16-year-old boy comes to clinic for the first time because of weight concerns. He was born full-term, and birth weight was 6 lb, 1 oz (2750 g). His mother reports that he had failure to thrive as an infant with severe diarrhea that required hospitalization and parenteral nutrition for many months. When he was a toddler, his weight increased rapidly, and he developed hyperphagia to the point that his parents had to put locks on cabinet doors. He has continued to gain weight despite ongoing issues with frequent diarrhea throughout childhood and adolescence. His current height is 67 in (170.2 cm) (32nd percentile), and weight is 242.5 lb (110 kg) (>99th percentile) (BMI = 37.9 kg/m^2).

Which of the following laboratory data would be anticipated for this patient?

A. Elevated ACTH, low cortisol
B. Elevated IGF-1
C. Elevated TSH, low free T_4
D. Low FSH, low LH, low testosterone
E. Low proinsulin, elevated insulin

31 A 2-day-old term male baby born in the United States is noted to have a goiter and irritability. The pregnancy was uncomplicated. His 28-year-old mother (G1, P1) was diagnosed with Graves disease at age 5 years. For many years, she was treated with methimazole before undergoing thyroidectomy at age 24 because she had multiple nodules and no remission of hyperthyroidism. She is chemically euthyroid on levothyroxine replacement. She takes no other prescription medications, but she does take a prenatal vitamin and a health-food store thyroid supplement. TRAb were negative when assessed during the second trimester. She has positive TPO antibodies.

On physical examination, the baby's heart rate is 178 beats/min. His weight is 4 lb, 10 oz (2100 g) (<1st percentile), length is 19.0 in (48.2 cm) (25th percentile), and head circumference is 12.6 in (32 cm) (3rd percentile). He has a palpable thyroid gland.

Laboratory test results:

TSH = <0.01 mIU/L (0.7-15.2 mIU/L)
Free T_4 = 5.1 ng/dL (0.9-2.5 ng/dL) (SI: 65.6 pmol/L [11.6-32.2 pmol/L])
TRAb = 0.94 IU/L (≤1.75 IU/L)

Which of the following is the most likely mechanism of this patient's goiter?

A. Activation of the TSH receptor
B. Iodine deficiency
C. Iodine excess
D. Iodide organification defect
E. Transplacental passage of maternal TPO antibodies

32 The parents of 12-year-old girl seek a second opinion for concern about her poor growth over the last 3 years. Her growth velocity is 4.2 cm/y. Midparental height is at the 50th percentile. Her mother had menarche at age 16 years, and her father had a growth spurt in the last year of high school.

On physical examination, her height is 54.7 in (139 cm) (25th percentile), weight is 110.2 lb (50 kg) (90th percentile), and BMI is 25.8 kg/m^2 (96th percentile). She has no hirsutism, acne, or stretch marks. She has normal external female genitalia with no signs of puberty.

Laboratory test results (sample drawn in the morning of the clinic visit):

IGF-1 = 150 ng/mL (97-332 ng/mL) (SI: 19.6 nmol/L [12.7-43.5 nmol/L])
TSH = 6.8 mIU/L (0.6-5.5 mIU/L)
Free T_4 = 1.2 ng/dL (0.93-1.60 ng/dL) (SI: 15.4 pmol/L [12.0-20.6 pmol/L])
Basic metabolic panel, normal
Total IgA = 30 mg/dL (42-378 mg/dL)
tTG IgA, negative
Liver function, normal

The peak GH value during clonidine-arginine GH-stimulation testing is 6.6 ng/mL (6.6 µg/L). Bone age is 10 years and 6 months. The endocrinologist she saw in the past had recommended starting GH therapy, but her parents are reluctant to initiate this unless it is absolutely needed to optimize growth.

Which of the following is the best next step in this patient's management?

A. Measure midnight salivary cortisol
B. Refer to gastroenterologist for endoscopic diagnosis of celiac disease
C. Repeat GH-stimulation testing after priming with β-estradiol
D. Start GH treatment
E. Start levothyroxine

33 A 13-year-old boy is followed by a nephrologist because of chronic kidney disease secondary to cystic dysplasia. He is referred for assessment of glycosuria that has persisted for the past 3 months. He has longstanding polyuria and polydipsia previously attributed to his kidney disease. Point-of-care testing in the office documents a glucose concentration of 280 mg/dL (15.4 mmol/L) and a hemoglobin A_{1c} value of 10.3% (89 mmol/mol). BMI is at the 34th percentile. His 8-year-old brother was born with a single kidney and is also followed by a nephrologist, but he has no evidence of hyperglycemia. His father died in his 40s due to complications of diabetes and nephropathy.

A basal-bolus insulin regimen is initiated. Diabetes autoantibodies (glutamic acid decarboxylase, zinc transporter 8, islet-cell, IA2, and insulin autoantibodies) are all undetectable.

Testing for pathogenic variants in which of the following genes will most likely lead to this patient's diagnosis?

A. *CEL*
B. *GCK*
C. *HNF1A*
D. *HNF1B*
E. *HNF4A*

34 The neonatal intensive care unit calls regarding a 3-month-old infant born at 34 weeks' gestation who was found to have multiple fractures (proximal femur, radial neck, distal ulna, lumbar vertebral compression fractures) and osteoporotic appearance of the bones on imaging done to evaluate the cause of bloody stool. Birth weight was 4 lb, 13.6 oz (2200 g). The baby has been in the intensive care unit since birth for continuous intravenous unfractionated heparin to treat a large inferior vena cava thrombus. Additional history includes dexamethasone in the immediate newborn period for respiratory distress and use of parenteral nutrition for the first 8 days of life before transition to enteral feeds. The infant currently receives ranitidine for gastric reflux and vitamin D supplementation.

Which of the follow risk factors most likely explains this patient's impaired bone health?

A. Dexamethasone
B. Heparin
C. Parenteral nutrition
D. Prematurity
E. Ranitidine

35 A 9-year-old girl (66 lb [30 kg]) with Chiari malformation and primary hypothyroidism undergoes Chiari decompression surgery. One week before the operation, free T_4 was normal and her TSH concentration was 7.1 mIU/L (0.7-4.2 mIU/L). Five hours after the operation begins, endocrinology is consulted because she has developed polyuria (10 cc/kg per h over the past 2 hours).

Laboratory test results:

Serum sodium = 149 mEq/L (136-145 mEq/L) (SI: 149 mmol/L [136-145 mmol/L])
Serum calcium = 10.9 mg/dL (8.8-10.7 mg/dL) (SI: 2.72 mmol/L [2.20-2.67 mmol/L])
Blood glucose = 92 mg/dL (70-106 mg/dL) (SI: 5.1 mmol/L [3.9-5.9 mmol/L])
Serum urea nitrogen, normal
Creatinine, normal

The operation had been proceeding uneventfully. She had been induced with sevoflurane and received multiple other medications intraoperatively, including midazolam, dexmedetomidine, remifentanil, ephedrine, piperacillin/tazobactam, and dopamine. She had received a total of 500 cc of intravenous fluids at the time polyuria was noted.

She requires a vasopressin infusion for 20 hours, during which her urine output decreases, and additional fluids to normalize her serum sodium. After the vasopressin infusion is ultimately discontinued, no further polyuria or hypernatremia develops.

Which of the following best explains this patient's presentation?

A. Cerebral salt-wasting
B. Dexmedetomidine-induced arginine vasopressin deficiency
C. Dopamine-induced polyuria
D. Hypercalcemia-induced diuresis
E. Undertreated hypothyroidism

36 A 6-week-old infant has atypical genitalia. Antenatal ultrasonography initially indicated a female fetus. Findings at birth were notable for a small phallus, proximal hypospadias, and bilateral descended testes. Weight and length at birth were at the 3rd percentile. He has otherwise been well; he is nursing frequently without vomiting, has the usual number of wet diapers each day, and is gaining weight appropriately. Family history is unremarkable, and he has a healthy 2-year-old sister.

Physical examination findings are notable for microcephaly, low muscle tone, penoscrotal hypospadias, partly bifid scrotum, phallus that measures 1.2 cm, and palpable testes in the scrotum bilaterally. There is some webbing between toes 2 and 3 bilaterally. Length and weight are slightly below the 3rd percentile.

On day 3 of life, the baby is determined to have a 46,XY karyotype, and the *SRY* gene is identified on fluorescence in situ hybridization testing.

Laboratory test results obtained on day 14 of life:

Cortisol = 11.9 μg/dL (3.4-22.5 μg/dL) (SI: 328.3 nmol/L [93.8-620.7 nmol/L])
17-Hydroxyprogesterone = 193.9 ng/dL (<199 ng/dL) (SI: 5.9 nmol/L [<6.0 nmol/L])
Total testosterone = 129 ng/dL (37-198 ng/dL) (SI: 4.5 nmol/L [1.3-6.9 nmol/L])
Dihydrotestosterone = 12.0 ng/dL (10-53 ng/dL) (SI: 0.41 nmol/L [0.34-1.83 nmol/L])
LH = 4.6 mIU/mL (1.5-9.3 mIU/mL) (SI: 4.6 IU/L [1.5-9.3 IU/L])
FSH = 9.3 mIU/mL (1.4-18.1 mIU/mL) (SI: 9.3 IU/L [1.4-18.1 IU/L])

No mullerian structures are identified on pelvic ultrasonography.

Which of the following is this patient's most likely diagnosis?

A. Denys-Drash syndrome
B. Frasier syndrome
C. *NR0B1* (*DAX1*) overexpression
D. Smith-Lemli-Opitz syndrome
E. WAGR syndrome

37 A medical student is present for the follow-up visit of a 17-year-old girl who has been recently diagnosed with type 2 diabetes mellitus. The patient's current hemoglobin A_{1c} value is 7.1% (54 mmol/mol). Her BMI is 41.7 kg/m^2 (>97th percentile for age and sex). The patient is considering the recommendation to start medication to help with glycemic control and weight loss. Possible pharmacotherapy options were discussed at her last clinic visit, and the patient reports that she is leaning towards starting one of the medications in particular, but she would like additional information regarding how the drug helps control blood glucose. The medical student asks if they can tackle the explanation and proceeds to tell the patient that one of the ways this medication helps glycemic control is by stimulating insulin release after food intake, which helps to lower blood glucose and suppress glucagon secretion by α cells.

Which of the following medications is most likely the patient's choice, based on her goals and the drug's mechanism of action?

A. Empagliflozin
B. Exenatide
C. Glyburide
D. Metformin
E. Sitagliptin

38 A 9-year-old boy presents for evaluation of tall stature. His parents state that he has always been tall, but they recently noted a few pubic hairs and became concerned.

On physical examination, his height is +2.5 SD, weight is +2.2 SD, and head circumference +2.5 SD. He has Tanner stage 2 pubic hair, and testicular volume is 4 cc bilaterally. There is no body asymmetry.

Bone age is interpreted to be 12 years.

His birth length and head circumference were both at the 98th percentile with a birth weight at the 75th percentile. His parents are of average height with a midparental height at the 50th percentile. There is no family history of tall stature. The patient has moderate intellectual disability and receives special education at school. He did not have neonatal hypoglycemia.

Which of the following is the best next step in this patient's clinical evaluation?

A. Measure 17-hydroxyprogesterone
B. Measure IGF-1
C. Measure LH and testosterone
D. Perform genetic testing for pathogenic variants in the *NSD1* gene
E. Perform kidney ultrasonography

39 A 15-month-old boy has a history of craniosynostosis with pyriform sinus aperture stenosis, depressed nasal bridge, and hypertelorism. The base of the skull has a coarse sclerotic appearance on imaging and scattered intracranial calcifications with mineralization along the intraorbital optic nerves. The child's primary teeth are small and yellow due to enamel hypoplasia.

Laboratory test results:

Calcium = 9.8 mg/dL (8.2-11.2 mg/dL) (SI: 2.5 mmol/L [2.1-2.8 mmol/L])
Phosphate = 3.0 mg/dL (4.2-7.4 mg/dL) (SI: 1.0 mmol/L [1.4-2.4 mmol/L])
FGF-23 = 280 RU/mL (<230 RU/mL)
PTH = 75 pg/mL (15-85 pg/mL) (SI: 75 ng/L [15-85 ng/L])
Alkaline phosphatase = 439 U/L (73-300 U/L) (SI: 7.3 μkat/L [1.2-5.0 μkat/L])
25-Hydroxyvitamin D = 36.9 ng/mL (20.0-60.0 ng/mL) (SI: 92.1 nmol/L [50-150 nmol/L])
1,25-Dihydroxyvitamin D = 34.8 pg/mL (47.1-151.0 pg/mL) (SI: 90.5 pmol/L [122.5-392.6 pmol/L])
Urinary protein, negative
Urinary blood, negative
Urinary glucose, negative
Tubular maximum reabsorption of phosphate-to-glomerular filtration rate = 2.99 mg/dL (3.25-5.51 mg/dL) (SI: 0.97 mmol/L [1.05-1.78 mmol/L])
Urinary calcium-to-creatinine ratio = 0.002 mg/dL (<0.2 mg/dL) (SI: 0.002 mmol/L [<0.2 mmol/L])

X-rays are shown (*see images*).

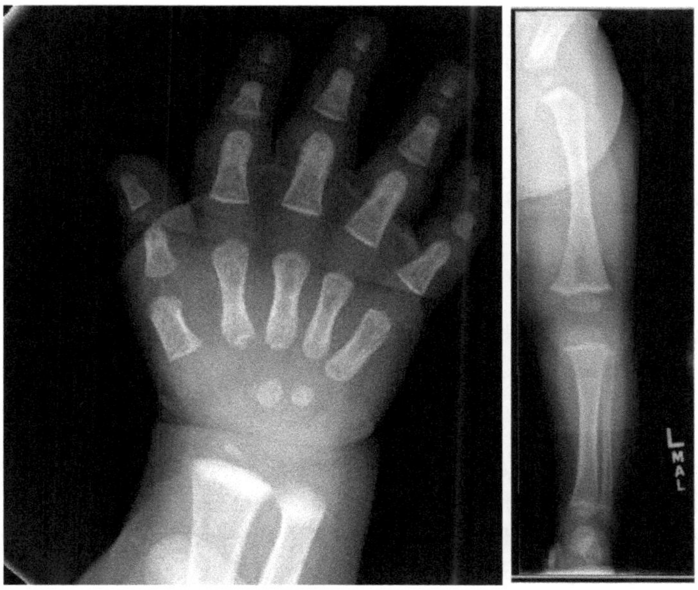

Based on these findings, pathogenic variants in which of the following genes most likely explain this child's condition?

A. *CLCN5* (Dent disease)
B. *DMP1* (autosomal recessive hypophosphatemic rickets type 1)
C. *ENPP1* (autosomal recessive hypophosphatemic rickets type 2)
D. *FAM20C* (Raine syndrome)
E. *SLC34A3* (hereditary hypophosphatemic rickets with hypercalciuria)

40 A 6-day-old male newborn is being evaluated for congenital hypothyroidism. He was born full-term after an uncomplicated pregnancy with a birthweight of 7 lb, 15.7 oz (3620 g), length of 20.9 in (53 cm), and head circumference of 13.7 in (34.7 cm). In the delivery room, he was noted to have a cleft lip and palate and bilateral choanal atresia. The rest of his physical examination findings were normal, and there was no palpable goiter.

His TSH-based newborn screening result was positive. Results of follow-up laboratory tests (day 6 of life):

TSH = 71.0 mIU/L (0.7-11.0 mIU/L)
Free T_4 = 1.2 ng/dL (0.9-2.2 ng/dL) (SI: 15.4 pmol/L [11.6-28.3 pmol/L])

This infant's clinical presentation is most likely due to pathogenic variant(s) in which of the following genes?

A. *FOXE1*
B. *NKX2-1*
C. *PAX8*
D. *POU1F1*
E. *TPO*

41 A 13-year-old girl with type 1 diabetes presents for a follow-up appointment. Diabetes was diagnosed 3 years ago after she presented in diabetic ketoacidosis. Her current hemoglobin A_{1c} value is 10.3% (89 mmol/mol), which is significantly increased compared with the past year's average of 8.2% (66 mmol/mol). Her BMI is stable at the 89th percentile with normal linear growth. She has not yet experienced menarche. Additionally, her mother has observed an escalating emotional struggle that has adversely affected the patient's diabetes self-management and academic performance. She has been skipping breakfast, stating that she is not hungry in the morning, and skipping lunch to avoid the school nurse. Her mother endorses concern about her eating habits, food choices, and meal timing. The patient declines to wear a glucose sensor despite the fear of hypoglycemia and she also refuses to try an insulin pump. Her self-reported total daily dose of insulin does not match her daily needs or elevated hemoglobin A_{1c} level.

Which of the following increases this patient's risk for an eating disorder?

A. BMI percentile
B. Duration of diabetes
C. Fear of hypoglycemia
D. History of diabetic ketoacidosis at the time of diagnosis
E. Refusal to try an insulin pump

42 A 14-year-old girl is being evaluated for poor growth and short stature. Anorexia nervosa was diagnosed at age 12 years. She was admitted for 7 months of inpatient nutritional rehabilitation and was discharged 9 months ago when her weight improved. Her height and BMI values are shown (*see table*). Breast and pubic hair development are both Tanner stage 3. She has not yet had menarche. Her midparental height is at the 75th percentile (0.67 SDS).

Time point	Height SDS	BMI SDS
Premorbid	−1.00	0.10
At hospital admission	−2.10	−2.38
At discharge	−1.80	−0.39
At 6-month follow-up	−1.62	−0.55

Laboratory test results at hospital admission:

IGF-1 = 188 ng/mL (199-537 ng/mL) (SI: 24.6 nmol/L [26.1-70.3 nmol/L])
TSH = 0.5 mIU/L (0.5-4.8 mIU/L)
Free T_4 = 0.7 ng/dL (0.90-1.67 ng/dL) (SI: 9 pmol/L [11.6-21.5 pmol/L])
Basic metabolic panel, normal
Celiac screen, negative

Which of the following most likely accounts for this patient's growth pattern?

A. Constitutional pubertal delay
B. GH resistance
C. Hypopituitarism
D. Hypothyroidism
E. Normal growth

43 An 18-year-old nonHispanic White girl presents for follow-up of obesity, prediabetes, and dyslipidemia. At the current visit with her pediatrician, her height is 64 in (162.6 cm) (50th percentile) and weight is 280 lb (127 kg) (>99th percentile). She previously participated in a lifestyle-based weight management program during which she was able to lose 8.8 lb (4 kg). Since the conclusion of the program, she has not been able to lose any more weight. She reports bullying at school related to her weight, and she is worried about her risk for developing type 2 diabetes mellitus, which affects several family members. She has noncommercial Medicaid insurance.

Which of the following represents the most significant barrier to this patient accessing bariatric surgery?

A. High risk of surgical complications
B. Lack of discussion initiated by her primary care physician about bariatric surgery
C. Less surgical efficacy given her race (compared with efficacy in racial minority patients)
D. Little benefit gained compared with a lifestyle-based weight-management program
E. Low likelihood of insurance approval because of her age

44 A 14-year-old girl presents for evaluation of infrequent menses. She had her first period at age 11 years, but she has had only 4 periods since then. Her periods last 7 to 10 days. Breast development started at age 9 years with normal progression through puberty. She has no fatigue, vision problems, headaches, abdominal pain, constipation, cold intolerance, excessive body or facial hair, acne, or recent weight change. She swims and plays field hockey. Family history is notable for hypothyroidism in her mother and maternal grandmother. Her mother underwent menarche at age 14 years and has no history of menstrual irregularity. The patient's midparental height is 63 in (160 cm).

Physical examination findings are unremarkable. Breast and pubic hair development are Tanner stage 5. Her height is 61.7 in (157 cm; 28th percentile), weight is 123 lb (55.7 kg; 72nd percentile), and BMI is 22.7 kg/m^2 (81st percentile).

Laboratory test results:

TSH, normal
Free T_4, normal
Complete blood cell count, normal
Complete metabolic profile, normal
Erythrocyte sedimentation rate, normal
Estradiol = 68.0 pg/mL (12.5-166.0 pg/mL [follicular]) (SI: 249.6 pmol/L [45.9-609.4 pmol/L (follicular)])
FSH = 6.3 mIU/mL (1.6-17.0 mIU/mL) (SI: 6.3 IU/L [1.6-17.0 IU/L])
LH = 8.4 mIU/mL (0.5-41.7 mIU/mL) (SI: 8.4 IU/L [0.5-41.7 IU/L])
Prolactin = 6.4 pg/mL (3.2-20.0 pg/mL) (SI: 0.28 nmol/L [0.14-0.87 nmol/L])
Total testosterone = 33 ng/dL (20-38 ng/dL) (SI: 1.1 nmol/L [0.7-1.3 nmol/L])
Androstenedione = 152 ng/dL (42-221 ng/dL) (SI: 5.3 nmol/L [1.5-7.7 nmol/L])

Which of the following is the best next step in this patient's management?

A. Complete a progesterone challenge test
B. Offer reassurance and continued monitoring
C. Perform pelvic ultrasonography
D. Refer to a dietician for weight management
E. Start a combined oral contraceptive pill

45 An 8-year-old girl with a diagnosis of congenital adrenal hyperplasia is being followed up in the pediatric endocrine clinic. She is currently receiving hydrocortisone replacement at a dosage of 14 mg/m^2 per day. Her parents report that they have noticed bruising of her skin, and she has been experiencing joint pain.

Which of the following is the best next step in this patient's management?

A. Assess for rheumatoid factor in a blood sample
B. Examine for hypermobility
C. Measure prothrombin time
D. Perform genetic testing for variants in the *VWF* gene
E. Reduce the hydrocortisone dosage

46

A male baby born at 38 weeks gestational age has a newborn screen performed on day 2 of life. On day 10 of life, the results return abnormal, and additional laboratory studies are performed on day 11 of life.

Newborn screen (day 2 of life):

Total T_4 = 1.3 µg/dL (>5.0 µg/dL) (SI: 16.7 nmol/L [>64.4 nmol/L])
TSH = 3.2 mIU/L (<20.0 mIU/L)

Serum (day 11 of life):

TSH = 2.5 mIU/L (1.7-9.1 mIU/L)
Free T_4 = 0.8 ng/dL (0.9-2.3 ng/dL) (SI: 10.30 pmol/L [11.6-29.6 pmol/L])

The baby's birth weight was 6 lb, 13 oz (3100 g) (45th percentile for gestational age), and he has been doing well at home. He is feeding and stooling normally and having 6 to 8 wet diapers per day. He has no hypothermia, signs of hypoglycemia, or prolonged jaundice. The pregnancy was uncomplicated, and there is no maternal history of thyroid disease. He receives no medications.

On physical examination, the infant has regained his birth weight and has normal vital signs and no dysmorphisms. He has normal red reflexes and no roving eye movements. The palate is normal. There is no umbilical hernia, the penis is normal in size and morphology, and both testes are descended. Muscle tone and reflexes are normal. The rest of the examination findings are normal.

Which of the following is the best next step in this patient's management?

A. Initiate levothyroxine treatment
B. Measure serum albumin
C. Measure serum free T_4 by equilibrium dialysis
D. Perform a cosyntropin-stimulation test
E. Perform MRI of the brain

47

A 15-year-old boy with type 1 diabetes presents for a follow-up visit. Diabetes was diagnosed at age 10 years. For the past year, he has used an automated hybrid closed-loop pump system, self-managing diabetes by using the system in automation 95% to 100% of the time. Today, his hemoglobin A_{1c} value is 7.8% (62 mmol/mol). His main concern is hypoglycemia after meals.

His pump report is reviewed:

- Total daily dose of insulin = 58 units (current weight, 62 kg; 0.93 unit/kg per day)
- Total daily basal dose of insulin = 35 units (60% of total daily dose)
- Sensor readings for a typical day for breakfast, late lunch, and dinner are shown (*see image*)

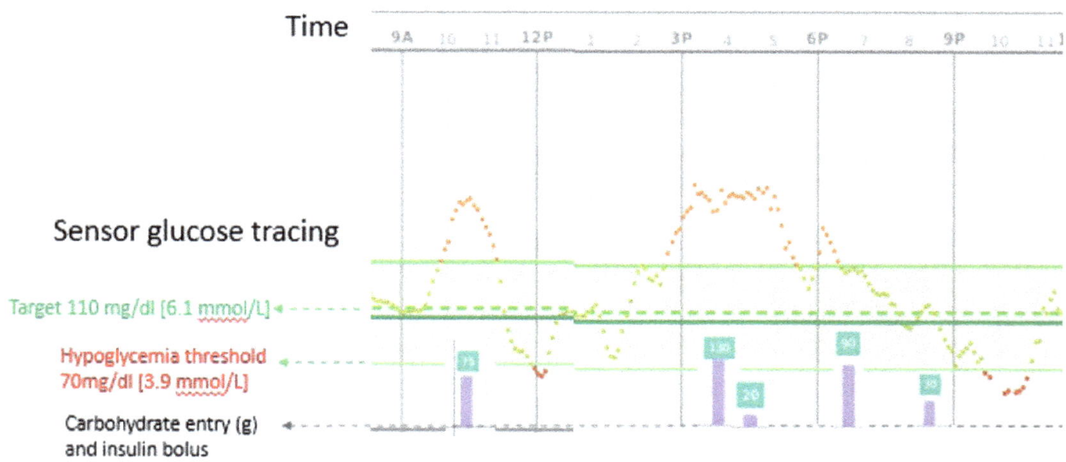

Which of the following interventions should be recommended to prevent this patient's postprandial hypoglycemia and improve his glycemic control?

A. Activate "exercise/activity" mode to elevate target glucose after meal bolus
B. Increase the insulin amount for all meals
C. Lower the basal rate in the postprandial period
D. Lower the insulin amount calculated by the correction (insulin sensitivity) factor
E. Re-educate about the timely entry of all carbohydrates before meal consumption

48

A 16-year-old girl seeks evaluation for a constellation of symptoms, including fatigue, headache, weight gain, irregular menses, and galactorrhea.

On physical examination, she has bradycardia, dry skin, and facial and peripheral edema.

Laboratory test results:

TSH = 1578 mIU/L (0.5-4.8 mIU/L)
Free T_4, undetectable
Prolactin = 113 ng/mL (4.8-23.3 ng/mL) (SI: 4.9 nmol/L [0.2-1.0 nmol/L]) (confirmed with serial dilution)

MRI of the brain and pituitary demonstrates a large sellar and suprasellar mass (23 × 23 × 10 mm) with associated compression of the cavernous sinus bilaterally and stretching of the optic chiasm.

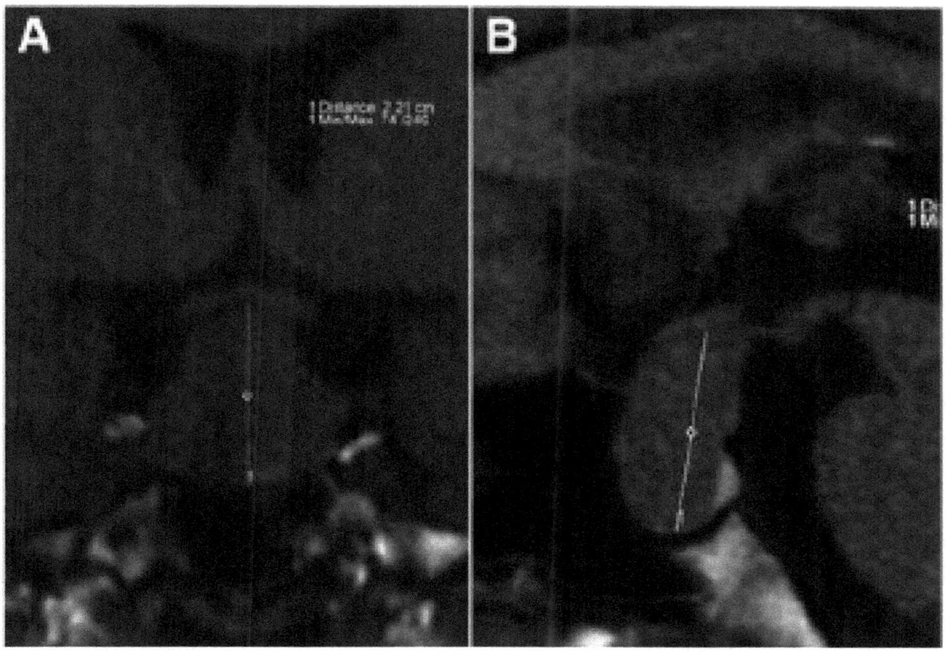

MRI of the brain and pituitary (postgadolinium, T1-weighted images). *Panel A*, coronal section; *Panel B*, sagittal section. Reprinted from Passeri, E et al. *J Clin Endocrinol Metab*, 2011; 96(1): 22–23. © The Endocrine Society.

Which of the following is this patient's most likely diagnosis?

A. Craniopharyngioma
B. Macroprolactinoma
C. Nonfunctioning pituitary macroadenoma
D. Pituitary hyperplasia
E. TSH-secreting pituitary adenoma

49 An 18-year-old girl presents to primary care because her friends noticed a change in the appearance of her eyes. Although she had not noticed anything herself, when she looks at old photographs she recognizes that her eyes now look more prominent. Her primary care physician notes that she has lid retraction and lid lag with conjunctival irritation. She has no diplopia or changes in visual acuity.

Her primary care physician orders thyroid function tests and refers her to pediatric endocrinology:

TSH = <0.01 mIU/L (0.5-4.3 mIU/L)
Free T_4 = 3.7 ng/dL (1.0-1.6 ng/dL) (SI: 47.6 pmol/L [12.9-20.6 pmol/L])
Thyroid-stimulating immunoglobulin = 412% (0%-139%)

On physical examination in the endocrinology clinic, she has lid lag, proptosis, swelling, and redness of the eyelids, and conjunctival redness and swelling. She has normal eye movements.

She is prescribed methimazole for management of hyperthyroidism. She is accompanied by her mother who has been reading about a new medication available to treat thyroid eye disease (teprotumumab). The patient is informed that treatment will depend on both her level of disease activity and severity.

Which of the following best reflects the clinical activity level, severity, and management recommendation for this patient's thyroid eye disease?

Answer	Clinical activity	Disease severity	Recommendation
A.	Active	Mild	Observation
B.	Active	Moderate	Teprotumumab
C.	Active	Severe	Orbital surgery
D.	Inactive	Mild	Observation
E.	Inactive	Moderate	Teprotumumab

50 A 4-year-old African American girl presents to her pediatrician for a yearly well-child visit. The pediatrician notes that her height has fallen from the 30th percentile (–0.5 SDS) at age 2 years to just under the 3rd percentile (–1.9 SDS). Her weight has stayed steady at the 40th percentile. She is otherwise healthy and has no notable findings on physical examination. Midparental height is at the 35th percentile, but there is a history of a grandmother who was "on the short side." The pediatrician reassures the parents that their daughter seems healthy and that she will likely end up growing fine in the next few years. The parents are not particularly concerned, as they state that being tall is not as important for girls as it is for boys.

The patient returns the following year for her 5-year well-child visit, and her height has fallen further (now –2.5 SDS). Her growth velocity is approximately 3.5 cm/y. The mother is becoming concerned about the girl's height and asks for a referral to a pediatric endocrinologist. The pediatrician provides the referral, and the patient is seen in endocrine clinic the following month. The history and physical examination are reviewed, and no additional relevant findings are noted. Her weight has continued to stay stable at the 40th percentile. Her body proportions are normal.

The endocrinologist orders a battery of tests. Results of complete blood cell count and complete metabolic panel are normal. Thyroid function is normal and a test for celiac disease is negative. Her IGF-1 concentration is –2.5 SD.

Which of the following is this patient's most likely diagnosis?

A. Constitutional delay of growth and development
B. Familial short stature
C. GH deficiency
D. *SHOX* deletion
E. Turner syndrome

51 A 12-year-old boy is being seen for follow-up of weight concerns. His current height is 59.3 in (150.5 cm) (56th percentile; Z-score, 0.16), and weight is 198.4 lb (90 kg) (>99th percentile; Z-score, 2.95). He reports having intermittent knee pain, and his mother notes that he occasionally limps. He has had no trauma or injury. He does not currently participate in structured sports, although he sometimes plays basketball with his friends.

On physical examination, he has genu varum.

Which of the following findings would be anticipated on this patient's knee radiographs?

A. Broadening of the medial tibial physis
B. Enlarged metaphysis and widened cupped physis
C. Lucency in the articular epiphysis
D. Swelling of the tibial tuberosity
E. Thickening of the proximal patellar tendon

52 A 17-year-old Hispanic boy is referred for management of prediabetes and obesity. Testing completed 3 months ago is notable for abnormal transaminase concentrations, dyslipidemia, and a hemoglobin A_{1c} value of 6.0% (42 mmol/mol). After being referred for weight management, he started going to the gym 2 to 3 times per week and plans to play football for school. He is now drinking water instead of soft drinks, but he frequently eats snack foods, eats big meal portions, and has a hard time making healthy choices. He has no polyuria or polydipsia.

On physical examination, his height is 72 in (182.9 cm) (88th percentile) and weight is 209 lb (95 kg) (94th percentile) (BMI = 28.4 kg/m^2 [Z-score = 1.57]). He has moderate acanthosis nigricans.

Laboratory test results:

Hemoglobin A_{1c} = 5.9% (4.8%-5.6%) (SI: 41 mmol/mol [29-38 mmol/mol])
AST = 33 U/L (0-40 U/L) (SI: 0.55 µkat/L [0-0.67 µkat/L])
ALT = 40 U/L (0-30 U/L) (SI: 0.67 µkat/L [0-0.50 µkat/L])
γ-Glutamyltransferase = 28 U/L (0-65 U/L) (SI: 0.47 µkat/L [0-1.1 µkat/L])
Total cholesterol = 203 mg/dL (<170 mg/dL) (SI: 5.26 mmol/L [<4.40 mmol/L])
Triglycerides = 255 mg/dL (<90 mg/dL) (SI: 2.88 mmol/L [<1.02 mmol/L])
HDL cholesterol = 37 mg/dL (>45 mg/dL) (SI: 0.96 mmol/L [>1.17 mmol/L])
LDL cholesterol (calculated) = 130 mg/dL (<110 mg/dL) (SI: 3.37 mmol/L [<2.85 mmol/L])

53 A 14-year-old boy is referred for evaluation of short stature. He is otherwise well with no concerning symptoms. He reports always being the shortest child in his peer group.

On physical examination, pubertal development is Tanner stage 3. His height is 53.9 in (136.8 cm) (Z-score, –3.18), and weight is 79.4 lb (36 kg) (Z-score, –2.32). Examination findings are normal, with no dysmorphic features. Specifically, he does not have Madelung deformity, scoliosis, or obvious limb shortening.

His father's height is 63 in (160 cm) (Z-score, –2.34), and mother's height is 60 in (152.4 cm) (Z-score, –1.68). Midparental height is 64 in (136.8 cm) (Z-score, –1.97).

Which of the following is the best next step in this patient's evaluation?

A. Calculation of sitting height-to-standing height ratio
B. Celiac disease screen
C. IGF-1 measurement
D. Reassurance with no further evaluation
E. Skeletal survey

54 An 8-day-old, full-term female baby is being evaluated for mild clitoromegaly that was first noted by her mother, who is a nurse, and confirmed by her primary care physician. Physical examination findings are notable for a prominent clitoris (length, 1.15 cm [normal <1 cm]). She has no hyperpigmentation, labial fusion, or urogenital sinus. There are no palpable gonads in the labia.

She has no history of neonatal hypoglycemia, and her newborn screening was normal, including a negative result for classic congenital adrenal hyperplasia (CAH) due to 21-hydroxylase deficiency.

Which of the following is the best first step in this patient's management?

A. Measure serum 17-hydroxyprogesterone, testosterone, electrolytes, and plasma renin
B. Perform a high-dose cosyntropin-stimulation test
C. Perform pelvic ultrasonography to evaluate for a uterus and gonads
D. Reassure the family that she does not have classic CAH
E. Refer for genetic counseling and order a gene panel to rule out differences of sex development

55 A 17-year-old girl presents with a lump in her right neck that has been noticeable for 3 weeks. She has no pain, dysphagia, voice changes, or symptoms of hyperthyroidism. She is otherwise healthy and takes no medications. Her family history is notable for autoimmune thyroiditis in her mother and Hirschsprung disease in her younger brother.

On physical examination, her pulse rate and blood pressure are normal. There is a 2-cm, firm nodule in her right thyroid lobe that moves with swallowing. An enlarged lymph node is palpable in her right lateral neck.

In addition to TSH measurement, which of the following is most important to measure as the next step in this patient's management?

A. Calcitonin
B. Free T_4
C. Radioiodine uptake
D. Thyroglobulin
E. TPO antibodies

56 A 4-day-old, full-term male newborn is referred due to concerns about a small penis. Birth weight was 6 lb 9 oz (3000 g) (Z-score, −1.12), and length was 19.7 in (50 cm) (Z-score, −0.45). Hypoglycemia was noted soon after birth, but he is currently feeding every 2 hours without prefeed hypoglycemia.

On physical examination, his penile length is 1.5 cm, and he has a cleft lip. The rest of his findings are normal.

Which of the following is the most appropriate next step in assessing whether this infant has GH deficiency?

A. Diagnostic fasting study to assess GH concentration during hypoglycemia
B. GH-stimulation test
C. IGFBP-1 measurement
D. IGF-1 measurement
E. Random GH measurement

57 An 11-year-old girl presents for endocrine evaluation following 2 episodes of galactorrhea in the past 2 months. She has been previously well, and her pediatrician has never expressed concerns about her growth. She has no headaches or vision changes. They have noticed some breast development and pubic hair, but no menarche yet. Her mother had menarche at age 15 years.

On physical examination, she is awake and alert, with normal vital signs. Pupils are equal, round, and reactive to light. There is no afferent pupillary defect and no papilledema. Breast development and pubic hair are Tanner stage 3.

Laboratory test results:

- Prolactin (confirmed on dilution) = 65.1 ng/mL (1.0-18.0 ng/mL) (SI: 2.83 nmol/L [0.04-0.78 nmol/L])
- Free T_4 = 0.8 ng/dL (1.0-1.7 ng/dL) (SI: 10.30 pmol/L [12.87-21.88 pmol/L])
- TSH = 3.18 mIU/L (0.7-4.2 mIU/L)
- IGF-1 = 231 ng/mL (197-642 ng/mL) (SI: 30.3 nmol/L [25.8-84.1 nmol/L]) (Z-score for Tanner stage = −0.5)
- LH = 1.65 mIU/mL (≤4.38 mIU/mL [<10-11 years]) (SI: 1.65 IU/L [≤4.38 IU/L])
- FSH = 7.39 mIU/mL (0.87-9.16 mIU/mL [10-13 years]) (SI: 7.39 IU/L [0.87-9.16 IU/L])
- Estradiol = 27 pg/mL (≤65 pg/mL) (SI: 99.1 pmol/L [≤238.6 pmol/L])
- ACTH = 36 pg/mL (9-57 pg/mL) (SI: 9.9 pmol/L [2.0-12.4 pmol/L])
- Cortisol (8 AM) = 27.8 μg/dL (3-25 μg/dL) (SI: 766.9 nmol/L [82.8-689.7 nmol/L])
- α-Subunit = 2.1 ng/mL (≤1.2 ng/mL [3 months-17 years]) (SI: 2.1 μg/L [≤1.2 μg/L])
- α-Fetoprotein = 3.1 ng/mL (<8.4 ng/mL) (SI: 3.1 μg/L [<8.4 μg/L])
- β-hCG = <1.0 mIU/mL (<1.0 mIU/mL) (SI: <1.0 IU/L [<1.0 IU/L])

Pituitary MRI documents a 3.2 × 2.5 × 2.1-cm sellar mass with suprasellar extension (*see image*).

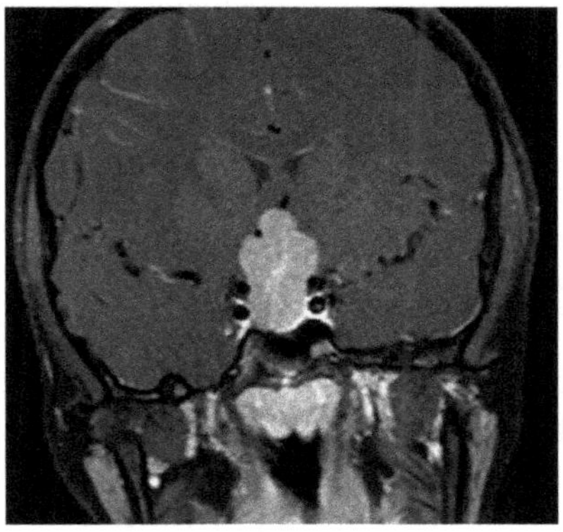

Formal neuro-ophthalmology evaluation demonstrates bilateral upper temporal visual field deficits (L>R), consistent with chiasmal compression (*see image*).

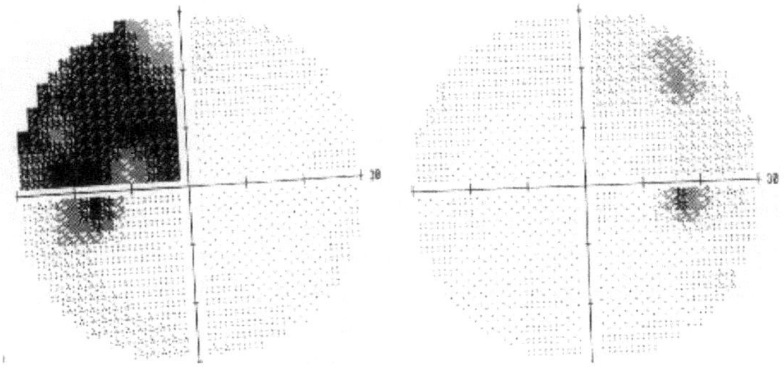

Visual fields via Humphrey visual field test. Left eye (*left panel*): moderate upper temporal visual field deficit; right eye (*right panel*): mild upper temporal visual field deficit.

She undergoes endoscopic endonasal resection of the mass. Histologic studies are consistent with an immature *PIT1* lineage adenoma/pituitary endocrine tumor (Pit-NET). Specifically, immunohistochemistry is positive for GATA3 and PIT1, negative for the estrogen receptor (not consistent with a well-differentiated lactotroph adenoma), negative for TSH, and negative for GH. Laboratory evaluation 6 weeks after the procedure demonstrates an intact hypothalamic-pituitary-adrenal axis, persistent central hypothyroidism, IGF-1 Z-score of 0.1, pubertal gonadotropin concentrations, and a prolactin concentration below the reference range. Follow-up pituitary MRI does not identify residual tumor.

Laboratory measurement of which of the following would be most useful with respect to surveillance for this particular tumor?

A. α-Subunit
B. 8-AM cortisol
C. hCG
D. IGF-1
E. TSH

58 A 17-year-old girl is referred for abnormal thyroid laboratory test results and ultrasonography findings. At her recent physical examination, she described significant fatigue. She has longstanding obesity, and her primary care physician has recommended initiation of semaglutide. She has not had any weight-loss success despite working on lifestyle modifications for more than a year. There is no family history of thyroid cancer or autoimmune conditions.

On physical examination, her height is 61.8 in (157.0 cm) and weight is 234.6 lb (106.4 kg) (BMI = 43.1 kg/m^2). Her blood pressure is 117/76 mm Hg. Her thyroid gland is palpable and smooth.

Laboratory test results:

TSH = 6.3 mIU/L (0.5-4.3 mIU/L)
Free T_4 = 1.1 ng/dL (1.0-1.6 ng/dL) (SI: 14.16 pmol/L [12.87-20.59 pmol/L]
TPO antibodies = 4.7 IU/mL (<9.0 IU/mL) (SI: 4.7 kIU/L [<9.0 kIU/L])
Thyroglobulin antibodies = 1.8 IU/mL (<4.0 IU/mL) (SI: 1.8 kIU/L [<4.0 kIU/L])

Thyroid ultrasonography shows mildly increased thyroid volume with loss of homogeneity and generalized hypoechogenicity suggestive of thyroiditis.

Which of the following is the best next step in this patient's management?

A. Explain that semaglutide is contraindicated due to abnormal findings on thyroid ultrasonography
B. Reassure her that no thyroid intervention is needed; semaglutide can be prescribed if indicated
C. Repeat thyroid ultrasonography in 6 months; if findings are stable, semaglutide can be considered
D. Repeat TSH, free T_4, and thyroid autoantibody measurement in 3 months; if stable, semaglutide can be considered
E. Start levothyroxine, 75 mcg daily; once TSH normalizes, semaglutide can be considered

59 A 15-year-old girl presents for evaluation of primary amenorrhea and short stature. Her height has remained the same for the last 2 years (58 in [147.3 cm]). Her primary care provider attributed her short stature to being a "late bloomer," and no previous workup was done. Breast development began 3 years ago; however, she is concerned that her breasts are small and that she still looks like a child. She is very bothered by her appearance and wants to look like her friends. She is also sexually active and usually uses condoms for contraception, but she admits often forgetting. There is no family history of delayed puberty. She has no nausea or fatigue and has had good weight gain in the last year. She takes ballet classes 3 times per week and dances for 2 hours in each session.

On physical examination, she has Tanner stage 3 pubic hair and early stage 3 breast development. Examination findings are otherwise unremarkable, with no acne or hirsutism. Her BMI is normal.

Her bone age is 14 years at the chronologic age of 15 years.

Laboratory test results:

IGF-1 = 156 ng/mL (160-640 ng/mL) (SI: 20.44 nmol/L [20.96-83.84 nmol/L])
LH = 4.5 mIU/mL (1.3-9.8 mIU/mL) (SI: 4.5 IU/L [1.3-9.8 IU/L])
FSH = 7.9 mIU/mL (1.6-17.0 mIU/mL) (SI: 7.9 IU/L [1.6-17.0 IU/L])
Testosterone = 10.0 ng/dL (10.7-15.4 ng/dL) (SI: 0.35 nmol/L [0.37-0.53 nmol/L])
Estradiol = 10.0 pg/mL (12.5-166.0 pg/mL) (SI: 36.7 pmol/L [45.9-609.4 pmol/L])

TSH = 2.0 mIU/L (0.45-4.5 mIU/L)
Free T_4 = 0.09 ng/dL (0.93-1.60 ng/dL) (SI: 1.16 pmol/L [11.97-20.59 pmol/L])
Cortisol = 9.0 µg/dL (6.2-19.4 µg/dL) (SI: 248.3 nmol/L [171.0-535.2 nmol/L])
Karyotype = 46,XX
Fluorescence in situ hybridization microarray, normal
Pregnancy test, negative

On pelvic ultrasonography, ovaries are not enlarged and there is no endometrial stripe. No cysts or anatomic abnormalities are noted.

Which of the following is the best next step in this patient's management?

A. Measure 17-hydroxyprogesterone
B. Offer reassurance; she is a late bloomer
C. Perform a cosyntropin-stimulation test
D. Perform MRI of her brain
E. Perform MRI to visualize her ovaries

60 A 2-year-old girl presents for an initial evaluation of severe short stature. Her mother reports that the pregnancy was uneventful except for intrauterine growth restriction. She did not take any medications during pregnancy. The patient was born at 38 weeks' gestation with a length of 14.4 in (36.5 cm) (–5 SD), weight of 3 lb 8 oz (1600 g) (–3.8 SD), and head circumference of 12.2 in (31 cm) (–1.8 SD). She has not demonstrated any catch-up growth, and her length is deviating further from the curve. She has had significant feeding difficulties and has required intermittent nasogastric tube feedings.

On physical examination, she has a prominent forehead and triangular-shaped face.

She previously had genetic testing, including methylation analysis of chromosome 11p15, and results are normal.

Laboratory testing documents normal results of a complete blood cell count, thyroid studies, celiac screen, and complete metabolic panel. Her IGF-1 concentration is at the mean for sex and age. Upon further questioning, the family discloses that there are additional relatives with a similar clinical presentation as depicted in the pedigree (*see image, proband noted with an arrow*).

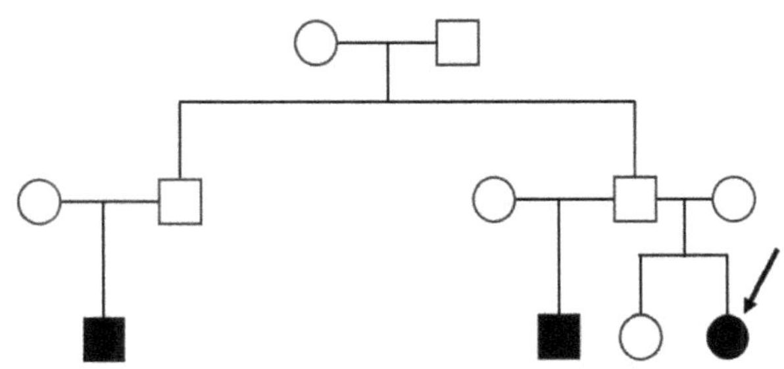

Which of the following is the best next test in this patient's diagnostic workup?

A. Assessing for uniparental disomy of chromosome 7
B. Karyotype analysis
C. Sequencing the *IGF1* gene
D. Sequencing the *IGF1R* gene
E. Sequencing the *IGF2* gene

61 A 14-year-old boy presents with a history of multiple fractures since early childhood, mostly in his lower extremities. He has required several orthopedic surgeries with rod and pin placement. He has chronic musculoskeletal pain and relies on analgesics almost daily. He has impaired mobility, necessitating the use of a cane or walker. He also has a history of premature loss of primary teeth. His midparental height is 70.5 in (179 cm).

On physical examination, he has significant short stature (height Z-score, –5.0) and leg deformities.

Laboratory test results (serum):

Calcium = 10.6 mg/dL (8.0-10.5 mg/dL) (SI: 2.7 mmol/L [2.0-2.6 mmol/L])
Phosphorus = 6.9 mg/dL (2.9-5.4 mg/dL) (SI: 2.2 mmol/L [0.9-1.7 mmol/L])
Alkaline phosphatase = <20 U/L (55-360 U/L) (SI: 0.33 μkat/L [0.92-6.01 μkat/L])
PTH = 25 pg/mL (10-65 pg/mL) (SI: 2.7 pmol/L [1.1-6.9 pmol/L])
25-Hydroxyvitamin D = 20 ng/mL (30-100 ng/mL) (SI: 49.9 nmol/L [74.9-249.6 nmol/L])
1,25-Dihydroxyvitamin D = 82 pg/mL (15-90 pg/mL) (SI: 213.2 pmol/L [39.0-234.0 pmol/L])

DXA demonstrates low bone mineral density at the lumbar spine (0.36 g/cm^2 [Z-score, −5.9]).

His bone radiograph is shown (*see image*).

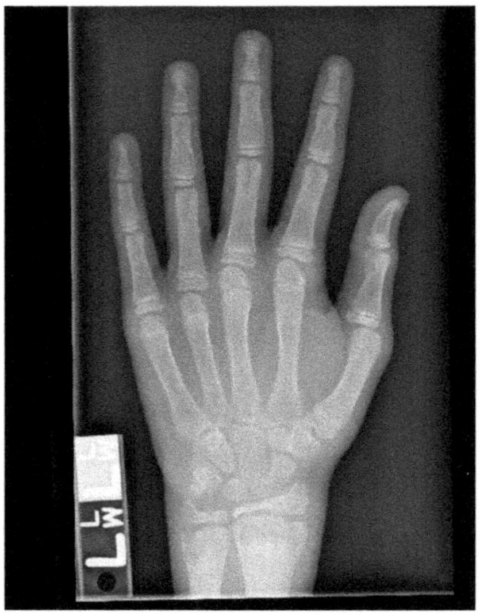

Reprinted from Bowden SA & Adler BH. Osteoporos *Int*, 2018; 29(2): 511-515.

Which of the following is the best next step in managing this patient's condition?

A. Measure serum pyridoxic acid
B. Order genetic testing for the *COL1A1* gene
C. Start a bisphosphonate
D. Start asfotase alfa
E. Start cholecalciferol

62 A 6-day-old girl remains in the hospital since birth for hypothermia and hyperbilirubinemia. She is sleepy and must be woken to feed. She was born at 38 weeks' gestation to a healthy woman (G1, P0) after an uncomplicated pregnancy.

On physical examination, her temperature is 98.3°F (36.8°C), and pulse rate and blood pressure are normal. Her fontanelles are mildly enlarged, and she is not dysmorphic. Red reflexes are normal, and she has no abnormal eye movements. Her palate is intact, her thyroid gland is not palpable, and the rest of the examination findings are normal.

Laboratory test results:

TSH = 5.4 mIU/L (1.7-9.1 mIU/L)
Free T_4 = 0.65 ng/dL (1.6-3.8 ng/dL) (SI: 8.4 pmol/L [20.6-48.9 pmol/L])
Total bilirubin = 16.2 mg/dL (0-12.0 mg/dL) (SI: 277.1 μmol/L [0-205.3 μmol/L])
Direct bilirubin = 0.8 mg/dL (0-0.6 mg/dL) (SI: 13.7 μmol/L [0-10.3 μmol/L])

Which of the following would be the most likely finding if this patient undergoes brain MRI?

A. Ectopic posterior pituitary
B. Normal findings
C. Optic nerve hypoplasia
D. Pituitary blastoma
E. Thickened pituitary stalk

63 A 2-year-old boy presents for follow-up after a recent hospital admission for new-onset diabetes. He had several weeks of excessive thirst and voracious appetite before hospital admission. His father, who was diagnosed with type 1 diabetes in childhood, checked the child's blood glucose, which read "high" on his home meter. Initial laboratory testing was notable for a blood glucose value of 407 ng/dL (22.6 mmol/L), hemoglobin A_{1c} value of 12.0% (108 mmol/mol), and negative urine ketones. A basal-bolus insulin regimen was initiated, and his hemoglobin A_{1c} value is now 7.8% (62 mmol/mol) on approximately 4 units of insulin daily. Subsequent testing was negative for diabetes autoantibodies. Genetic testing identified a likely pathogenic variant in the insulin gene (*INS*).

Which of the following is the best management of this patient's diabetes?

A. Continue basal-bolus insulin
B. Eliminate mealtime insulin dosing and continue basal insulin
C. Taper insulin and monitor blood glucose levels
D. Transition to a sulfonylurea
E. Transition to oral repaglinide

64 A 4-year-old boy is being seen for follow-up of rapid weight gain. His current BMI is 29 kg/m^2. His mother read a news article about plastics exposure and the potential impact on risk for overweight/obesity, as well as other health problems, during childhood and beyond. She would like to make some changes to their home environment, but she feels overwhelmed since she notes that "there are plastics everywhere she looks" in their home.

Which of the following is the best recommendation to reduce the most abundant source of microplastics exposure for this child?

A. Limit amount of fresh produce consumed
B. Limit use of topical body lotions
C. Replace cotton bedding with linen sheets
D. Reduce synthetic clothing items
E. Swap bottled shampoo for a shampoo bar

65 A 13-year-old prepubertal boy with a history of type 1 diabetes diagnosed at age 8 years presents with fatigue, faltering growth, skin hyperpigmentation, behavioral problems, and a decline in school performance. His diabetes control has been good (hemoglobin A_{1c} ranging from 7.3%-8.2% [56-66 mmol/mol]).

Laboratory test results:

Celiac disease screening, negative
Thyroid function, normal
ACTH (8 AM) = 1200 pg/mL (<47 pg/mL) (SI: 264.0 pmol/L [<10.3 pmol/L])
Cortisol (8 AM) = 2.1 µg/dL (5-25 µg/dL) (SI: 57.9 nmol/L [137.9-689.7 nmol/L])
Plasma renin = 24 ng/mL per h (0.5-3.3 ng/mL per h)
Adrenal androgens, undetectable
21α-Hydroxylase antibodies, undetectable

Of note, his 15-year-old brother has behavioral problems and was diagnosed with attention-deficit/hyperactivity disorder 1 year ago.

Which of the following tests is the best next step in this patient's evaluation?

A. *ABCD1* gene testing
B. *AIRE* gene testing
C. Brain MRI
D. Cosyntropin-stimulation testing
E. Measurement of very long-chain fatty acids

66 A 17-year-old girl is referred for evaluation and management of thyrotoxicosis. She presented to her physician after an early pregnancy loss and was noted to have hyperthyroidism. She is otherwise healthy with no notable medical history. There is no family history of thyroid disease or other autoimmune disease.

On physical examination, her blood pressure is 136/87 mm Hg and pulse rate is 108 beats/min. Her height is 69.3 in (176.0 cm), and weight is 126.3 lb (57.3 kg) (BMI = 18.5 kg/m^2). She has a smooth goiter. The rest of her examination findings are normal.

Laboratory test results:

TSH = <0.01 mIU/L (0.5-4.3 mIU/L)
Free T_4 = 3.4 ng/dL (1.0-1.6 ng/dL) (SI: 23.17 pmol/L [12.87-20.59 pmol/L])
Total T_3 = 278 ng/dL (91-218 ng/dL) (SI: 4.28 nmol/L [1.40-3.36 nmol/L])
TRAb = 11.2 IU/L (0-1.75 IU/L)

The 3 treatment modalities available to her (methimazole, radioactive iodine therapy, thyroidectomy) are discussed. She asks specifically about pregnancy complications associated with therapy in the event that she wants to conceive again very soon.

Assuming she responds quickly to therapy and becomes euthyroid, which of the following therapies conveys the greatest risk for fetal Graves disease if she becomes pregnant within the next 2 years?

A. Medical therapy with methimazole
B. Radioactive iodine
C. Radioactive iodine or methimazole (equal risk)
D. Thyroidectomy
E. Thyroidectomy or methimazole (equal risk)

67 A 12-week-old male infant, born at 27 weeks' gestation, had an eventful course in the neonatal intensive care unit that included respiratory distress syndrome, sepsis, and medical necrotizing enterocolitis with a 3-week duration of total parenteral nutrition. He developed chronic lung disease and has been on inhaled budesonide and oral furosemide since 10 weeks of age. He also had apnea of prematurity that improved with caffeine. He is fed with fortified expressed breast milk. At 12 weeks of age, he was noted to have decreased bilateral leg movement. Radiographs show femoral shaft fractures (*see image, arrows*), generalized osteopenia, and metaphyseal changes indicative of rickets (cupping, fraying, and splaying).

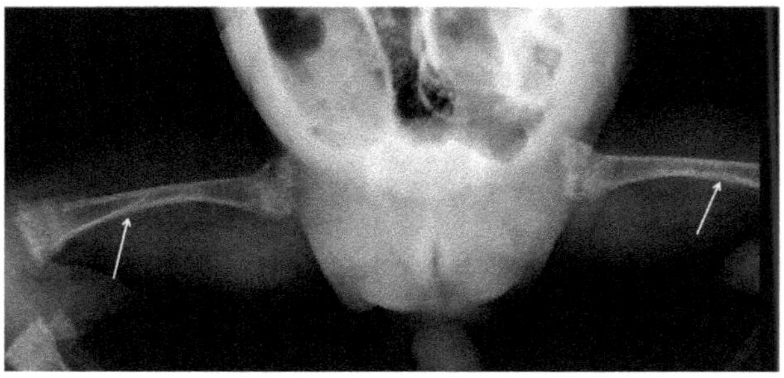

Laboratory test results (serum):

Calcium = 9.4 mg/dL (9.0-11.0 mg/dL) (SI: 2.4 mmol/L [2.3-2.8 mmol/L])
Phosphorus = 3 mg/dL (4-8 mg/dL) (SI: 0.97 mmol/L [1.29-2.58 mmol/L])
Alkaline phosphatase = 1300 U/L (150-420 U/L) (SI: 21.71 µkat/L [2.51-7.01 µkat/L])
25-Hydroxyvitamin D = 28 ng/mL (20-80 ng/mL) (SI: 69.9 nmol/L [49.9-199.7 nmol/L])
PTH = 215 pg/mL (10-65 pg/mL) (SI: 22.8 pmol/L [1.1-6.9 pmol/L])
Tubular reabsorption of phosphorus = 70% (78%-91%)

Which of the following is the best therapeutic intervention?

A. Calcium and calcitriol
B. Phosphate alone
C. Phosphate and calcitriol
D. Phosphate and cholecalciferol
E. Phosphate, cholecalciferol, and fortified human milk with calcium-to-phosphate ratio of 1:2

68 An 11-year-old boy is referred by his pediatrician to address a concern of rapid growth. The child is healthy with no known chronic medical conditions. He takes no medications. Review of his growth charts documents a growth velocity of 10.5 cm/y over the past 1 year. At today's visit, his height is 57.9 in (147 cm) (68th percentile). At his 10-year checkup, his height was 53.7 in (136.5 cm) (36th percentile). His BMI has stayed at the 50th percentile. Both parents' heights are at the 35th percentile.

On physical examination, his blood pressure is 110/70 mm Hg and pulse rate is 65 beats/min. His thyroid gland is not enlarged, and he has no palpable nodules. Pubic hair is Tanner stage 3, and testicular volume is 12 cc bilaterally.

His IGF-1 concentration is 550 ng/mL (123-497 ng/mL) (SI: 72.1 nmol/L [16.1-65.1 nmol/L]).

Which of the following is the best next step in this patient's management?

A. Brain MRI
B. GH-suppression test
C. Gonadotropin and testosterone measurements
D. Reassurance with no further testing
E. Thyroid function tests

69 An 8-year-old boy presents with penile enlargement (3.5 in [9 cm]), testicular volume of 4 cc bilaterally, Tanner stage 3 pubic hair, and linear growth acceleration in the last 6 months. His parents were not initially concerned because the father reports he also had early puberty, but he does not recall exactly how old he was at the time. His mother's height is 63 in (160 cm), and father's height is 71 in (180 cm). There is no history of exogenous testosterone exposure at home. The patient's primary care physician referred the child for further evaluation after performing some initial laboratory tests.

Laboratory test results (sample drawn at 8 AM):

LH = 0.01 mIU/mL (<0.02-0.50 mIU/mL) (SI: 0.01 IU/L [<0.02-0.50 IU/L])
FSH = 0.20 mIU/mL (≤2.30 mIU/mL) (SI: 0.20 IU/L [≤2.30 IU/L])
Total testosterone = 200 ng/dL (<2.5-10.0 ng/dL) (SI: 7.0 nmol/L [0.1-0.3 nmol/L])
DHEA-S = 150 µg/dL (18-194 µg/dL) (SI: 4.07 µmol/L [0.49-5.26 µmol/L])
17-Hydroxyprogesterone= 70 ng/dL (10-138 ng/dL) (SI: 2.1 nmol/L [0.3-4.18 nmol/L])

Bone age is determined to be 11 years at the chronologic age of 8 years.

Which of the following is the best next step in this patient's management?

A. Measure β-hCG
B. Measure LH again
C. Perform brain MRI
D. Perform genetic testing for pathogenic variants in the kisspeptin 1 gene (*KISS1*)
E. Perform genetic testing for pathogenic variants in the LH receptor gene (*LHCGR*)

70 An 8-year-old boy presents for growth concerns. His height has been consistently between the fifth and tenth percentile since age 2 years, and his parents are concerned about his height because they are tall (midparental height = 71 in [180.3 cm]). He was born at term after an uncomplicated pregnancy, with normal birth weight and length. He had delayed speech development and receives supports at school for speech and writing. He has longstanding severe constipation managed by a gastroenterologist.

On physical examination, his blood pressure is 82/51 mm Hg and pulse rate is 64 beats/min. His upper-to-lower segment ratio is elevated for age. He has a broad face, flattened nasal bridge, thickened lips, and a large tongue. His muscle tone is low, and he walks slowly, with a wide-based gait. The rest of the examination findings are normal.

Laboratory test results:

TSH = 1.1 mIU/L (0.5-5.0 mIU/L)
Free T_4 = 0.7 ng/dL (0.8-1.9 ng/dL) (SI: 9.01 pmol/L [10.30-24.45 pmol/L])
Total T_3 = 205 ng/dL (80-210 ng/dL) (SI: 3.16 nmol/L [1.23-3.23 nmol/L])
Hematocrit = 32% (34%-43%) (SI: 0.32 [0.34-0.43])
Mean corpuscular volume = 82.1 fL (77.8-86.5 fL)

Bone age is between 5 and 6 years.

A pathogenic variant in which of the following genes is most likely responsible for this patient's findings?

A. *ALB* (albumin)
B. *IGSF1* (immunoglobulin subfamily 1)
C. *SLC16A2* (solute carrier family 16 member 2)
D. *TBL1X* (transducing beta-like 1)
E. *THRA* (thyroid hormone receptor alpha)

71 A 14-year-old girl with type 2 diabetes presents for follow-up. When new-onset diabetes was diagnosed a year ago, her hemoglobin A_{1c} value was 8.3% (67 mmol/mol), she had negative ketones, and autoantibodies were negative. Her BMI at that time was 35.9 kg/m^2 (99th percentile). Metformin was prescribed, and she has tolerated a dosage of 1000 mg twice daily. However, she has been unable to lower her BMI and her hemoglobin A_{1c} has only decreased to 7.2% (55 mmol/mol). Her mother has seen advertisements for SGLT-2 inhibitors and would like to know more about this medication class.

In counseling this adolescent, which of the following should she expect with the addition of an SGLT-2 inhibitor?

A. Occasional mild hypoglycemia
B. 1% to 2% reduction in hemoglobin A_{1c}
C. Sustained increase in urination frequency
D. Transient gastrointestinal symptoms, including nausea, vomiting, and diarrhea
E. 2% to 4% reduction in body weight

72 A 10-year-old boy is referred for evaluation of slow growth. He has autism with an extremely restricted diet. Over the past few months, he has had intermittent loose stools. His height is 48.5 in (123.2 cm) (Z-score, −2.41), and weight is 49.6 lb (22.5 kg) (Z-score, −2.51). His midparental height is 70 in (179 cm) (Z-score, 0.3).

On physical examination, he is prepubertal and findings are normal, except for a rash on his face (*see image*).

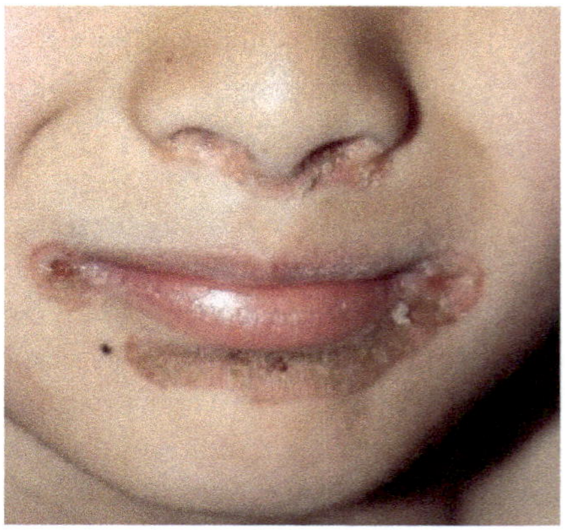

Laboratory test results:

IGF-1 = 80 ng/mL (100-449 ng/mL) (SI: 10.5 nmol/L [13.1-58.8 nmol/L])
Celiac disease screen, negative
Thyroid function, normal

Which of the following investigations is most likely to identify the cause of this boy's faltering growth?

A. Copper measurement
B. GH-stimulation testing
C. Iron measurement
D. Vitamin C measurement
E. Zinc measurement

73 A 19-year-old previously healthy girl presents with a 5-month history of irregular menses, weight gain (26.5 lb [12 kg] over the same interval), and blurred vision. Menarche was at age 12 years, and periods were regular until the development of these more recent symptoms. Her growth charts are shown (*see images*). Despite having grown less than 1 cm during the 2 years before presentation, she has grown another 2.5 cm in the past 12 months. Her hands have increased in size, and she has also gained a shoe size.

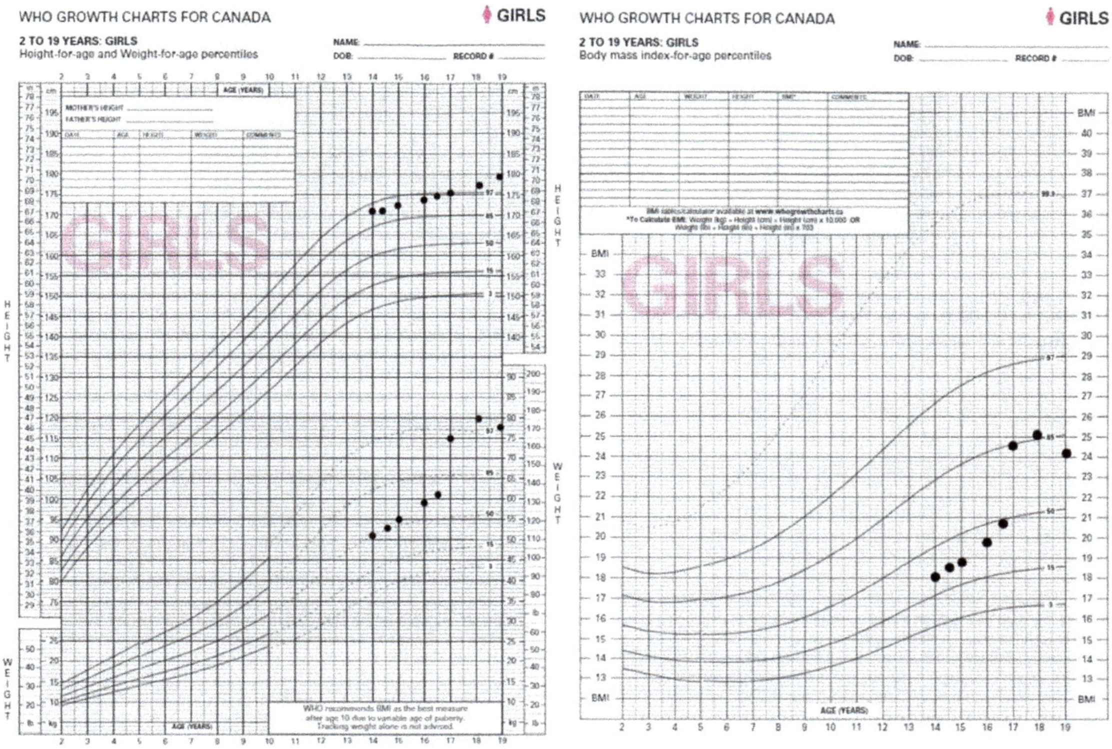

Reprinted from Galbiati F & Kaiser UB. *JCEM Case Rep*, 2023; 1(2): luad030. © The Authors. Published by Oxford University Press on behalf of the Endocrine Society.

There is no family history of pituitary, parathyroid, pancreatic, or adrenal tumors and no history of kidney stones. She is performing well in school. She takes no medications.

On physical examination, her height is 70 in [177.8 cm] (>99th percentile, with a midparental height at the 75th percentile), blood pressure is 131/90 mm Hg, and BMI is 23.7 kg/m^2. She has coarse facial features (enlarged tongue, widened nose) and decreased visual fields to confrontation on the right side.

Laboratory test results:

Electrolytes, normal
Kidney function, normal
IGF-1 = 1285 ng/mL (188-512 ng/mL) (SI: 168.3 nmol/L [24.6-67.1 nmol/L])
Random GH = 54 ng/mL (0.01-3.61 ng/mL) (SI: 54 µg/L [0.01-3.61 µg/L])
Prolactin = 43 ng/mL (3.8-20.1 ng/mL) (SI: 1.87 nmol/L [0.17-0.87 nmol/L])
Random cortisol = 22.8 µg/dL (6.2-19.4 µg/dL) (SI: 629.0 nmol/L [171.0-535.2 nmol/L])
Free T_4 = 0.8 ng/dL (0.8-1.8 ng/dL) (SI: 10.3 pmol/L [10.3-23.2 pmol/L])
TSH = 1.43 mIU/L (0.4-4.2 mIU/L)
LH = 1.36 mIU/mL (0.4-11.7) (SI: 1.36 IU/L [0.4-11.7 IU/L])
FSH = 2.97 mIU/mL (1.0-9.2) (SI: 2.97 IU/L [1.0-9.2 IU/L])

Estradiol = 18 pg/mL (15-350 pg/mL) (SI: 66.1 pmol/L [55.1-1284.9 pmol/L])
Pregnancy test, negative

MRI of the pituitary gland with and without contrast shows a 4.2 × 2.5 × 3.5-cm enhancing mass centered within the sella turcica (*see image, stars*), causing pituitary and infundibulum displacement. There is extrasellar extension and involvement of the left cavernous sinus (*arrow*), prepontine cistern, sphenoid sinus, and optic chiasm (*ovals*).

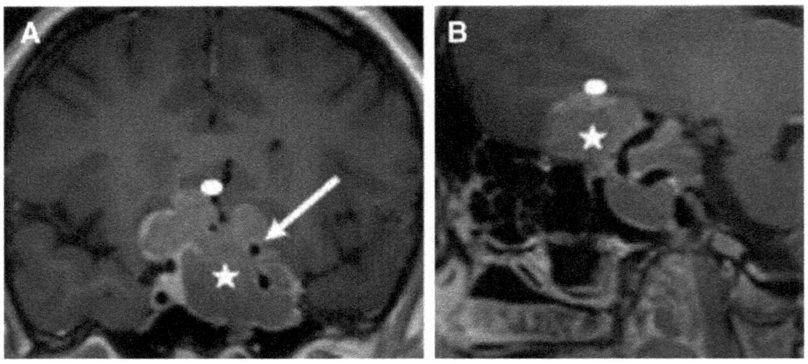

A pathogenic variant in which of the following genes is the most likely etiology of this patient's presentation?

A. *AIP*
B. *GNAS*
C. *GPR101*
D. *MEN1*
E. *NF1*

74 An 11-year-old girl is referred for concerns of weight gain and abnormal thyroid function. Her current height is 55.1 in (140 cm) (32.6th percentile), and weight is 159 lb (72.1 kg) (>99th percentile) (BMI = 36.8 kg/m² [>99th percentile for age]). Growth charts indicate that she has gained more than 30 lb (>13.6 kg) in the past 12 months. Her mother is very worried that her abnormal thyroid status is contributing to her rapid weight gain. There is no known family history of thyroid disorders. She was previously healthy and has no acute symptoms, apart from some fatigue. She does not have a goiter on examination.

Laboratory test results:

TSH = 5.9 mIU/L (0.5-4.3 mIU/L)
Free T_4 = 1.1 ng/dL (0.9-1.4 ng/dL) (SI: 14.2 pmol/L [11.6-18.0 pmol/L])

Which of the following is the most appropriate next step in addressing the laboratory results?

A. Measure free T_3
B. Measure thyroglobulin antibodies
C. Measure TSH in 4 to 6 months
D. Recommend Ashwagandha supplement
E. Start levothyroxine, 50 mcg daily

75 A 4-year-old boy with X-linked hypophosphatemia has been treated with oral phosphate and calcitriol since his diagnosis at age 3 years, when the family was living overseas. After recently returning to the United States, he is evaluated at a pediatric endocrinology clinic. His weight is 35.3 lb (16 kg) (Z-score, −0.3), and height is 37.3 in (94.8 cm) (Z-score, −2.5). He has genu varum with bilateral distal tibial torsion.

Laboratory test results (serum):

Calcium = 9.1 mg/dL (8.5-10.5 mg/dL) (SI: 2.28 mmol/L [2.13-2.63 mmol/L])
Phosphorus = 2.9 mg/dL (4-8 mg/dL) (SI: 0.94 mmol/L [1.29-2.58 mmol/L])
Alkaline phosphatase = 492 U/L (151-342 U/L) (SI: 8.22 μkat/L [2.52-5.71 μkat/L])
PTH = 84.1 pg/mL (18.4-80.1 pg/mL) (SI: 8.92 pmol/L [1.95-8.29 pmol/L])

Switching from conventional therapy with phosphate and calcitriol to a newer therapy with burosumab, an anti–FGF-23 antibody, is discussed with the patient's parents.

Which of the following is the best management plan?

A. Discontinue phosphate and calcitriol 1 week before starting burosumab
B. Discontinue phosphate and calcitriol on the day burosumab is initiated
C. Start burosumab and continue phosphate and calcitriol; measure serum phosphorus weekly; discontinue phosphate and calcitriol once serum phosphorus is normalized
D. Start burosumab and discontinue calcitriol and phosphate in 1 week
E. Start burosumab, discontinue phosphate, and continue calcitriol; measure serum phosphorus and PTH in 2 weeks; discontinue calcitriol when PTH is normalized

76 A 14-year-old boy is referred for evaluation of short stature. His medical history is otherwise unremarkable. He has no concerns. Review of his growth charts demonstrate that he has been consistently growing below the third percentile for many years with a normal growth velocity for the last 5 years resulting in no progressive decrement in height standard deviations. His height is currently at −2.4 SDS with a normal BMI. The family members' height percentiles and standard deviation scores can be seen in the pedigree (*see image, patient is noted with an arrow*).

He has no dysmorphic features on physical examination. He is prepubertal with a testicular volume of 3 cc bilaterally.

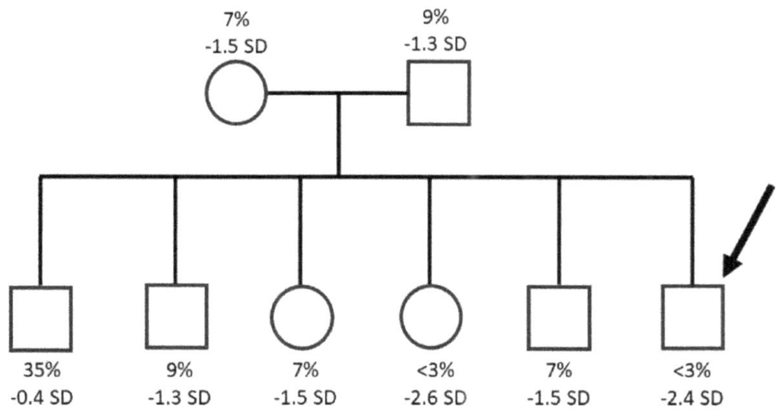

Laboratory test results:

Thyroid function, normal
Complete blood cell count, normal
Kidney function, normal
IGF-1 = 32 ng/mL (187-599 ng/mL) (SI: 4.2 nmol/L [24.5-78.5 nmol/L]) (−5 SD)
IGFBP-3 = 0.22 μg/mL (2.58-6.27 μg/mL) (SI: 0.22 mg/L [2.58-6.27 mg/L]) (−9 SD)

A GH-stimulation test demonstrates a peak GH value of 30 ng/mL (SI: 30 μg/L).

Which of the following is the most likely diagnosis?

A. Bioinactive GH (Kowarski syndrome)
B. Heterozygous pathogenic variant in the IGF-1 gene (*IGF1*)
C. Recessive pathogenic variants in the GH receptor gene (*GHR*) (Laron syndrome)
D. Recessive pathogenic variants in the IGF acid-labile subunit gene (*IGFALS*)
E. Recessive pathogenic variants in the STAT5b gene (*STAT5B*)

77 A 3-year-old boy presents for evaluation of genu varum that was noticeable after he started walking at age 1 year. He was born to nonconsanguineous parents at 38 weeks' gestation with a birth weight of 7 lb, 0.9 oz (3200 g). He has attained normal developmental milestones.

On physical examination, his height is 33.5 in (85 cm) (Z-score, −2.3) and weight is 24.3 lb (11 kg) (Z-score, −1). He has a waddling gait and significant varus deformities of bilateral lower extremities.

Laboratory test results (serum):

Calcium = 9.6 mg/dL (8.0-10.5 mg/dL) (SI: 2.4 mmol/L [2.0-2.6 mmol/L])
Phosphorus = 2.6 mg/dL (4.2-6.5 mg/dL) (SI: 0.8 mmol/L [1.4-2.1 mmol/L])
Alkaline phosphatase = 472 U/L (150-342 U/L) (SI: 7.88 µkat/L [2.51-5.71 µkat/L])
25-Hydroxyvitamin D = 33 ng/mL (30-100 ng/mL) (SI: 82.4 nmol/L [74.9-249.6 nmol/L])
1,25-Dihydroxyvitamin D = 48 pg/mL (15-90 pg/mL) (SI: 124.8 pmol/L [39.0-234 pmol/L])
PTH = 75 pg/mL (10-65 pg/mL) (SI: 8.0 pmol/L [1.1-6.7 pmol/L])
FGF-23 = 234 RU/mL (≤230 RU/mL)
Tubular resorption of phosphate = 83% (≥85%)
Urinary calcium-to-creatinine ratio = 0.02 (<0.42 mg calcium/mg creatinine)

Radiograph of the lower extremities shows bilateral tibia vara with metaphyseal flaring of the proximal tibia, distal tibia, and distal femur (*see image*).

The hypophosphatemia gene panel identifies homozygous nonsense pathogenic variants in the ectonucleotide pyrophosphatase/phosphodiesterase 1 (*ENPP1*) gene. No pathogenic variants are found in *PHEX, FGF23,* or *DMP1.*

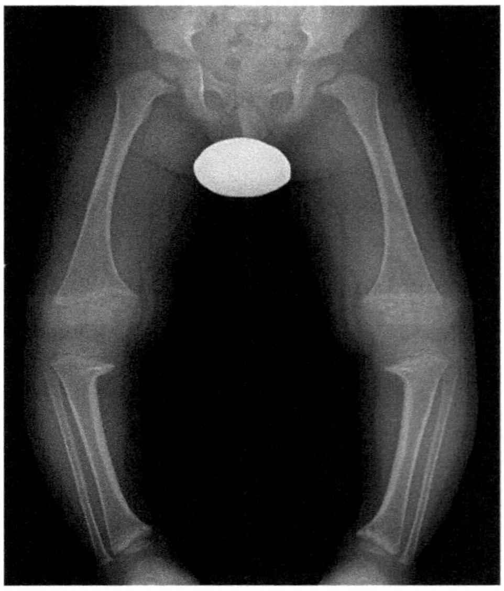

Reprinted from Choe Y et al. *Front Endocrinol* (Lausanne). 2022; 13: 911672. © The Authors. Published by Frontiers Media S.A.

Which of the following is the best treatment for an optimal outcome in this patient?

A. Burosumab
B. Cinacalcet
C. High-dosage cholecalciferol
D. Pamidronate
E. Phosphate and calcitriol

78 A 16-year-old girl is accompanied by her parents for evaluation of a lump she noticed on the left side of her neck. Her primary care physician checked thyroid function and arranged for neck ultrasonography. TSH and free T_4 concentrations are normal. Ultrasonography shows a 3.2-cm, solid, hypoechoic nodule in the lower portion of the left thyroid lobe. The nodule has smooth margins and is not taller than wide. There are no internal echogenic foci and no increased internal vascularity. The background thyroid tissue has heterogenous echotexture. There is no suspicious cervical lymphadenopathy. FNA biopsy is recommended because of the concerning ultrasonography features. Cytology documents atypia of undetermined significance with nuclear atypia.

These findings are most consistent with which of the following?

Answer	Bethesda category	Risk of malignancy
A.	II	5%-15%
B.	III	10%-20%
C.	III	>50%
D.	IV	28%-100%
E.	IV	65%-100%

79 A 16-year-old boy with delayed puberty presents for a follow-up visit to discuss recent laboratory test results and next steps in management. He is self-conscious about being physically less developed than his peers. His academic performance is good overall, although he has some difficulties in English class.

His height is 71.3 in (181cm) (75th percentile), and he has been growing well along this percentile. His BMI is at the 50th percentile. His midparental height is 69.3 in (176 cm).

On physical examination, testicular volume is 8 cc bilaterally, pubic hair is early Tanner stage 3, and he has gynecomastia (Tanner stage 2 breast development).

His bone age is interpreted to be 15 years and 6 months.

Laboratory test results (sample drawn at 8 AM):

Total testosterone = 70 ng/dL (100-320 ng/dL) (SI: 2.4 nmol/L [3.3-11.1 nmol/L])
FSH = 30.0 mIU/mL (1.2-12.9 mIU/mL) (SI: 30.0 IU/L [1.2-12.9 IU/L])
LH = 10.0 mIU/mL (1.3-9.8 mIU/mL) (SI: 10.0 IU/L [1.3-9.8 IU/L])
Karyotype = 47,XXY

Which of the following is the best next step in this patient's management?

A. Perform testicular ultrasonography
B. Provide reassurance and recommend follow-up in 1 year
C. Refer for cognitive evaluation
D. Start intramuscular testosterone enanthate injections, 100 mg once monthly
E. Start intramuscular testosterone, 25 mg once monthly

80 An 8-year-old girl with a history of relapsed acute lymphoblastic leukemia status post matched-sibling donor bone marrow transplant 2 years ago presents to her primary care physician with 2 days of fever. Testing for influenza A is positive, and she is prescribed oseltamivir. She vomits several times and has diarrhea over the next 2 days. She is nauseated and unable to tolerate enteral intake or medications, so she is admitted to the hospital.

Her medical history is notable for conditioning with total-body irradiation (1200 cGy), thiotepa (208 mg), and cyclophosphamide (4120 mg). Her course is complicated by graft-vs-host disease (last prednisone dose administered 1.5 years ago) and poor weight gain, for which she takes megestrol. She also has asthma treated with inhaled budesonide-formoterol. She takes oral cholecalciferol for bone health.

Laboratory test results:

Sodium = 129 mEq/L (136-145 mEq/L) (SI: 129 mmol/L [136-145 mmol/L])
Glucose = 52 mg/dL (70-140 mg/dL) (SI: 2.9 mmol/L [3.9-7.8 mmol/L])
Kidney function, no change from baseline

Subsequent laboratory testing is performed to evaluate persistent hyponatremia:

Cortisol (8 AM) = <1 µg/dL (7-25 µg/dL) (SI: <28 nmol/L [193-690 nmol/L])

Which of the following is the most likely cause of this patient's adrenal insufficiency?

A. Current treatment with daily budesonide/formoterol
B. Current treatment with megestrol
C. Previous treatment with cyclophosphamide
D. Previous treatment with prednisone
E. Previous total-body irradiation

81 A 14-year-old girl presents with a history of delayed puberty and primary amenorrhea. She has been growing along the 50th percentile for height and 75th percentile for weight. She has been healthy and has had no hospitalizations. There is no family history of delayed puberty.

On physical examination, she has Tanner stage 1 breast development and female external genitalia but no pubic or axillary hair. Her blood pressure is 135/90 mm Hg.

Laboratory test results:

Karyotype = 46,XY
Total testosterone = 33 ng/dL (SI: 1.1 nmol/L)
Androstenedione = 20 ng/dL (SI: 0.70 nmol/L)
DHEA-S = 50 μg/dL (108-441 μg/dL) (SI: 1.36 μmol/L [2.93-11.95 μmol/L])
Estradiol = <10 pg/mL (0-20 pg/mL) (SI: 36.7 pmol/L [0-73.4 pmol/L])
Progesterone = 7.0 ng/mL (0.3-0.7 ng/mL) (SI: 22.3 nmol/L [1.0-2.2 nmol/L])
FSH = 24.0 mIU/mL (SI: 24.0 IU/L)
LH = 40.0 mIU/mL (SI: 40.0 IU/L)

Pelvic ultrasonography shows no uterus or ovarian structures. Testicular ultrasonography shows inguinal testes.

Which of the following is this patient's most likely diagnosis?

A. 46,XY difference of sex development due to heterozygous pathogenic variant in the *NR5A1 (SF-1)* gene
B. Lipoid adrenal hyperplasia
C. 17α-Hydroxylase/17,20-lyase deficiency (P450c17)
D. 17β-Hydroxysteroid dehydrogenase type III deficiency
E. 3β-Hydroxysteroid dehydrogenase deficiency type II

82 A 14-year-old boy is referred for evaluation of short stature. He has been generally healthy throughout childhood but has always been shorter than his peers.

His height is 40.6 in (103 cm) (<1st percentile). Height velocity is 3 cm/y, and his sitting height-to-standing height ratio is 0.47 (<1st percentile). His mother's height is at the 50th percentile, and his father's is at the 75th percentile.

On physical examination, he had no dysmorphic features or Madelung deformity. His testicular volume is 20 cc bilaterally.

His bone age is 15 years.

Which of the following is the most appropriate next assessment in this patient's evaluation?

A. DNA methylation studies
B. IGF-1 measurement
C. *SHOX* gene testing
D. Skeletal survey
E. Whole-exome sequencing

83 A consultation is requested to evaluate a 4-day-old female baby born at 36 weeks' gestation who has had hypoglycemia since birth. Birth weight and length were appropriate for gestational age (length, 18.1 in [46 cm]; weight, 7.2 lb [3.28 kg]; head circumference, 12.4 in [31.5 cm]). She developed hypoglycemia shortly after birth, which required a high glucose infusion rate of 22 mg/kg per min.

Laboratory test results (sample drawn at the time of hypoglycemia):

Plasma glucose = 42 mg/dL (70-99 mg/dL) (SI: 2.3 mmol/L [3.9-5.5 mmol/L])
Insulin = 3.9 μIU/mL (2.6-24.9 μIU/mL) (SI: 27.1 pmol/L [18.1-172.9 pmol/L])
Cortisol = 27.3 μg/dL (6.2-19.4 μg/dL) (SI: 753 nmol/L [171-535 nmol/L])
Carbon dioxide = 17 mEq/L (21-31 mEq/L) (SI: 17 mmol/L [21-31 mmol/L])
GH = 13.7 ng/mL (<10 ng/mL) (SI: 13.7 μg/L [<10 μg/L])
Free fatty acids = 7.9 mg/dL (<0.8 mg/dL) (SI: 0.28 mmol/L [<0.03 mmol/L])

She is prescribed diazoxide and hydrochlorothiazide after normal findings on echocardiography and has been able to transition off intravenous fluids to a normal feeding pattern.

On physical examination, a geneticist notes low-set ears, long palpebral fissures, and abnormal finger spacing.

Whole-exome sequencing has documented a pathogenic variant in the causative gene.

This patient's presentation is most consistent with which of the following syndromes?

A. Beckwith-Wiedemann syndrome
B. Costello syndrome
C. Kabuki syndrome
D. Sotos syndrome
E. Usher-congenital hyperinsulinism syndrome

84 A 15-year-old girl presents for evaluation of a lump in her left neck that has been present for 1 month. The lump has been stable in size, and she has no dysphagia or voice changes. She has no symptoms of hypothyroidism or hyperthyroidism.

On physical examination, her blood pressure is 110/74 mm Hg and pulse rate is 95 beats/min. Her eyes are normal. Her thyroid gland has a 3-cm, mobile, nontender nodule in the left lobe; the right lobe is small. There is no cervical lymphadenopathy. Heart examination findings are normal. Reflexes are normal and there is no tremor.

Laboratory test results:

TSH = 0.18 mIU/L (0.5-5.0 mIU/L)
Free T_4 = 1.5 ng/dL (0.8-1.9 ng/dL) (SI: 19.3 pmol/L [10.3-24.5 pmol/L])
Total T_3 = 199 ng/dL (80-210 ng/dL) (SI: 3.06 nmol/L [1.23-3.23 nmol/L])
TPO antibodies = 167 IU/mL (0-60 IU/mL) (SI: 167 kIU/L [0-60 kIU/L])
TRAb = 0.3 IU/L (≤2.0 IU/L)

In addition to thyroid ultrasonography, which of the following is the most appropriate next step in this patient's management?

A. Initiate atenolol
B. Initiate methimazole
C. Obtain FNA
D. Perform thyroid scintigraphy
E. Refer for surgical consultation

85 A 12-year-old previously healthy boy is seen as a new patient in clinic. His current height is 59 in (149.9 cm) (53th percentile for age and sex; Z-score, 0.07), weight is 180.8 lb (82 kg) (99th percentile for age and sex; Z-score, 2.7), and BMI is 36.6 kg/m^2 (99th percentile for age and sex; Z-score, 2.58). When the medical assistant is obtaining vital signs, his blood pressure is elevated at 119/77 mm Hg (with the automatic cuff blood pressure measurement device). His blood pressure is measured once more using the auscultatory technique after sitting quietly in the exam room for 5 minutes, and similar measurements are documented.

Which of the following is the best next step in addressing the blood pressure concerns?

A. Determine the average of 2 auscultatory measurements
B. Order ambulatory blood pressure monitoring
C. Perform electrocardiography
D. Prescribe a low-dosage ACE inhibitor (eg, lisinopril)
E. Recommend a low-salt diet

86 A 13-year-old girl with multiple endocrine neoplasia type 2A presents for follow-up. She has a pathogenic variant in codon 634 of the *RET* gene, and she underwent prophylactic total thyroidectomy at age 6 years. Pathologic examination of her thyroid gland revealed a 2-mm focus of C-cell hyperplasia. She is on levothyroxine, 125 mcg daily. She has been growing and gaining weight normally, and calcitonin levels have remained undetectable. She presents today with her mother to discuss concerns of fatigue, difficulty concentrating, and constipation. She has already seen her primary care provider who has documented normal laboratory results for complete blood cell count, complete metabolic panel, ferritin, erythrocyte sedimentation rate, and celiac serology. Her mother has a history of total thyroidectomy and had similar symptoms while on levothyroxine therapy. Her mother reports that her own symptoms resolved when she switched to a "natural thyroid" product, and she asks about making the same switch for her daughter.

Laboratory test results:
TSH = 1.8 mIU/L (0.5-4.3 mIU/L)
Free T_4 = 1.6 ng/dL (1.0-1.6 ng/dL) (SI: 20.59 pmol/L [12.87-20.59 pmol/L])
Total T_3 = 95 ng/dL (91-218 ng/dL) (SI: 1.46 nmol/L [1.40-3.36 nmol/L])

The patient and her mother are aware that desiccated thyroid products are not approved by the US FDA for treatment of hypothyroidism, but they feel well informed and want to make the switch.

After discussing the lack of studies in pediatric patients and engaging in shared decision-making, which of the following would be the most reasonable approach?

A. Advise that desiccated thyroid extract is not recommended as it has been proven to be harmful
B. Measure reverse T_3 to determine whether a treatment change should be considered
C. Suggest a therapeutic trial of combination therapy with levothyroxine, 100 mcg daily, and liothyronine, 25 mcg daily
D. Recommend that she continue current therapy; a normal TSH result confirms that there is no role for alternative treatment
E. Suggest a therapeutic trial of combination therapy with levothyroxine, 112 mcg daily, and liothyronine, 2.5 mcg twice daily

87 A 3-month-old baby presents for evaluation of growth concerns and possible skeletal dysplasia. She was born at 40 weeks' gestation via spontaneous vaginal delivery. Her birth weight was 6 lb, 6.3 oz (2900 g), and birth length was 19.3 in (49 cm). Short limbs had been documented on prenatal ultrasonography. There is no family history of skeletal dysplasia. The parents report no consanguinity.

On physical examination, her weight is 11.3 lb (5.11 kg) (12th percentile; Z score, −1.16), length is 22.0 in (56 cm) (5th percentile; Z-score, −1.7), and head circumference is 16.5 in (41.8 cm) (96th percentile). She has frontal bossing, depressed nasal bridge, and protuberant abdomen. There is bilateral, symmetric rhizomelic shortening of the upper and lower limbs and short fingers.

Skeletal survey demonstrates generalized platyspondyly (*see image, panels A and B*) leading to an increased height of the intervertebral spaces. The pelvis shows a squared configuration with a horizontalized acetabular roof and narrowing of the sacrosciatic notch. The proximal femora have an oval-shaped lucent appearance. The long tubular bones (*panel A*) are shorter with metaphyseal "flaring" irregularity, and the fibulae are longer than the tibiae. The cranium (*panel C*) is large, and both frontal and occipital regions are prominent. The hands (*panel D*) have shortening of all tubular bones—metacarpals and phalanges.

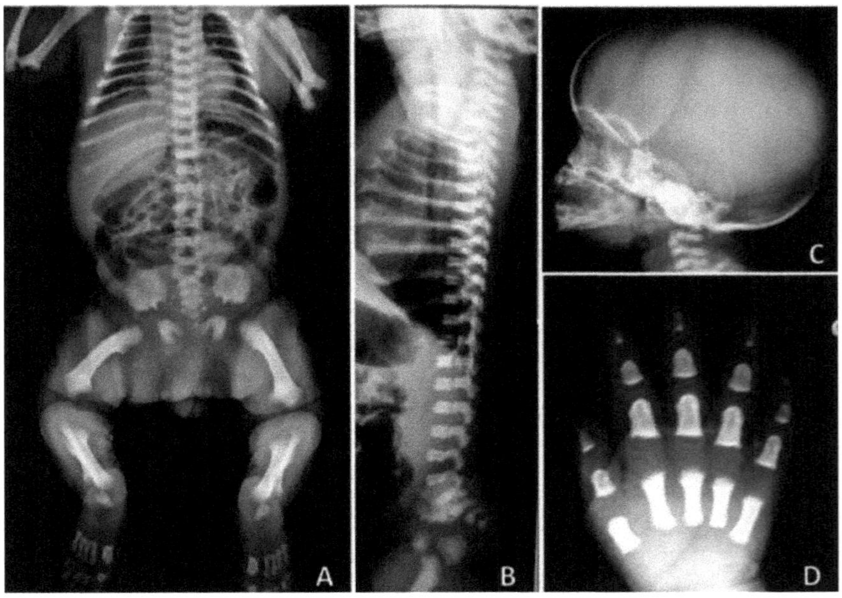

Reprinted from Llerena Jr J et al. *BMC Pediatr*, 2022; 22(1): 492. © The Authors. Published by BioMed Central Ltd., a part of Springer Nature.

Which of the following best describes the molecular basis of this condition?

A. Gain-of-function pathogenic variant in the *FGFR3* gene (fibroblast growth factor receptor 3)
B. Gain-of-function pathogenic variant in the *FGF23* gene (fibroblast growth factor 23)
C. Gain-of-function pathogenic variant in the *NPR2* gene (natriuretic peptide receptor 2)
D. Loss-of-function pathogenic variant in the *FGFR3* gene (fibroblast growth factor receptor 3
E. Loss-of-function pathogenic variant in the *NPR2* gene (natriuretic peptide receptor 2)

88 A 3-year-old boy presents for evaluation of short stature. He was born by spontaneous vaginal delivery at a gestational age of 38 weeks, and there were no perinatal complications. His birth weight was 5 lb 5 oz (2410 g) (<3rd percentile; SDS, −2.1), and length was 17.5 in (44.5 cm) (<1st percentile; SDS, −2.9). His height has followed a consistent curve but has always remained below the third percentile. He is appropriately meeting developmental milestones.

Both parents are healthy. His father's height is 68 in (172.7 cm). He had later timing of puberty and completed growth at 19 years. His mother's height is 62 in (157.5 cm). Menarche was at age 13 years.

On physical examination, the patient's height is 34.7 in (88.2 cm) (<1st percentile; SDS, −2.48) and weight is 27 lb (12.3 kg) (3rd percentile; SDS, −1.82). Examination findings are unremarkable. There are no dysmorphic features or asymmetry, and his sitting-to-standing height ratio is 0.54.

His bone age is 3 years.

Laboratory test results:

IGF-1 = 58 ng/mL (39-205 ng/mL) (SI: 7.6 nmol/L [5.1-26.9 nmol/L])
IGFBP-3 = 1.9 mg/L (1.6-4.5 mg/L)
TSH = 3.7 mIU/L (0.6-5.5 mIU/L)
Free T_4 = 1.95 ng/dL (0.8-2.2 ng/dL) (SI: 25.10 pmol/L [10.30-28.32 pmol/L])
Erythrocyte sedimentation rate = 12 mm/h (0-20 mm/h)
Celiac screening, negative
Complete blood cell count, normal
Comprehensive chemistry panel, normal

Which of the following is the best next step in this patient's management?

A. Assess height velocity over 6 months
B. Perform a GH-stimulation test
C. Perform testing for SHOX deficiency
D. Request a consultation with gastroenterology
E. Start GH treatment

89 A 10-year-old girl with type 1 diabetes recently started using a hybrid closed-loop insulin pump (automated insulin delivery system). She reports her continuous glucose monitor functions reliably for 8 to 10 days at a time and pump sites last 3 days without site failures. She consistently boluses before eating and demonstrates accurate carbohydrate counting. She is active in after-school gymnastics. Before pump use, she was able to prevent exercise-induced hypoglycemia by bringing her blood glucose up to 180 mg/dL (10.0 mmol/L) with a snack before gymnastics. Since starting pump therapy, she has been using activity/exercise mode during gymnastics but has had frequent episodes of hypoglycemia late at night. She and her parents would like to know how to best manage her nighttime hypoglycemia after gymnastics.

Which of the following is the best recommendation?

A. Consume 15 to 20 g of carbohydrates before gymnastics and use activity/exercise mode during gymnastics
B. Continue activity/exercise mode until bedtime on gymnastics days
C. Enter half the carbohydrates at lunch on gymnastics days
D. Reassure her that the pump algorithm will adjust to her pattern and no change is needed
E. Set a temporary basal rate during exercise and for 1 to 2 hours after exercise

90 Twin male babies present for a newborn visit at 7 days of age. They were born at term to a 32-year-old woman (G2, P1) after an uncomplicated pregnancy. Their mother has autoimmune hypothyroidism that was diagnosed at age 22 years. She takes levothyroxine, and her TSH concentration was normal throughout the pregnancy. The babies are doing well and are feeding and stooling normally. They have a healthy older sibling.

On physical examination, both babies are well-appearing, and they have regained their birth weight. Their fontanelles are normal in size. They have no jaundice, macroglossia, or umbilical hernia. Muscle tone is normal. The rest of the examination findings are normal.

Newborn screening results are normal.

Which of the following is the most appropriate next step in the management of these newborns?

A. Measure TPO antibodies in the babies
B. Measure TRAb in the babies
C. Measure TRAb in the mother
D. Provide routine newborn care
E. Repeat newborn screening at 2 weeks of age

91 An 18-year-old woman with type 2 diabetes presents for a follow-up visit. Previously, pharmacotherapeutic options for weight management and blood glucose control were discussed. Her current BMI is 37.0 kg/m^2. Her most recent hemoglobin A_{1c} value is 7.3% (56 mmol/mol). She was prescribed semaglutide at her last visit, and she has been tolerating it well. However, due to changes in insurance coverage, she is now inquiring about switching to tirzepatide. She knows that it targets 2 different receptors in the body, although she is uncertain what to expect from this dual-action agent compared with semaglutide. After further discussion, she elects to start weekly tirzepatide.

Which of the following is most likely to occur if she switches to tirzepatide?

A. Enhanced bone resorption
B. Enhanced glucagon secretion
C. Glucose-independent insulin secretion
D. Increased glucose-dependent insulinotropic polypeptide secretion in the duodenum
E. Similar reductions in body weight

92 A 5-year-old girl with neurofibromatosis type 1 and bilateral optic pathway gliomas presents for follow-up endocrine evaluation after being seen in the neuro-oncology clinic. Neurofibromatosis type 1 was diagnosed in infancy after a dermatologist evaluated her for multiple café-au-lait macules. At 2 years of age, bilateral optic pathway gliomas with associated visual threat were identified, and she thus received chemotherapy (carboplatin and vincristine). There has been no additional progression of her tumors on serial MRI, and findings on neuro-ophthalmological examination have been stable.

Her neuro-oncologist is concerned, however, about height acceleration over the past year, with a height Z-score of 2.4 (midparental height at the 75th percentile) and a height velocity Z-score of 2.8. In the past, her BMI was consistently at the 75th percentile; it has increased to the 95th percentile.

On physical examination, she appears well and has multiple café-au-lait macules and axillary freckling. Breast development and pubic hair are Tanner stage 1.

Laboratory test results (sample drawn at 8 AM):

IGF-1 = 466 ng/mL (46-243 ng/mL) (SI: 61.0 nmol/L [6.0-31.8 nmol/L])
LH = 0.04 mIU/mL (0.02-0.18 mIU/mL) (SI: 0.04 IU/L [0.02-0.18 IU/L])
FSH = 1.60 mIU/mL (1.0-4.2 mIU/mL) (SI: 1.60 IU/L [1.0-4.2 IU/L])

GH-suppression testing (via a 2-hour oral glucose tolerance test) reveals a 2-hour glucose value of 152 mg/dL (8.4 mmol/L) and nadir GH value of 2.7 ng/mL (2.7 μg/L).

Which of the following is the most appropriate next step in this patient's management?

A. Germline genetic testing for X-linked acrogigantism
B. Gonadotropin-releasing hormone analogue therapy
C. Resumption of chemotherapy
D. Somatostatin analogue therapy
E. Surgical resection of optic pathway gliomas

93 A 2-week-old full-term male newborn presents to the emergency department with a 1-week history of poor feeding and vomiting. He has lost 10% of his body weight since birth.

On physical examination, the baby is lethargic, hypotensive, and tachycardic. He has normal external genitalia and no hyperpigmentation.

He has a negative newborn screening result for congenital adrenal hyperplasia due to 21-hydroxylase deficiency. There is no history of consanguinity.

Laboratory test results:

Sodium = 121 mEq/L (135-145 mEq/L) (SI: 121 mmol/L [135-145 mmol/L])
Potassium = 6.7 mEq/L (3.5-5.0 mEq/L) (SI: 6.7 mmol/L [3.5-5.0 mmol/L])
Blood glucose = 80 mg/dL (60-100 mg/dL) (SI: 4.4 mmol/L [60-100 mmol/L])
Plasma bicarbonate =12 mEq/L (17-25 mEq/L) (SI: 12 mmol/L [17-25 mmol/L])
Plasma renin activity = 150 ng/mL per h (1.4-7.8 ng/mL per h)
Aldosterone = 400 ng/dL (17-154 ng/dL) (SI: 11,096 pmol/L [472-4272 pmol/L])

Which of the following is this patient's most likely diagnosis?

A. Aldosterone synthase deficiency type 1
B. Lipoid congenital adrenal hyperplasia
C. Pseudohypoaldosteronism type 1, autosomal dominant
D. Pseudohypoaldosteronism type 1, autosomal recessive
E. Pseudohypoaldosteronism type 2

94 A 10-year-old boy is referred for evaluation of short stature. He has a diagnosis of attention-deficit/hyperactivity disorder and has been treated with methylphenidate for the past 2 years. His mother asks about the effects of this medication on his growth and maturation.

Which of the following is the most likely effect of this treatment on his growth and development?

A. Acceleration of linear growth
B. Earlier pubertal onset
C. Later peak height velocity
D. No effect on growth during breaks from treatment
E. Reduced peak height velocity

95 A 3-year-old boy presents with pubic hair, growth acceleration, and penile enlargement. He has no history of fractures. Family member heights are average for his mother, father, maternal grandmother, paternal grandfather, and paternal grandmother. His maternal grandfather's height is 60 in (152.4 cm).

On physical examination, he has 5-cc, soft testes bilaterally, an enlarged phallus (3.5 in [8 cm]), and Tanner stage 3 pubic hair. There are no café-au-lait spots.

Bone age is interpreted to be 7 years. Findings on skeletal survey are normal.

Laboratory test results (sample drawn at 8 AM):

LH = 0.20 mIU/mL (0.02-0.30 mIU/mL) (SI: 0.20 IU/L [0.02-0.30 IU/L])
FSH = 0.40 mIU/mL (0.02-2.80 mIU/mL) (SI: 0.40 IU/L [0.02-2.80 IU/L])

Testosterone = 200 ng/dL (≤30 ng/dL) (SI: 6.9 nmol/L [≤1.0 nmol/L])
17-Hydroxyprogesterone = 15 ng/dL (0-90 ng/dL) (SI: 0.45 nmol/L [0-2.73 nmol/L])
β-hCG, undetectable
DHEA-S = 30.0 μg/dL (0.1-56.0 μg/dL) (SI: 0.81 μmol/L [0.01-1.52 μmol/L])

Results of GnRH-stimulation testing:

Measurement	Basal	Peak
LH	0.20 mIU/mL (SI: 0.20 IU/L)	0.50 mIU/mL (SI: 0.50 IU/L)
FSH	0.40 mIU/mL (SI: 0.40 IU/L)	2.60 mIU/mL (SI: 2.60 IU/L)

Findings on testicular ultrasonography are normal.

Which of the following is the best next step in this patient's management?

A. Adrenal CT
B. Brain MRI
C. Genetic testing for pathogenic variants in the LH receptor gene (*LHCGR*)
D. GnRH-stimulation test in 6 months
E. Karyotype analysis

96 An endocrine consultation is requested for a 6-year-old boy in the intensive care unit after abnormal thyroid function test results were documented. He was previously healthy and was admitted to the hospital 4 days ago with fever, headache, and confusion. He was hypotensive, and despite initial fluid resuscitation, his condition deteriorated. He is intubated and ventilated with multiorgan dysfunction. He is currently receiving intravenous fluids, intravenous antibiotics (cefotaxime and vancomycin), and vasopressors (milrinone and dobutamine). Blood cultures are positive for *Streptococcus pneumoniae.*

Laboratory test results (ordered because of ongoing tachycardia):
TSH = 0.35 mIU/L (0.6-4.8 mIU/L)
Free T_4 = 0.7 ng/dL (1.0-1.7 ng/dL) (SI: 9.01 pmol/L [12.87-21.88 pmol/L])
Total T_3 = 57 ng/dL (93-231 ng/dL) (SI: 0.88 nmol/L [1.43-3.56 nmol/L])

On physical examination, the patient is sedated, intubated, and ventilated. His height is 45.5 in (115.5 cm), and weight is 45.6 lb (20.7 kg). His pulse rate is 114 beats/min, and blood pressure is 96/54 mm Hg. There is no thyromegaly or palpable thyroid nodules.

Which of the following mechanisms is most likely contributing to this child's thyroid function profile?

A. Downregulation of hypothalamic iodothyronine deiodinase type 2
B. Induction of hypothalamic iodothyronine deiodinase type 3
C. Induction of skeletal muscle iodothyronine deiodinase type 3
D. Induction of TSH secretion by dobutamine
E. Increased hypothalamic thyrotropin-releasing hormone expression

97 A 7-year-old girl with elevated BMI (86th percentile) is referred for evaluation of increased weight gain, pubic hair development, and headaches. Her family history is notable for hypertension in her mother that has not been well controlled with different combinations of antihypertensive drugs. Similarly, her maternal grandmother has suboptimal control of her hypertension and had a stroke at age 50 years. The patient's 4-year-old sister does not have hypertension.

On physical examination, her blood pressure is 154/96 mm Hg.

Laboratory test results:

Sodium = 140 mEq/L (135-145 mEq/L) (SI: 140 mmol/L [135-145 mmol/L])
Potassium = 3.0 mEq/L (3.5-5.0 mEq/L) (SI: 3.0 mmol/L [3.5-5.0 mmol/L])
Free T_4 = 1.0 ng/dL (1.0-6.0 ng/dL) (SI: 12.87 pmol/L [12.87-77.23 pmol/L])
TSH = 0.6 mIU/L (0.5-4.3 mIU/L)
Progesterone = <0.35 ng/mL (<0.35 ng/mL) (SI: <1.11 nmol/L [<1.11 nmol/L])
17-Hydroxypregnenolone = 631.8 ng/dL (<549.0 ng/dL) (SI: 19.0 nmol/L [<16.5 nmol/L])
17-Hydroxyprogesterone = 67 ng/dL (<100 ng/dL) (SI: 2.0 nmol/L [<3.0 nmol/L])
Cortisol = 19 μg/dL (5-15 μg/dL (SI: 524.1 nmol/L [137.9-413.8 nmol/L])
11-Deoxycortisol = 183 ng/dL (20-151 ng/dL) (SI: 5.29 nmol/L [0.58-4.36 nmol/L])
11-Deoxycorticosterone = 24 ng/dL (2-34 ng/dL) (SI: 0.73 nmol/L [0.06-1.03 nmol/L])
Androstenedione = 27 ng/dL (10-17 ng/dL) (SI: 0.94 nmol/L [0.35-0.59 nmol/L])
Aldosterone = 18 ng/dL (<15 ng/dL) (SI: 499 pmol/L [<416.1 pmol/L])
Plasma renin = 0.3 ng/mL per h (1.2-2.4 ng/mL per h)
Aldosterone-to-plasma renin ratio = 60

Which of the following is this patient's most likely diagnosis?

A. Apparent mineralocorticoid excess
B. 11β-hydroxylase deficiency
C. Glucocorticoid-remediable hyperaldosteronism
D. Liddle syndrome
E. 17α-hydroxylase deficiency/17,20-lyase deficiency

98 A 14-year-old boy has been followed in the pediatric endocrinology clinic for multiple pituitary hormone deficiencies (GH, TSH, ACTH, arginine-vasopressin) resulting from partial resection and radiation for craniopharyngioma that was diagnosed at age 9 years. His bone age is delayed by 2 years, and pubic hair and testicular volume are Tanner stage 1. Laboratory testing documents prepubertal-range values for 8-AM gonadotropins (high-sensitivity assay) and testosterone.

After careful discussion of the available options and evidence, the family elects to proceed with pubertal initiation using hCG. hCG is started at a dosage of 250 international units twice weekly and is increased over the next 2 years to a total dosage of 750 international units 3 times weekly. The patient is pleased with the overall effects of this treatment.

On physical examination, he has evidence of virilization (increased facial and body hair, more muscle mass), pubic hair is Tanner stage 3, and testicular volume is 8 cc bilaterally.

His current 8-AM testosterone concentration is 614 ng/dL (21.3 nmol/L).

With the support of his family, he now wishes to address his future fertility and pursue sperm analysis and cryopreservation.

Which of the following is the most appropriate next step in this patient's management?

A. Add recombinant FSH
B. Add testosterone
C. Continue hCG at the same dosage until testicular volume reaches 12 to 15 cc
D. Increase the hCG dosage
E. Pause hCG to evaluate for spontaneous pubertal development

99 A 20-year-old man is referred to a pediatric endocrinologist for evaluation of low bone density. The patient recently tripped and fell on a sidewalk while running and broke his humerus. In the emergency department, x-rays showed that his growth plates were not yet fused. The orthopedist also noted that the bones appeared osteopenic, and she suggested that the patient see an endocrinologist.

He follows a regular diet with adequate calcium and vitamin D intake. He is unaware of any medical problems. When asked about a family history of hormonal disorders, his mother says that her hormones were "all out of whack" during pregnancy, with increased hair growth and acne. Her symptoms went away after the patient was born. Otherwise, she is not aware of hormonal problems in the family. The patient's growth chart is shown (*see image*).

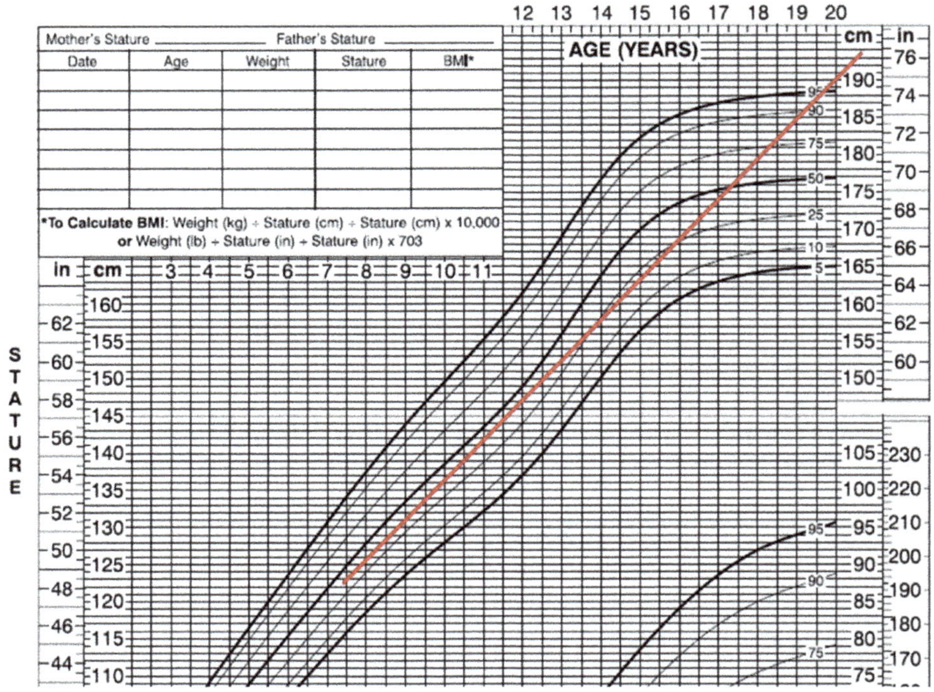

On physical examination, he is tall and has mild abdominal adiposity. His arm span is 4.7 in (12 cm) greater than his height. He has Tanner stage 5 pubic hair, a fully virilized phallus, and 30-cc testes bilaterally. He has mild genu valgum.

Bone age is interpreted to be 14 years.

Which of the following hormonal profiles is most characteristic of this patient's condition?

Answer	Testosterone	Estradiol	LH	FSH
A.	Low	Low	Low	Low
B.	Low	Low	High	High
C.	Normal	Low	Normal	High
D.	Normal	High	High	High
E.	High	Normal	High	Normal

100 A 12-year-old girl with Turner syndrome presents for evaluation because she has had no breast development. She is treated with GH for short stature, and she is currently growing at the 50th percentile of the Turner syndrome growth chart. Her midparental height is at the 60th percentile. Her parents ask if treatment should be started now or whether it is best to see if she will start puberty on her own.

On physical examination, breast development is Tanner stage 1 and pubic hair is Tanner stage 2.

Laboratory test results (sample drawn at 8 AM):

FSH = 30.0 mIU/mL (2.1-11.0 mIU/mL) (SI: 30.0 IU/L [2.1-11.0 IU/L])
LH = 20.0 mIU/mL (0.2-11.9 mIU/mL) (SI: 20.0 IU/L [0.2-11.9 IU/L])
Estradiol = 10 pg/mL (21-85 pg/mL) (SI: 36.7 pmol/L [77.1-312.0 pmol/L])
DHEA-S = 250.0 µg/dL (67.8-328.6 µg/dL) (SI: 6.78 µmol/L [1.84-8.91 µmol/L])
Testosterone = 15 ng/dL (5-58 ng/dL) (SI: 0.5 nmol/L [0.2-2.0 nmol/L])
Karyotype = 45,X

Findings on pelvic ultrasonography are consistent with prepuberty, and anatomy is normal.

Which of the following is the best next step in this patient's management?

A. Determine bone age to estimate her final adult height
B. Initiate treatment with a combined estradiol/progesterone pill
C. Initiate treatment with an estradiol patch, 50 mcg twice weekly
D. Initiate treatment with an estradiol patch, 6.25 mcg daily (one-quarter of 25 mcg patch)
E. Observe until she is 15 years old

ANSWERS

PEDIATRIC ENDOCRINE SELF-ASSESSMENT PROGRAM 2025-2026

Part II

1 ANSWER: A) Autoimmune polyglandular syndrome type 1

Autoimmune polyglandular syndrome (APS) type 1 (Answer A), also known as autoimmune polyendocrinopathy-candidiasis-ectodermal dystrophy (APECED), is characterized by the triad of chronic mucocutaneous candidiasis, hypoparathyroidism, and adrenal insufficiency. Clinically, the condition is diagnosed if 2 of the 3 features are present. In general, candidiasis of the skin and mucous membranes manifests in early childhood (usually before age 5 years), hypoparathyroidism (usually before age 10 years), and Addison disease (usually before age 15 years). Chronic candidiasis is reported as the most frequent nonendocrine manifestation (82%-100%). Hence, obtaining a careful medical history is essential. The condition is highly heterogeneous, and the onset of features can be variable (*table*). The disease can proceed in a monocomponent manner, making it difficult to diagnose clinically. In this vignette, the presence of enamel dysplasia and adrenal insufficiency points to a diagnosis of APS type 1. Enamel dysplasia is reported in up to 77% of patients with APS type 1. Aldosterone deficiency is not always present and can be an evolving problem that requires continued screening.

Table. Common Features in Autoimmune Polyglandular Syndrome Type 1

Classic triad	Adjunct triad	Other features seen
• Chronic mucocutaneous candidiasis • Hypoparathyroidism • Adrenal insufficiency	• Enamel hypoplasia • Urticaria • Intestinal malabsorption	• Gastritis • Hepatitis • Sjogren syndrome • Pneumonitis • Premature ovarian insufficiency • Vitiligo • Alopecia • Vitamin B_{12} deficiency • Keratoconjunctivitis • Hypothyroidism • Type 1 diabetes • Testicular insufficiency

Adapted from Squire JD & Leiding JW. Primary immune deficiency disease with prominent autoimmunity. In Sullivan KE & Stiehm ER, eds. Stiehm's Immune Deficiencies: Inborn Errors of Immunity. 2nd ed. Academic Press, 2020, pp. 633-642.

APS type 1 is due to biallelic loss-of-function variants in the *AIRE* (autoimmune regulator) gene and is thus inherited in an autosomal recessive manner. Approximately 500 to 700 affected patients have been described worldwide and more than 126 *AIRE* pathogenic variants have been reported. *AIRE* encodes the AIRE protein, which is a transcription factor responsible for orchestrating expression of thousands of proteins expressed in the body (tissue-restricted antigens) and in medullary thymic epithelial cells (mTECs). Ordinarily, the naïve thymocytes (naïve T cells) that recognize these antigens with high affinity undergo apoptosis. In this way, T cells that respond to antigens normally produced in the body never enter the circulation, a process called negative selection. This establishes self-tolerance, a critical step for the induction of immunologic self-tolerance. Pathogenic variants in the *AIRE* gene lead to a breakdown in self-tolerance and the development of multiorgan autoimmune diseases.

Adrenal insufficiency is part of sphingosine phosphate lyase insufficiency syndrome (Answer D), but the process is not autoimmune driven and is not associated with the associated features seen in APS type 1.

X-linked adrenoleukodystrophy (Answer E) is a X-linked recessive disorder that affects boys, but it is not associated with enamel dysplasia. Of note, female carriers of X-linked adrenoleukodystrophy can also be affected with neurological symptoms.

APS type 2 (Answer B), also known as Schmidt syndrome, and IPEX syndrome (Answer C) are autoimmune polyendocrine syndromes. APS type 2 is a polygenic disorder that has a complex inheritance pattern with strong linkage to the human leukocyte antigen locus. APS type 2 is characterized by at least 2 of the following 3 endocrinopathies: type 1 diabetes, adrenal insufficiency, and autoimmune thyroid disease. APS type 2 occurs at any age and in both sexes, but it is most common in middle-aged women and is very rare in childhood. Chronic candidiasis and enamel dysplasia are not present. IPEX syndrome is an X-linked recessive disorder that commonly presents with chronic diarrhea, type 1 diabetes, and eczematous dermatitis. It is caused by pathogenic variants in the *FOXP3* gene, resulting in hyperactive T cells with both autoimmune and allergic manifestations. Typically,

IPEX syndrome presents within the first year of life in boys. Without aggressive immunosuppression or bone marrow transplant, most affected individuals die before age 2 years. Several patients with a milder phenotype have been described to survive into the second or third decade of life.

Educational Objective

Diagnose autoimmune polyglandular syndrome type 1 due to pathogenic variants in the *AIRE* gene.

Reference(s)

Abramson J, Husebye ES. Autoimmune regulator and self-tolerance - molecular and clinical aspects. *Immunol Rev.* 2016;271(1):127-140. PMID: 27088911

Ahonen P, Myllärniemi S, Sipilä I, Perheentupa J. Clinical variation of autoimmune polyendocrinopathy-candidiasisectodermal dystrophy (APECED) in a series of 68 patients. *N Engl J Med.* 1990;322(26):1829-1836. PMID: 2348835

Bjørklund G, Pivin M, Hangan T, Yurkovskaya O, Pivina L. Autoimmune polyendocrine syndrome type 1: clinical manifestations, pathogenetic features, and management approach. *Autoimmun Rev.* 2022;21(8):103135. PMID: 35690244

Husebye ES, Anderson MS. Autoimmune polyendocrine syndromes: clues to type 1 diabetes pathogenesis. *Immunity.* 2010;32(4):479-487. PMID: 20412758

2 ANSWER: B) Chromosomal microarray

The girl in this vignette has Turner syndrome mosaicism, which is the likely explanation for her short stature. Her karyotype findings are sufficient to diagnose Turner syndrome. However, based on her karyotype, it is unclear whether any Y-chromosome material is present. Because the ring chromosome may have been derived from either an X or Y chromosome, the patient in this vignette requires chromosomal microarray (Answer B) to determine the origin of the ring. This is important because prophylactic gonadectomy should be recommended at the time of diagnosis for patients with Turner syndrome who have Y-chromosome material. Approximately 10% of individuals with Turner syndrome have a karyotype containing Y-chromosome material. Several genes on the Y chromosome, including octamer-binding transcription factor 3/4 (*POU5F1*) and testis-specific protein Y-linked 1 (*TSPY1*), may contribute to gonadoblastoma formation.

In a study of a large cohort of patients with Turner syndrome and a 45,X/46,XY karyotype without atypia of the external genitalia, 58 patients had undergone gonadectomy at a mean age of 15 ± 8 years. Gonadoblastoma was present in 9 patients, and 2 of these tumors were malignant (discovered at 14 and 32 years of age). While the prognosis for gonadoblastoma is generally favorable, there is a risk of malignant degeneration. Fluorescence in situ hybridization (FISH) for *SRY* (Answer E) only detects the presence of the *SRY* gene and may not detect other Y-chromosome material related to risk of gonadoblastoma.

Current Turner syndrome guidelines recommend screening for cardiovascular abnormalities with transthoracic echocardiography, not cardiac MRI (Answer A).

While kidney ultrasonography at the time of diagnosis is recommended to identify associated kidney abnormalities, pelvic ultrasonography (Answer D) to assess internal female anatomy is not required.

Individuals with Turner syndrome should have DXA (Answer C) after adult hormone replacement has been initiated. Thus, DXA is not needed now for this patient.

Other appropriate assessments at diagnosis include audiometric testing; a comprehensive ophthalmologic examination; dental evaluation; thyroid function testing; screening for celiac disease, transaminitis, and inflammatory bowel disease; and surveillance for scoliosis and melanocytic nevi.

Educational Objective

Identify the risks associated with Y-chromosome material in a girl with Turner syndrome.

Reference(s)

Karila D, Donadille B, Léger J, et al. Prevalence and characteristics of gonadoblastoma in a retrospective multi-center study with follow-up investigations of 70 patients with Turner syndrome and a 45,X/46,XY karyotype. *Eur J Endocrinol.* 2022;187(6):873-881. PMID: 36305565

Shankar RK, Backeljauw PF. Current best practice in the management of Turner syndrome. *Ther Adv Endocrinol Metab.* 2018;9(1):33-40. PMID: 29344338

3 ANSWER: B) Perform oral glucose tolerance testing every 6 months

Type 1 diabetes (T1D) is an autoimmune disease characterized by progressive pancreatic β-cell loss resulting in insulin deficiency and hyperglycemia. The disorder represents a disease continuum that begins before its symptomatic manifestations. The risk of developing symptomatic T1D can be identified and quantified, the disease can be characterized into well-defined stages, and the rate of progression to symptomatic disease can be predicted with appreciable accuracy (*see figure*).

T1D has 3 proposed stages that have been widely adopted.

- Stage 1 represents individuals who have developed 2 or more islet autoantibodies associated with T1D but have normoglycemia. For children who are screened for genetic risk at birth and reach this stage, the 5- and 10-year risks of symptomatic disease are approximately 44% and 70%, respectively, and the lifetime risk approaches 100%.
- Stage 2, like stage 1, includes individuals with 2 or more islet autoantibodies but whose disease has progressed to glucose intolerance, or dysglycemia, from loss of functional β-cell mass. The 5-year risk of symptomatic disease at this stage is approximately 75%.
- Stage 3 represents the typical clinical symptoms and signs of diabetes, which may include polyuria, polydipsia, weight loss, fatigue, diabetic ketoacidosis, and others.

Figure. Probability of Progression in Islet Autoantibody-Positive Relatives of Individuals With Type 1 Diabetes Stratified for Number of Autoantibodies

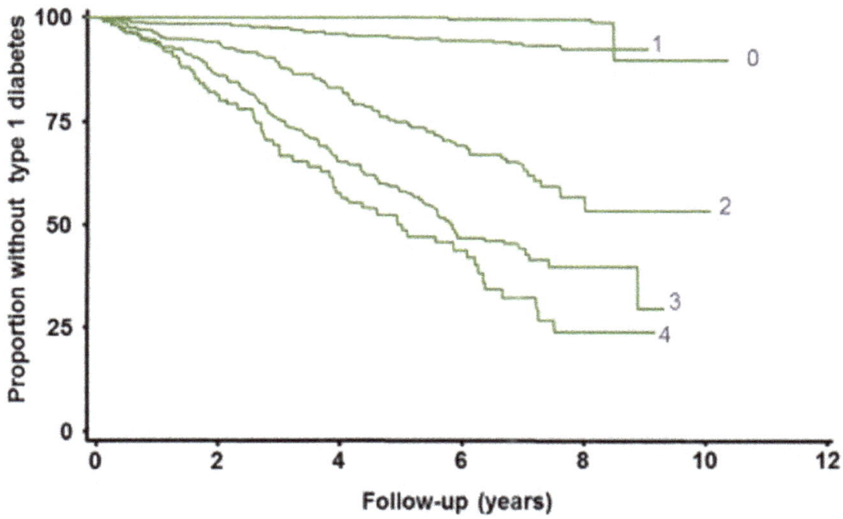

In relatives of individuals with T1D, β-cell glucose sensitivity, as measured by oral glucose tolerance testing, declines up to 1.45 years before the onset of symptomatic disease. This decline is associated with the progression of T1D, independent of factors such as sex, age, BMI, and clinical risk. Consequently, it is advisable to monitor this patient with regular oral glucose tolerance testing (Answer B), clinical follow-up, and hemoglobin A_{1c} measurement every 6 months.

Baseline insulin sensitivity, fasting insulin, C-peptide secretion (Answer A), and total postglucose insulin output do not demonstrate predictive value for disease progression.

The HLA region on chromosome 6 accounts for 30% to 50% of the genetic risk of T1D, with the greatest association with HLA class II haplotypes DRB1*0301-DQB1*0201 (DR3-DQ2) and DRB1*0401-DQB1*0302 (DR4-DQ8) (Answer C). HLA haplotypes are useful to identify prestage 1 genetic susceptibility and to help with genetic risk detection. However, this will not add any predictive benefits for this patient's risk of developing clinical diabetes.

There have been many approaches to prevent progression and onset of symptomatic disease, including oral nicotinamide, oral insulin, nasal insulin (Answer E), and parenteral and low-dosage subcutaneous insulin (Answer D), without any substantial benefit in preventing progression.

Presently, the staging classification system is used for clinical research where it aids in design of risk screening, clinical trial subject stratification, and design of natural history and intervention clinical trials. The application for clinical practice is limited, but patients can be offered effective glucose screening and the only currently available FDA-approved therapy, anti-CD3 (teplizumab), to delay disease progression.

Educational Objective

Assess the stages of type 1 diabetes mellitus and estimate the risk of disease progression.

Reference(s)

Ferrannini E, Mari A, Nofrate V, Sosenko JM, Skyler JS; DPT-1 Study Group. Progression to diabetes in relatives of type 1 diabetic patients: mechanisms and mode of onset. *Diabetes.* 2010;59(3):679-685. PMID: 20028949

Krischer JP; Type 1 Diabetes TrialNet Study Group. The use of intermediate endpoints in the design of type 1 diabetes prevention trials. *Diabetologia.* 2013;56(9):1919-1924. PMID: 23744306

Orban T, Sosenko JM, Cuthbertson D, et al; Diabetes Prevention Trial-Type 1 Study Group. Pancreatic islet autoantibodies as predictors of type 1 diabetes in the Diabetes Prevention Trial-Type 1. *Diabetes Care.* 2009;32(12):2269-2274. PMID: 19741189

Steck AK, Vehik K, Bonifacio E, et al; TEDDY Study Group. Predictors of progression from the appearance of islet autoantibodies to early childhood diabetes: The Environmental Determinants of Diabetes in the Young (TEDDY). *Diabetes Care.* 2015;38(5):808-813. PMID: 25665818

Ziegler AG, Rewers M, Simell O, et al. Seroconversion to multiple islet autoantibodies and risk of progression to diabetes in children. *JAMA.* 2013;309:2473-2479. PMID: 23780460

4 ANSWER: A) Continue the current treatment plan with no changes

Lonapegsomatropin is a once-weekly formulation of GH in which somatropin (recombinant human GH) is linked with a polyethylene glycol carrier. The linker dissolves over time, allowing for the slow release of GH into the circulation. The apparent half-life of somatropin that is released from lonapegsomatropin is approximately 25 hours, which allows for once-weekly dosing.

A phase 3 clinical trial of lonapegsomatropin in patients with GH deficiency demonstrated a first-year annualized growth velocity of 11.2 cm/y in the lonapegsomatropin-treated group with an average annualized growth velocity of 13.3 cm/y at week 13, similar to that of the patient in this vignette. The patient's clinical characteristics mirror those of the average trial participant. In patients receiving lonapegsomatropin, IGF-1 concentrations vary greatly over the course of the week, with maximum levels achieved approximately 48 hours postinjection, which is the time that the patient in this vignette has his IGF-1 level measured. A mathematical model has been created to help estimate the average IGF-1 concentration based on the timing of the blood sampling relative to the most recent injection (*see table*). A sample checked at 4.5 days after injection gives the best representation of average IGF-1 levels over the week. Similar mathematical models exist for the other weekly formulations of GH.

Table 1. The predicted difference between observed IGF-1 SDS and average IGF-1 SDS by time with 90% prediction intervals (PI)

Day	Mean	RSD	Lower limit of 90% PI	Upper limit of 90% PI
0.0	-1.22	0.35	-1.80	-0.65
0.5	-0.12	0.20	-0.46	0.22
1.0	0.39	0.28	-0.07	0.86
1.5	0.60	0.27	0.16	1.04
2.0	0.67	0.21	0.32	1.02
2.5	0.68	0.15	0.43	0.93
3.0	0.62	0.10	0.45	0.78
3.5	0.46	0.08	0.33	0.59
4.0	0.21	0.09	0.06	0.36
4.5	**-0.09**	**0.14**	**-0.31**	**0.13**
5.0	-0.39	0.18	-0.68	-0.09
5.5	-0.64	0.23	-1.01	-0.26
6.0	-0.85	0.27	-1.29	-0.42
6.5	-1.07	0.30	-1.57	-0.57
7.0	-1.22	0.33	-1.77	-0.68

Bold text indicates the day when sampling time for IGF-1 was coincident with the average IGF-1 SDS. Abbreviation: RSD, residual standard deviation.

In the current case, 2 days after injection, the measured IGF-1 SDS is approximately 0.67 SD above the average. Thus, in this patient, the weekly mean IGF-1 value is approximately +1.63 SD (+2.3 – 0.67 = +1.63). Therefore, this patient has an average IGF-1 concentration within the normal range and there is no indication to decrease the dosage of lonapegsomatropin (Answers B and C). Given the patient's excellent growth response and normal estimated mean IGF-1 concentration, continuing current therapy (Answer A) is correct. Measurement of IGF-1 on day 6 (Answer D) would represent a trough value.

There is no indication to switch to daily GH (Answer E) in a patient whose response to therapy is excellent, who has had no adverse events, and who has needle phobia.

Educational Objective

Explain how the timing of IGF-1 measurement affects result interpretation in patients receiving once-weekly, long-acting GH therapy.

Reference(s)

Lin Z, Shu AD, Bach M, Miller BS, Rogol AD. Average IGF-1 prediction for once-weekly lonapegsomatropin in children with growth hormone deficiency. *J Endocr Soc.* 2021;6(1):bvab168. PMID: 34913019

Thornton PS, Maniatis AK, Aghajanova E, et al. Weekly lonapegsomatropin in treatment-naïve children with growth hormone deficiency: the phase 3 heiGHt Trial. *J Clin Endocrinol Metab.* 2021;106(11):3184-3195. PMID: 34272849

5 ANSWER: A) Initiate intravenous levothyroxine

This infant has primary hypothyroidism. Based on his young age and the importance of thyroid hormone on brain development, he should be treated as soon as possible (Answer A). The oral dosage recommended for infants with congenital hypothyroidism is 10 to 15 mcg/kg daily. In this case, due to his critical illness and the relatively mild degree of hypothyroidism, a dosage at the lower end of this range is recommended. This infant is critically ill (on ECMO), and doses will need to be given intravenously. The conversion from oral to intravenous levothyroxine is not 1:1. The intravenous dose should be 75% of the oral dose. For this infant weighing 4.2 kg, a dose of 30 mcg intravenously (10*4.2*0.75) would be reasonable.

This infant has had cardiac catheterization and cardiac surgery with an open wound. He was exposed to intravenous iodinated contrast during cardiac catheterization and likely has ongoing exposure to topical iodine for wound management (although this information was not shared). Excess iodine can lead to hypothyroidism of varying duration. The mature thyroid gland responds to excess iodine exposure by acutely decreasing thyroid hormone production (Wolff-Chaikoff effect). In a mature thyroid gland, there is "escape" from this phenomenon and resumption of normal thyroid hormone production within 1 to 2 weeks, even in the face of ongoing excess iodine exposure. This ability to escape the Wolff-Chaikoff effect develops in the fetal gland between 36 and 40 weeks' gestation.

In 2022, the US FDA issued a warning that children younger than 3 years who are exposed to intravenous iodinated contrast are at risk of thyroid dysfunction and should be monitored. They subsequently revised their recommendation to state that the risk was most likely significant only for younger children, especially those with additional risk factors.

The limited literature suggests that iodinated contrast–induced thyroid dysfunction is more likely to occur in:

- Premature infants
- Infants with very low birth weight
- Infants with congenital heart disease
- Infants with decreased renal clearance
- Infants with repeated exposures

This infant has congenital heart disease and has had repeated exposures to iodine. He is at risk for iodine-induced thyroid dysfunction, and therefore checking thyroid function was appropriate after exposure.

Measurement of urinary iodine (Answer D) could be performed, but it should not delay treatment initiation for this infant. The evidence of iodine exposure is available in the history; urinary iodine excretion will not change the management plan. The most accurate determination of iodine status is by 24-hour urinary iodine measurement. A spot urine iodine-to-creatinine ratio may also be assessed. These tests can be considered if confirmation of excess iodine exposure is sought, but they are more useful for population studies of iodine exposure than for individual patients.

In this infant with a TSH value greater than 20.0 mIU/L and a borderline free T_4 value, it is inappropriate to wait 2 weeks to repeat testing (Answer E). Assuming iodine excess caused the dysfunction, the initial iodine exposure occurred 3 weeks ago during cardiac catheterization and recovery should have happened by now (another reason to avoid waiting 2 more weeks to recheck). He also has ongoing exposure to iodine transdermally. This infant should not need long-term thyroid hormone replacement. There are no long-term studies, but based on the likely cause in this case, a trial off therapy may be considered several months after all excess iodine exposure is removed.

This infant has a critical illness and thyroid laboratory values typically change in these situations (nonthyroidal illness syndrome [NTIS]). The classic pattern seen in NTIS is low free T_4, normal or slightly low TSH, and high reverse T_3. TSH can increase significantly during the recovery phase of NTIS, although not typically to the magnitude described in this infant. He is not in the recovery phase of NTIS. Measurement of reverse T_3 levels (Answer C) is rarely needed to diagnose NTIS and is not appropriate in this case. Changes in thyroid laboratory values have also been shown in neonates on ECMO. Within 1 hour of ECMO initiation, TSH, total T_4, T_3, and reverse T_3 all decrease. TSH quickly recovers to baseline pre-ECMO levels, and total T_4, T_3, and reverse T_3 recover within 48 hours. The free T_4 concentration does not change significantly during ECMO.

Measurement of free T_4 by equilibrium dialysis (Answer B) is not appropriate. The diagnosis of primary hypothyroidism is made based on the elevated TSH concentration, not free T_4. Waiting for this result would delay treatment initiation.

Educational Objective

Identify the potential risk of hypothyroidism after intravenous iodinated contrast exposure and guide management.

Reference(s)

Leeuwen L, van Heijst AFJ, van Rosmalen J, et al. Changes in thyroid hormone concentrations during neonatal extracorporeal membrane oxygenation. *J Perinatol.* 2017;37(8):906-910. PMID: 28448064

Kubicki R, Grohmann J, Kunz K-G, et al. Frequency of thyroid dysfunction in pediatric patients with congenital heart disease exposed to iodinated contrast media - a long-term observational study. *J Pediatr Endocrinol Metab.* 2020;33(11):1409-1415. PMID: 33001853

Rose SR, Wassner AJ, Wintergerst KA, et al; Section on Endocrinology Excecutive Committee; Council on Genetics Executive Committe. Congenital hypothyroidism: screening and management. *Pediatrics.* 2022;151(1):e2022060420. PMID: 36827521

Williams FLR, Watson J, Day C, et al. Thyroid dysfunction in preterm neonates exposed to iodine. *J Perinat Med.* 2017;45(1):135-143. PMID: 27564693

6 ANSWER: E) Whole-exome sequencing

This patient has a form of combined pituitary hormone deficiency (CPHD), which typically refers to the combination of GH deficiency and at least 1 other anterior pituitary hormone deficiency. He has pituitary stalk interruption syndrome (ORPHA95496). Pituitary stalk interruption syndrome most often presents with anterior pituitary hormone deficiencies in the setting of characteristic imaging findings also present in this patient: (1) thin or interrupted pituitary stalk; (2) ectopic (or absent) posterior pituitary gland; and (3) hypoplasia (or aplasia) of the anterior pituitary gland. Genetic causes (eg, transcription factors involved in developmental programming or genes expressed in hypothalamus or pituitary relevant for function), environmental causes (eg, exposures during critical windows of embryonic development, infection, trauma), and complex interactions between genes and environment have been implicated in the pathogenesis of CPHD. CPHD can be syndromic, associated with other anomalies typically related to shared disrupted developmental processes, or nonsyndromic, when the disorder is confined to pituitary hormone production. Although next-generation genetic sequencing (Answer E) continues to offer new insights, a genetic diagnosis is not made in most children with CPHD. Assigning causality to candidate variants identified in next-generation sequencing is often challenging and adds complexity to establishing a genetic diagnosis. However, some variants are clearly associated with CPHD. Of the options available, whole-exome sequencing is the most likely to yield a cause, even though this testing currently still only identifies a genetic culprit in a small proportion of patients.

In individuals with pituitary stalk interruption syndrome, pathogenic variants have been identified in genes affecting embryonic development of these structures, including *HESX1, LHX3, LHX4, POUF1, PROP1, OTX2, SOX3, PROKR2, GLI2*, and *GPR161.* However, in multiple familial studies, the phenotype does not seem to segregate with the pathogenic variant identified in the manner that might be expected for a typical monogenic disorder. Thus, alternative patterns of inheritance have been considered, as in this patient, in whom a known loss-of-function variant in *PROKR2* (c.253C.T;p.R85C) was inherited from an unaffected mother, and a functionally relevant variant in *WDR11* (c.1306A.G;p.I436V) was inherited from an unaffected father.

In a different study, whole-exome sequencing in 3 children with congenital CPHD (combination of GH deficiency and at least 1 other hormone deficiency) also identified multiple heterozygous pathogenic variants in genes affecting development and/or function of the hypothalamus and pituitary, suggesting that this spectrum of condition may be oligogenic or monogenic. In one representative series, of the minority of cases where genetic causes of CPHD were implicated, equal numbers of putative genetic culprits were monogenic and polygenic.

Sanger sequencing of the *GH1* gene (Answer C) is not appropriate because pathogenic variants in this gene are associated with isolated GH deficiency, not CPHD and/or anatomic pituitary abnormalities.

Microarray testing (Answer A) can detect chromosomal anomalies and deletions, but it is less likely to disclose the specific genetic variants associated with CPHD and is thus incorrect.

In the absence of other abnormalities on physical examination, skeletal survey (Answer D) is unlikely to generate other insights with respect to the possibility of syndromic CPHD. Individuals with pathogenic variants in some genes may have pituitary hormone deficiencies along with skeletal manifestations, including cervical spine rigidity with pathogenic *LHX3* variants and hypoplastic sella turcica with *LHX4* variants. These disorders may also be more definitively diagnosed via genetic testing.

Exposures such as alcohol (Answer B) have been implicated in the development of midline anomalies, but establishing causality is more challenging in the absence of other features (eg, neurodevelopmental abnormalities). Genetic testing can offer a more definitive diagnosis.

Educational Objective

Recognize the potential for monogenic and polygenic inheritance in individuals with congenital hypopituitarism.

Reference(s)

Bando H, Urai S, Kanie K, Sasaki Y, et al. Novel genes and variants associated with congenital pituitary hormone deficiency in the era of next-generation sequencing. *Front Endocrinol (Lausanne)*. 2022;13:1008306. PMID: 36237189

Fang Q, George AS, Brinkmeier ML, et al. Genetics of combined pituitary hormone deficiency: roadmap into the genome era. *Endocr Rev.* 2016;37(6):636-675. PMID: 27828722

McCormack SE, Li D, Kim YJ, et al. Digenic inheritance of PROKR2 and WDR11 mutations in pituitary stalk interruption syndrome. *J Clin Endocrinol Metab.* 2017;102(7):2501-2507. PMID: 28453858

Sertedaki A, Tatsi EB, Vasilakis IA, et al. Whole exome sequencing points towards a multi-gene synergistic action in the pathogenesis of congenital combined pituitary hormone deficiency. *Cells.* 2022;11(13). PMID: 35805171

7 ANSWER: A) Adopt a low-fat, carbohydrate-appropriate diet

The American Academy of Pediatrics recommends universal lipid screening (nonfasting lipid panel) for all children aged 9 to 11 years and 17 to 21 years. However, additional risk factors (BMI >85th percentile, parent with known dyslipidemia, personal history of diabetes, etc) should prompt consideration of screening for any child 2 years or older. Hypertriglyceridemia refers to a fasting triglyceride value that is above the 95th percentile for age and sex. This corresponds to a triglyceride concentration of 100 mg/dL or higher (≥1.13 mmol/L) for children aged 0 to 9 years and to 130 mg/dL or higher (≥1.47 mmol/L) for children aged 10 to 19 years. Approximately 10% of children in the United States between the ages of 12 and 19 years have fasting triglyceride values greater than 150 mg/dL (>1.70 mmol/L).

Definitions of fasting hypertriglyceridemia in adults:

- Moderate = 150-199 mg/dL (1.70-2.26 mmol/L)
- Moderate to high = 200-499 mg/dL (2.26-5.64 mmol/L)
- Very high = 500-999 mg/dL (5.65-11.29 mmol/L)
- Severe = 1000-1999 mg/dL (11.30-22.59 mmol/L)
- Very severe = >2000 mg/dL (>22.60 mmol/L)

In children, the most common hypertriglyceridemia pattern is moderately elevated triglyceride levels in conjunction with low HDL-cholesterol levels in those with obesity. Often referred to as combined dyslipidemia, the pattern of a triglyceride concentration between 150 and 400 mg/dL (1.70-4.52 mmol/L) and an HDL-cholesterol concentration less than 40 mg/dL (<1.04 mmol/L) is present in 30% to 60% of adolescents with obesity. Initiation of a heart-healthy lifestyle (low-fat, carbohydrate-appropriate diet [Answer A]) with increased dietary fiber and increased dietary omega-3 intake, as well as weight loss in the setting of obesity, and 30 to 60 minutes of moderate-vigorous physical activity daily is recommended for all patients with hypertriglyceridemia, regardless of etiology. For those with moderate hypertriglyceridemia and low HDL cholesterol, seen with obesity, lifestyle modifications are typically the only treatment needed and are successful in those who adhere to them.

Currently, no medications to treat hypertriglyceridemia are FDA-approved specifically for children younger than 18 years. Statins (Answer D) are recommended for patients with persistently elevated LDL-cholesterol levels due to familial hypercholesterolemia or for those with combined dyslipidemia. Statins typically decrease triglyceride levels by 10% to 15%. Current recommendations from the National Heart, Lung, and Blood Institute suggest that statin therapy be considered in children whose fasting triglyceride levels are between 200 and 499 mg/dL (2.26-5.64 mmol/L) and who also have non–HDL-cholesterol levels greater than 145 mg/dL (>3.76 mmol/L). A statin would not be the most appropriate recommendation for this patient because his non–HDL-cholesterol concentration is less than 145 mg/dL (<3.76 mmol/L). Additionally, lifestyle modifications would still be the first-line recommendation for at least 3 to 6 months prior to considering statin therapy, even in those with elevated non–HDL cholesterol.

The main goal of treating severe hypertriglyceridemia is to avoid the risk for acute pancreatitis. Rates of acute pancreatitis related to hypertriglyceridemia are not well established in pediatric populations. Best estimates are that 2% to 7% of acute pancreatitis cases in pediatric patients are due to metabolic causes, including hypertriglyceridemia. Additionally, the degree of hypertriglyceridemia required to cause acute pancreatitis is still debated, although data from adult populations suggest that triglyceride concentrations close to or greater than 1000 mg/dL (>11.30 mmol/L) place patients at higher risk for acute pancreatitis. The initial management of severe hypertriglyceridemia focuses on trying to acutely decrease triglyceride levels to 1000 mg/dL or lower (≤11.30 mmol/L) to avoid acute pancreatitis. In addition to other treatment modalities, aggressive restriction of dietary fats to less than 10% to 15% of daily caloric intake (<20 g daily) is needed. Given that the patient in the vignette does not meet criteria for severe hypertriglyceridemia, aggressive restriction of dietary fat intake (Answer C) is not appropriate.

While fasting can minimize variation in laboratory test results, insisting on fasting is not necessary when ordering initial lipid screening. For most children, postprandial triglyceride levels remain less than 150 mg/dL (<1.70 mmol/L); therefore, it would be inaccurate to tell the family that the elevated triglycerides are erroneous (Answer B). As an initial screen, nonfasting lipid samples are appropriate and may reduce barriers to screening by eliminating the need for fasting. There is also increasing evidence from data in adults that nonfasting triglyceride levels may be predictive of acute pancreatitis and premature cardiovascular risk. When hypertriglyceridemia is suspected or known, asking that subsequent measurements be undertaken while fasting is reasonable because fasting measurement reduces variation and helps the provider better understand the impact of lifestyle modifications and/or triglyceride-lowering medications.

Prescription omega-3 fatty acids (up to 4 g daily) have been used with variables outcomes in adult and pediatric patients. Over-the-counter omega-3 supplements (Answer E) are not recommended because most are not FDA-regulated and often contain inadequate amounts of eicosapentaenoic and docosahexaenoic acid. While triglyceride-lowering medications such as prescription omega-3 fatty acids could be considered for off-label use in patients with triglyceride concentrations of 500 mg/dL or higher (≥5.65 mmol/L) to decrease risk for acute pancreatitis, the patient in this vignette has only moderately elevated triglyceride levels and thus pharmacotherapy would not be indicated now.

Educational Objective

Summarize the management and treatment goals for hypertriglyceridemia in pediatric patients.

Reference(s)

Grisham JM, Tran AH, Ellery K. Hypertriglyceridemia-induced acute pancreatitis in children: a mini-review. *Front Pediatr.* 2022;10:931336. PMID: 36110119

Valaiyapathi B, Sunil B, Ashraf AP. Approach to hypertriglyceridemia in the pediatric population. *Pediatr Rev.* 2017;38(9):424-434. PMID: 28864733

Wilson DP, Williams L, Kavey R-EW. Hypertriglyceridemia in youth. *J Pediatr.* 2022;243:200-207. PMID: 34929246

8 **ANSWER: B) Euthyroidism**

In pregnant individuals with Graves disease, transplacental passage of stimulatory TRAb can cause hyperthyroidism in the fetus and newborn. Neonatal hyperthyroidism occurs in 1% to 5% of babies born to individuals with Graves disease. The risk of fetal and neonatal hyperthyroidism is directly associated with the concentration and activity of stimulatory TRAb in the maternal circulation. Neonatal hyperthyroidism is most likely when maternal TRAb concentrations are more than 5 times the upper limit of the reference range, whereas maternal TRAb concentrations less than 3 times the upper limit are very unlikely to cause neonatal hyperthyroidism (Answers C or E). When the mother has positive TRAb, the risk of neonatal hyperthyroidism can also be assessed by measuring TRAb in cord blood at birth. Infants without detectable TRAb are at negligible risk of hyperthyroidism, whereas those with significantly elevated TRAb require close monitoring of thyroid function for the possibility of evolving hyperthyroidism. One literature-based review suggests measurement of TSH, free T_4, and total T_3 on day of life 3 to 5 and on day of life 10 to 14 in newborns with positive TRAb.

In pregnant individuals with Graves disease who are treated with methimazole, transplacental passage of methimazole can lead to hypothyroidism in the fetus or in the neonate immediately after birth. The risk of fetal or neonatal hypothyroidism is directly related to the methimazole dosage and is unlikely when the maternal dosage of methimazole is below 10 mg daily. In addition, because the fetal thyroid is more sensitive to methimazole than is the maternal thyroid, fetal or neonatal hypothyroidism is likely if the mother is treated with methimazole to full euthyroidism (normal TSH and normal free T_4). For this reason, current guidelines recommend that pregnant individuals with Graves disease be treated to a target free T_4 concentration slightly above the reference range, rather than to normal. Finally, high dosages of methimazole transmitted through breastmilk can cause neonatal hypothyroidism, but this is unlikely with dosages below 20 or 30 mg daily. In this vignette, the risk of neonatal hypothyroidism (Answers D and E) is low based on the mother's low dosage of methimazole and the fact that her free T_4 remained above the reference range while on treatment.

In mothers with high-activity stimulatory TRAb who are treated with methimazole, the presence of methimazole may mask the effect of TRAb transmitted to the infant. In this situation, the neonate may be hypothyroid or euthyroid at birth but develop hyperthyroidism (Answer E) over the next 1 to 2 weeks as methimazole is cleared from the neonatal circulation. Since this patient is at low risk of both neonatal hyperthyroidism and methimazole-induced hypothyroidism, this scenario is unlikely.

Central hypothyroidism (Answer A) can occur in babies born to individuals with Graves disease who are exposed to persistent fetal hyperthyroidism, presumably due to changes in the central portion of the thyroid axis during gestation. If it occurs, such central hypothyroidism is usually transient, although rare cases of persistent central hypothyroidism have been reported. In this case, maternal hyperthyroidism appears to have been well controlled during pregnancy, so the likelihood of this infant developing central hypothyroidism is low.

Since the risk is low of both neonatal hypothyroidism and hyperthyroidism, the most likely outcome is that the patient will remain euthyroid (Answer B).

Educational Objective

Assess the risk of neonatal thyroid dysfunction in babies born to mothers with Graves disease.

Reference(s)

Ross DS, Burch HB, Cooper DS, et al. 2016 American Thyroid Association guidelines for diagnosis and management of hyperthyroidism and other causes of thyrotoxicosis. *Thyroid.* 2016;26(10):1343-1421. PMID: 27521067

van der Kaay DC, Wasserman JD, Palmert MR. Management of neonates born to mothers with Graves' disease. *Pediatrics.* 2016;137(4):e20151878. PMID: 26980880

van Dijk MM, Smits IH, Fliers E, Bisschop PH. Maternal thyrotropin receptor antibody concentration and the risk of fetal and neonatal thyrotoxicosis: a systematic review. *Thyroid.* 2018;28(2):257-264. PMID: 29325496

Yoshihara A, Noh JY, Inoue K, et al. Incidence of and risk factors for neonatal hypothyroidism among women with Graves' disease treated with antithyroid drugs until delivery. *Thyroid.* 2023;33(3):373-379. PMID: 36680759

9 **ANSWER: C) *HSD11B1* (hydroxysteroid 11-beta dehydrogenase 1)**

The gene *HSD11B1* (Answer C) encodes the enzyme 11-hydroxysteroid dehydrogenase type 1 (11β-HSD1). The ketoreductase activity of the enzyme is responsible for the conversion of cortisone (*E*) to cortisol (*F*) shown in *figure A*. In contrast, the conversion of cortisol to cortisone is performed by 11β-HSD2. The balance of cortisone and cortisol is therefore maintained by the action of these 2 enzymes. Pathogenic variants in *HSD11B1* (hence 11β-HSD1 deficiency) have been shown to cause "true" cortisone reductase deficiency. This results in an increase in cortisol to cortisone conversion and decrea3se in cortisol feedback to the hypothalamic-pituitary-adrenal axis to increase cortisol. Although cortisol in blood is maintained in this way, androgen production is increased. This proposed mechanism of action is supported by enlargement of the adrenal glands seen in male *11β-HSD1*$^{-/-}$ mice. Reported phenotypes in humans vary and can include pseudoprecocious puberty (in boys), premature adrenarche, hirsutism, obesity, infertility, and polycystic ovary syndrome (in girls).

Figure. 11β-HSD1 action and consequences of 11β-HSD1 deficiency

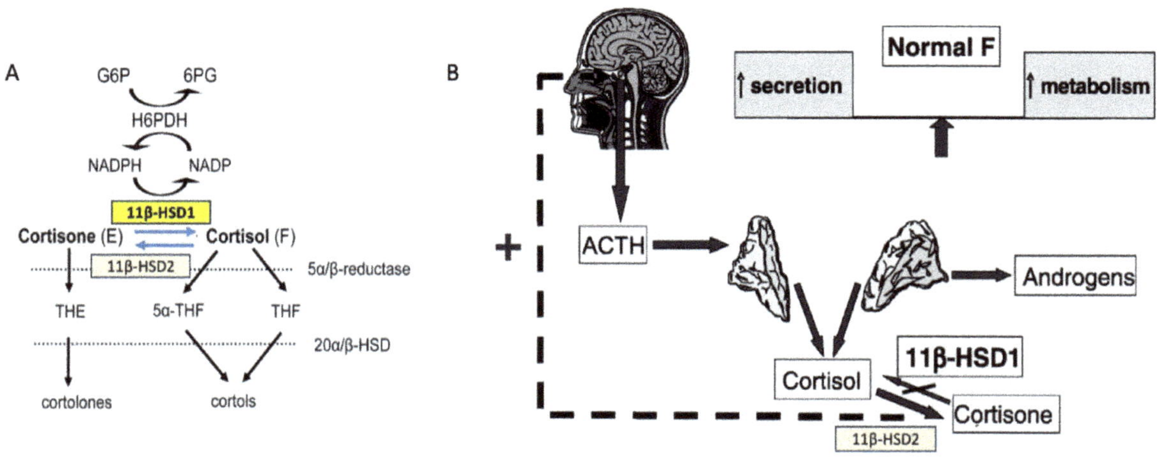

Schematic representation of 11β-HSD1 action at the level of the endoplasmic reticulum in adrenal cells (*Panel A*) and the overall consequence of 11β-HSD1 deficiency (*Panel B*). Equilibrium of cortisone and cortisol is maintained by enzymes 11β-HSD1 and 11β-HSD2. 11β-HSD1 deficiency leads to excess cortisol clearance to cortisone and is proposed to lead to hypothalamic-pituitary-adrenal activation, which drives adrenal androgen excess. *Panel A*: Reprinted with permission from Lawson AJ et al. *Proc Natl Acad Sci U S A*, 2011; 108(10): 4111-4116. © The National Academy of Sciences. *Panel B*: Reprinted with permission form Draper N & and Stewart PM. *Journal of Endocrinology*, 2005; 186(2): 251-271. © The Society for Endocrinology.

While serum cortisol levels are normal in persons with cortisone reductase deficiency, metabolites detected in the urine serve as excellent biomarkers of 11β-HSD1 activity. Cortisone and cortisol are metabolized by 5α-reductases to produce tetrahydrocortisone and 5β-reductases to produce 5α-tetrahydrocortisol and tetrahydrocortisol. The 20α- and 20β-HSDs further metabolize these to cortolones and cortols. Overall, in patients with 11β-HSD1, there is a decrease in the ratio of cortisol-to-cortisone metabolites and an overall increase in adrenal steroid metabolites. Typically, the ratio of tetrahydrocortisol plus 5α-tetrahydrocortisol to tetrahydrocortisone and the ratio of cortols to cortolones can be used as markers of cortisone reductase deficiency, with values of the tetrahydrocortisol + 5α-tetrahydrocortisol-to-tetrahydrocortisone ratio less than 0.1 (reference range, 0.7-1.3). For 24-hour urine collection, cortisone metabolites are elevated relative to cortisol metabolites, together with a decrease in 5α- and 5β-tetrahydrocortisol. Additionally, metabolites of the androgenic precursors androsterone, etiocholanolone, and DHEA-S are pathologically elevated.

Pathogenic variants in *HSD3B1* (Answer D), *CYP11B1* (Answer A), *CYP17A1* (Answer B), and *HSD3B2* (Answer E) would not give rise to such characteristic findings on urinary steroid profiles.

Of note, apparent cortisone reductase deficiency can also be caused by pathogenic variants in hexose-6-phosphate dehydrogenase, which encodes the enzyme known by the same name that generates NADPH by the conversion of glucose-6-phosphate transported via the G6P translocase, to 6-phosphogluconate within the endoplasmic reticulum. 11β-HSD1 uses NADPH as a cofactor, allowing conversion of cortisone to cortisol. Hence, H6PDH deficiency can lead to clinical features similar to those seen in 11β-HSD1 deficiency.

Educational Objective

Diagnose 11-hydroxysteroid dehydrogenase type 1 deficiency and explain the underlying pathophysiology.

Reference(s)

Draper N, Stewart PM. 11β-Hydroxysteroid dehydrogenase and the pre-receptor regulation of corticosteroid hormone action. *J Endocrinol.* 2005;186(2):251-271. PMID: 16079253

Lavery GG, Idkowiak J, Sherlock M, et al. Novel H6PDH mutations in two girls with premature adrenarche: 'apparent' and 'true' CRD can be differentiated by urinary steroid profiling. *Eur J Endocrinol.* 2013;168(2):K19-K26. PMID: 23132696

Lavery GG, Walker EA, Tiganescu A, et al. Steroid biomarkers and genetic studies reveal inactivating mutations in hexose-6-phosphate dehydrogenase in patients with cortisone reductase deficiency. *J Clin Endocrinol Metab.* 2008;93(10):3827-3832. PMID: 18628520

Lawson AJ, Walker EA, Lavery GG, et al. Cortisone-reductase deficiency associated with heterozygous mutations in 11beta-hydroxysteroid dehydrogenase type 1. *Proc Natl Acad Sci U S A.* 2011;108(10):4111-4116. PMID: 21325058

Małunowicz EM, Tomer TE, Urban M, Bossowski A. 11β-Hydroxysteroid dehydrogenase type 1 deficiency ('apparent cortisone reductase deficiency') in a 6-Year-old boy. *Horm Res.* 59(4):205-210. PMID: 12649576

10 ANSWER: C) Methylation testing of chromosome 11p15

The patient described in this vignette has classic features of Russell-Silver syndrome. The Netchine-Harbison Clinical Scoring System has been developed to help identify patients with this syndrome. Russell-Silver syndrome should be strongly considered in any patient who has 4 or more of the 6 clinical criteria:

- Being born small-for-gestational-age with either a birth weight or birth length ≤ −2 SDS for gestational age
- Postnatal growth failure defined as a height at 24 months of ≤ −2 SDS or 2 SD below the midparental target height
- Relative macrocephaly at birth with a head circumference ≥1.5 SDS above the birth weight and/or length SDS
- Protruding forehead
- Body asymmetry defined as a leg length discrepancy of ≥0.5 cm; if smaller than that, there must be at least 2 other asymmetric body parts
- Feeding difficulties and/or low BMI at age 24 months. Use of a feeding tube or appetite stimulant meets this criterion

The patient in this vignette meets 5 of the criteria with no comment on a protruding forehead, thus raising the clinical suspicion of Russell-Silver syndrome. Children with Russell-Silver syndrome can have many additional clinical features such as a triangular face, fifth-finger clinodactyly, and speech delay, all of which are present in this patient. Approximately 20% of children with Russell-Silver syndrome have a history of hypoglycemia.

The most common genetic etiology of Russell-Silver syndrome is hypomethylation of the imprinted region on chromosome 11p15 (Answer C). This hypomethylation causes loss of paternal *IGF2* expression and gain of maternal *H19* expression, which leads to growth restriction. There are other genetic etiologies of Russell-Silver syndrome, including copy number variants in this region, uniparental disomy of chromosome 7, and specific variants in the *CDKN1C* or *IGF2* genes, although these are less common. The most often used first test is a methylation-specific multiplex ligation-mediated PCR amplification (MS-MLPA) that assesses for both copy number changes and DNA methylation in this region and can be combined with testing for uniparental disomy of chromosome 7.

Karyotype analysis (Answer B), chromosomal microarray (Answer A), or whole-exome sequencing (Answer E) would not identify the methylation disturbance that is the most common etiology of Russell-Silver syndrome. Pathogenic variants in the *PTPN11* gene (Answer D) are the most common cause of Noonan syndrome.

Educational Objective

Identify the clinical features of Russell-Silver syndrome and explain how specific methylation analysis is necessary for the diagnosis.

Reference(s)

Fuke T, Nakamura A, Inoue T, et al. Role of imprinting disorders in short children born SGA and Silver-Russell syndrome spectrum. *J Clin Endocrinol Metab.* 2021;106(3):802-813. PMID: 33236057

Wakeling EL, Brioude F, Lokulo-Sodipe O. Diagnosis and management of Silver-Russell syndrome: first international consensus statement. *Nat Rev Endocrinol.* 2017;13(2):105-124. PMID: 27585961

11 ANSWER: B) Total body less head, lumbar spine, proximal femur for the 11-year-old and total body less head, lumbar spine for the 4-year-old

The International Society for Clinical Densitometry (ISCD) is regarded as a leader in skeletal health assessment. According to the ISCD recommendations, DXA is recommended for patients with primary bone disease when the patient "may benefit from interventions to decrease their elevated risk of a clinically significant fracture, and DXA results will influence that management." Pathogenic variants in *COL1A1* and *COL1A2* are the most common causes of osteogenesis imperfecta, and disease-causing variants lead to reduced quantity or impaired quality of type 1 collagen. Children and adults with osteogenesis imperfecta have an increased risk for fracture due to reduced bone mass and bone size, as well as increased bone turnover. DXA aids in bisphosphonate management decisions in these individuals. The 2019 pediatric position statement supports the acquisition of lumbar spine and total body less head scans as the preferred sites in children, noting that additional sites may be useful depending on clinical need. Specifically, the proximal femur (sometimes referred to as the total hip) can be used in children at risk for bone fragility who would benefit from continuity of DXA measurements into adulthood. Answer B recommends obtaining the preferred DXA sites of the total body less head and the lumbar spine in both children and includes the proximal femur for the 11-year-old child. At this time, no reference ranges are available for the proximal femur in children younger than 5 years.

Answer A represents prior guidance from the 2007 and 2013 official pediatric position statements when the proximal femur scan was not recommended because of concerns about the reliability of the machine to detect bone margins and the variability in development of hip geometry. While scan precision and analysis concerns may improve as growth plates and the lesser trochanter develop, the precision estimates for the proximal femur in children are similar to those of the total body less head and lumbar spine.

Answer C includes a distal radius scan for both children. Most commonly, bone density is measured at the 33% distal radius site. While reference ranges are available for this skeletal site in children 1 year of age and older, this scan site has poorest precision and thus is only recommended if the preferred skeletal sites cannot be obtained. The distal radius can be an important scan site in individuals with osteogenesis imperfecta if spinal hardware or other orthopedic hardware impair the ability to obtain the preferred skeletal sites.

Answer D refers to the 2007 recommendations where total body less head DXA measurement was only recommended in children older than 5 years. In 2022, Kalkwarf et al published additional reference data for children aged 1 to 5 years, which were combined with the Bone Mineral Density in Childhood Study data to smooth the age-, sex-, and race-specific reference curves for the lumbar spine, total body less head, and distal radius. Reference ranges for the total body less head were limited to those older than 3 years given difficulty in scan acquisition due to movement artifacts in younger children.

Answer A omits the opportunity to assess bone density at the proximal femur in the 11-year-old child and bone density of the total body less head in the 4-year-old child.

Answer E lists the recommended scan sites for adults. The total body less head is not a preferred skeletal site to assess fracture risk in adults.

Educational Objective

Identify the skeletal sites from which DXA scans can provide valid and reliable data regarding bone density in pediatric patients.

Reference(s)

Gordon CM, Leonard MB, Zemel BS, International Society for Clinical Densitometry. 2013 Pediatric Position Development Conference: executive summary and reflections. *J Clin Densitom.* 2014;17(2):219-224. PMID: 24657108

Kalkwarf HJ, Shepherd JA, Fan B, et al. Reference ranges for bone mineral content and density by dual energy x-ray absorptiometry for young children. *J Clin Endocrinol Metab.* 2022;107(9):e3887-e3900. PMID: 35587453

Liu W, Lee B, Nagamani SCS, et al. Approach to the patient: pharmacological therapies for fracture risk reduction in adults with osteogenesis imperfecta. *J Clin Endocrinol Metab.* 2023;108(7):1787-1796. PMID: 36658750

Weber DR, Boyce A, Gordon C, et al. The utility of DXA assessment at the forearm, proximal femur, and lateral distal femur, and vertebral fracture assessment in the pediatric population: 2019 ISCD official position. *J Clin Densitom.* 2019;22(4):567-589. PMID: 31421951

12 **ANSWER: C) Monomorphous pituitary neuroendocrine tumor with a single cellular population**
Management of suspected prolactin-secreting pituitary neuroendocrine tumors (PitNETs) includes consideration of the possibility of GH co-secretion, according to Endocrine Society guidelines. Specifically, measuring IGF-1 is recommended when this type of tumor is suspected or diagnosed. In addition, as in this case, the possibility of GH co-secretion should be revisited based on the clinical course. Acromegaly can develop in individuals with prolactin-secreting PitNETs that seem initially amenable to medical control. In a report of 2 illustrative cases, acromegaly developed more than a decade after the initial presentation. The co-occurrence in patients with pituitary tumors is most likely because somatotrophs and lactotrophs share a common developmental origin: cells derived from the oral epithelium under the regulation of specific transcription factors such as Pit1.

GH and prolactin co-secreting tumors have been dissected and explored both clinically and in vitro. The fifth edition of the World Health Organization classification of endocrine tumors and NETs related to the pituitary gland bases histological subtyping on tumor features, including cell lineage (based on pituitary transcription factor expression), cell type, and cell characteristics. Several types of co-secreting tumors can be identified on pathology:

- Mixed NETs (bimorphous, ie, 2 cell types), originating from both well-differentiated somatotroph and lactotroph populations. The 2 separate cell types are distinguishable via immunohistochemical staining, and each cell produces its respective hormone. Most often, GH excess leads to clinical attention and diagnosis. Prolactin excess is typically a later development in affected patients (thus, Answer B is incorrect).
- Monomorphous NETs (ie, 1 cell type), originating from mature mammosomatotroph cells, where both GH and prolactin are secreted from the same cells. Patients with this type of tumor most often present with symptoms of acromegaly, not with prolactin excess as in this case.
- Monomorphous NETs (ie, 1 cell type), originating from primitive acidophilic stem cells, where both GH and prolactin are secreted from the same cells. These tumors are believed to represent tumors of precursor cells that may retain the capacity to produce multiple hormones and lack features of terminal differentiation. As in this patient, prolactin excess is most often what initially brings an affected patient to clinical attention, and GH excess becomes apparent later (Answer C). Unfortunately, serial operative resections and/or adjuvant therapies are typically required. These are very rare tumors.

Evolution from prolactin-only to prolactin-plus-GH co-secretion can also be accompanied by oncogenic transformation (eg, *GNAS* gene) that may be absent from the initial tumor specimen, but present in subsequent sections.

Hyperplasia of prolactin-producing cells (Answer D) can be physiologic, as in pregnancy, or a secondary effect (eg, from stalk compression), but neither of these is the cause of this patient's condition.

Infiltration of chronic inflammatory cells into the adenohypophysis (Answer A) is most characteristic of lymphocytic hypophysitis, not a GH-prolactin co-secreting tumor. While inflammation can occur in the setting of pituitary tumors, it is not to the same extent as in hypophysitis.

The description of a tumor with 3 components, including blastemal cells, Rathke pouch epithelium, and adenohypophyseal neuroendocrine cells (Answer E), is characteristic of a pituitary blastoma, a rare embryonal sellar tumor often associated with DICER1 syndrome. Neuroendocrine cells in pituitary blastomas tend to demonstrate corticotroph differentiation, most likely because this is the first anterior pituitary cell type to develop antenatally. This is inconsistent with the GH and prolactin co-secretion observed in this patient.

Educational Objective

Describe the pathologic correlation of prolactin and GH co-secreting pituitary adenomas.

Reference(s)

Asa SL, Mete O, Perry A, Osamura RY. Overview of the WHO 2022 classification of pituitary tumors. *Endocr Path.* 2022;33(1):6-26. PMID: 35291028

Lania AG, Ferrero S, Pivonello R, et al. Evolution of an aggressive prolactinoma into a growth hormone secreting pituitary tumor coincident with GNAS gene mutation. *J Clin Endocrinol Metab.* 2010;95(1):13-17. PMID: 19890024

Lopes MBS. Growth hormone-secreting adenomas: pathology and cell biology. *Neurosurg Focus.* 2010;29(4):E2. PMID: 20887127

Manuylova E, Calvi LM, Hastings C, et al. Late presentation of acromegaly in medically controlled prolactinoma patients. *Endocrinol Diabetes Metab Case Rep.* 2016;16:0069. PMID: 27855229

Melmed S, Casanueva FF, Hoffman AR, et al. Endocrine Society. Diagnosis and treatment of hyperprolactinemia: an Endocrine Society clinical practice guideline. *J Clin Endocrinol Metab.* 2011;96(2):273-288. PMID: 21296991

13 ANSWER: C) Age, 4 years; pH, 7.0; bicarbonate, 7.0 mEq/L; glucose, 425 mg/dL; serum urea nitrogen, 23 mg/dL; Pco_2, 15 mm Hg

Depending on the geographic region, diabetic ketoacidosis occurs in 20% to 80% of children presenting with newly diagnosed type 1 diabetes. Cerebral edema occurs in 0.5% to 1.0% of diabetic ketoacidosis episodes in children, and its mortality rate is 25% to 30%. The pathophysiologic mechanism underlying cerebral edema associated with diabetic ketoacidosis is controversial; however, some risk factors have been identified:

- Elevated serum urea nitrogen concentration (>20 mg/dL [>7.1 mmol/L])
- Severe acidosis (pH <7.1)
- Severe hypocapnia (Pco_2 <21 mm Hg)
- Age <5 years

Answer C includes all these risk factors and therefore represents the patient who would be at highest risk for cerebral edema. However, any patient with new-onset diabetes presenting in diabetic ketoacidosis is at risk of cerebral edema, depending on other factors associated with medical management, specifically bicarbonate treatment for correction of acidosis or insulin bolus administration.

Neuroimaging studies have led to the appreciation that cerebral edema is not a rare phenomenon in children with diabetic ketoacidosis, but rather that it occurs frequently and with varying severity.

Clinically significant cerebral injury usually develops within the first 12 hours after treatment has started, but it can occur before treatment has begun or, rarely, may develop as late as 24 to 48 hours after treatment has started. Symptoms and signs are variable. Mild to moderate headache at presentation is not unusual in children with diabetic ketoacidosis. However, development of headache or substantial worsening of headache after commencing treatment is concerning.

The International Society for Pediatric and Adolescent Diabetes guidelines suggest diagnostic criteria for diagnosing cerebral edema. Patients without the diagnostic criteria can be observed for the listed symptoms under major and minor criteria. Two major or 1 major and 2 minor criteria have a sensitivity of 92% and a false-positive rate of only 4%. Signs that occur before treatment should not be considered in the diagnosis. Neuroimaging is not required for diagnosis of cerebral injury.

Diagnostic criteria:

- Abnormal motor or verbal response to pain
- Decorticate or decerebrate posture
- Cranial nerve palsy (especially III, IV, and VI)
- Abnormal neurogenic respiratory pattern (eg, grunting, tachypnea, Cheyne-Stokes respiration, apneusis)

Major criteria:

- Altered mentation, confusion, fluctuating level of consciousness
- Sustained heart rate deceleration (decrease more than 20 beats/min) not attributable to improved intravascular volume or sleep state
- Age-inappropriate incontinence

Minor criteria:

- Vomiting
- Headache
- Lethargy or not easily arousable
- Diastolic blood pressure >90 mm Hg
- Age <5 years

Educational Objective

Identify risk factors for cerebral edema in the setting of diabetic ketoacidosis.

Reference(s)

Bello FA, Sotos JF. Cerebral oedema in diabetic ketoacidosis in children. *Lancet.* 1990;336(8706):64. PMID: 1973254

Duck SC, Wyatt DT. Factors associated with brain herniation in the treatment of diabetic ketoacidosis. *J Pediatr.* 1988;113(1 Pt 1):10-4. PMID: 3133455

Glaser N, Fritsch M, Priyambada L, et al. ISPAD clinical practice consensus guidelines 2022: diabetic ketoacidosis and hyperglycemic hyperosmolar state. *Pediatr Diabetes.* 2022;23(7):835-856. PMID: 36250645

Krane EJ, Rockoff MA, Wallman JK, Wolfsdorf JI. Subclinical brain swelling in children during treatment of diabetic ketoacidosis. *N Engl J Med.* 1985;312(18):1147-1151. PMID: 3920521

Rosenbloom AL. Intracerebral crises during treatment of diabetic ketoacidosis. *Diabetes Care.* 1990;13(1):22-33. PMID: 2105195

14 ANSWER: D) Hispanic female

Prevalence studies show that the rates of congenital hypothyroidism are highest in individuals of Hispanic ethnicity and higher in females than in males. Thus, compared with the infant in this vignette, a Hispanic female child (Answer D) would be at higher risk for congenital hypothyroidism.

Variations in prevalence of congenital hypothyroidism exist based on sex and ethnicity. Numerous studies have shown the highest rates of congenital hypothyroidism in Hispanic and Asian individuals and the lowest rates in Black individuals. There is also an overall female preponderance with a female-to-male ratio of 2.0:1 to 2.5:1. One large study documented female preponderance to be greatest in the Hispanic population. Ascertainment bias in these prevalence studies is limited because of universal newborn screening programs.

African American female and African American male (Answers A and B) are incorrect because studies have consistently shown the lowest rates of congenital hypothyroidism in Black infants. The female-to male-preponderance of congenital hypothyroidism is also not observed in the Black population. One Canadian study assessed the prevalence of congenital hypothyroidism based on its etiology (thyroid dysgenesis vs dyshormonogenesis) and found that thyroid dysgenesis is far less prevalent in the Black population than it is in other ethnic groups.

In the overall population, thyroid dysgenesis accounts for most cases of congenital hypothyroidism. Thyroid dysgenesis is typically not inherited. There is a high discordance rate among monozygotic twins (92%), yet the rate of thyroid dysgenesis among relatives is 15-fold higher than expected from chance alone, so some genetic influence clearly exists. In contrast, dyshormonogenesis is inherited, typically in an autosomal recessive manner, and no differences are seen in rates between males and females. It is postulated that the lack of female preponderance and the decreased rates of congenital hypothyroidism overall may be related to decreased prevalence of thyroid dysgenesis in the Black population.

Limited data are available regarding the prevalence of congenital hypothyroidism in the American Indian population, but one Californian study that included them as a separate ethnic group found they had rates of congenital hypothyroidism higher than rates in the White population but lower than rates in the Hispanic population (thus, Answer C is incorrect).

The prevalence of congenital hypothyroidism in the White population is lower than in the Hispanic population. Female preponderance of congenital hypothyroidism is observed among White infants, so the prevalence in White male children is lower than in the general White population (thus, Answer E is incorrect).

Table. Rates of Congenital Hypothyroidism (From Most to Least Prevalent)

Race	Rates of congenital hypothyroidism according to sex
Hispanic	Females > males
American Indian	Unknown
White	Females > males
African American	Females = males

Educational Objective

Describe race and sex differences in the prevalence of congenital hypothyroidism.

Reference(s)

Stoppa-Vaucher S, Van Vliet G, Deladoey J. Variation by ethnicity in the prevalence of congenital hypothyroidism due to thyroid dysgenesis. *Thyroid.* 2011;21(1):13-18. PMID: 21054242

Waller DK, Anderson JL, Lorey F, Cunningham GC. Risk factors for congenital hypothyroidism: an investigation of infant's birth weight, ethnicity, and gender in California, 1990-1998. *Teratology.* 2000;62(1):36-41. PMID: 10861631

15 ANSWER: A) Enhancement of the GH/IGF-1 axis

This patient has recent accelerated growth, weight loss, no signs of puberty, and a small goiter. This constellation of findings is suggestive of hyperthyroidism as the underlying diagnosis. There is complex interplay between the TSH-T_4 axis and the GH–IGF-1 axis. Excessive thyroid hormone in prepubertal patients with hyperthyroidism enhances the effect of GH and IGF-1 on their target tissues (Answer A), thereby promoting growth.

She has no clinical signs or symptoms suggestive of puberty. Therefore, she is not expected to have pulsatile secretion of GnRH (Answer D).

Thyroid hormone speeds up (not slows [Answer E]) the maturation of growth plates. Bone age is frequently advanced compared with the chronologic age in growing children at the time hyperthyroidism is diagnosed.

Even though exogenous obesity (Answer B) can cause accelerated growth and bone age advancement in prepubertal children, the presence of goiter and recent increase in growth velocity despite weight loss indicate hyperthyroidism as the cause of accelerated growth in this child.

Similarly, a normal growth pattern in children with familial tall stature (Answer C) does not include the sudden increase in prepubertal growth and other features noted in this patient.

Educational Objective

Identify hyperthyroidism as the cause of growth acceleration and explain the mechanism of thyroid hormone in regulating growth.

Reference(s)

Lazar L, Kalter-Leibovici O, Pertzelan A, Weintrob N, Josefsberg Z, Phillip M. Thyrotoxicosis in prepubertal children compared with pubertal and postpubertal patients. *J Clin Endocrinol Metab.* 2000;85(10):3678-3682. PMID: 11061522

Smith TJ. Insulin-like growth factor pathway and the thyroid. *Front Endocrinol (Lausanne).* 2021;12:653627. PMID: 34149612

Tarım Ö. Thyroid hormones and growth in health and disease. *J Clin Res Pediatr Endocrinol.* 2011;3(2):51-55. PMID: 21750631

16 ANSWER: E) Venous thromboembolism

The patient in this vignette meets diagnostic criteria for gender dysphoria and use of gender-affirming treatment according to Endocrine Society and American Academy of Pediatrics guidelines. Risks of gender-affirming hormone therapy (GAHT) are less clear for adolescents than for adults, for whom a substantial amount of data indicates similar risks associated with sex hormone replacement. There is particular concern for risk of venous thromboembolism (VTE) (Answer E) with GAHT. Several large retrospective studies have found a higher risk of VTE in transgender women receiving GAHT compared with risk in natal males and in the general population, primarily in patients treated with ethinyl estradiol. Studies in which individuals were treated with 17β-estradiol have not found an increased risk. As such, Endocrine Society guidelines recommend against the use of ethinyl estradiol specifically and recommend monitoring hormone levels during treatment to ensure that serum estradiol levels are maintained in the normal physiological range of 100 to 200 pg/mL (367.1-734.2 pmol/L). Given the lack of data regarding the risk of VTE in adolescents treated with estrogen for GAHT, the most prudent approach would be to screen for risk of thrombotic disease before starting GAHT and to avoid use of ethinyl estradiol in this patient population.

Studies in adults suggest that GAHT may have an adverse effect on cardiometabolic health, potentially increasing risk of stroke, myocardial infarction, type 2 diabetes, and low bone mineral density. However, these risks may not be a concern in transgender and gender-diverse youth. A multicenter, retrospective, cross-sectional study was conducted using PEDSnet data from 4172 transgender and gender-diverse youth and 16,648 matched control participants. The adjusted odds of obesity and dyslipidemia were higher among transgender and gender-diverse youth than in control participants. However, among the transgender and gender-diverse youth in the study, treatment with estradiol was not associated with an increased risk of overweight/obesity (Answer D), dyslipidemia (Answer A), liver dysfunction (Answer B), or dysglycemia. While the study included youth with type 1 diabetes, this subgroup was not analyzed alone, so conclusions cannot be drawn regarding altered glycemic control in transgender and gender-diverse youth with type 1 diabetes.

The risk of low bone density (Answer C) in transgender and gender-diverse youth is primarily due to the use of GnRH agonists to suppress pubertal hormones, not due to the use of GAHT. Any adverse effects of GnRH agonists for pubertal suppression are likely reversed with sex hormone treatment.

Educational Objective

Appropriately manage cardiometabolic risk factors in transgender youth.

Reference(s)

Hembree WC, Cohen-Kettenis PT, Gooren L, et al. Endocrine treatment of gender-dysphoric/gender-incongruent persons: an Endocrine Society clinical practice guideline. *J Clin Endocrinol Metab.* 2017;102(11):3869-3903. PMID: 28945902

Valentine A, Davis S, Furniss A, et al. Multicenter analysis of cardiometabolic-related diagnoses in transgender and gender-diverse youth: a PEDSnet study. *J Clin Endocrinol Metab.* 2022;107(10):e4004-e4014. PMID: 35945152

17 ANSWER: D) Oxcarbazepine

This patient's laboratory testing shows a pattern of central hypothyroidism, with low free T_4 and lack of TSH elevation. Anticonvulsant medications can alter thyroid function, with different medications causing characteristic patterns of thyroid alterations. Oxcarbazepine (Answer D) can cause central hypothyroidism, as seen in this case, although the mechanism for this effect is unclear. In most cases, central hypothyroidism caused by oxcarbazepine is mild and asymptomatic, but in some cases it may be severe enough to cause symptoms, including fatigue, constipation, and slow growth velocity, that improve with levothyroxine treatment. Levetiracetam (Answer C) generally has no effect on thyroid function. Valproic acid (Answer E) can cause primary hypothyroidism that is usually mild and subclinical, but it does not cause central hypothyroidism.

Although the differential diagnosis of central hypothyroidism includes a structural lesion of the central nervous system (Answer B), this is less likely in a patient with another known cause of central hypothyroidism (oxcarbazepine) and no central nervous system signs or symptoms.

Large dosages of biotin (Answer A) (greater than 5 to 10 mg daily) can confound the laboratory assessment of thyroid function due to interference with some competitive-binding assays whose design depends on the binding of biotin to the protein avidin. The direction of confounding of each analyte (falsely high or falsely low) depends on the specific assay, but most commonly, biotin causes falsely low TSH and falsely high total and free T_4, total and free T_3, and TRAb. The pattern of central hypothyroidism in this patient generally is not observed in cases of biotin interference. In any case, discontinuation of biotin intake for 48 to 72 hours before blood sampling is sufficient to avoid assay interference, so biotin would not explain the thyroid function pattern in this patient.

Educational Objective

Diagnose central hypothyroidism associated with oxcarbazepine treatment.

Reference(s)

Han Y, Yang J, Zhong R, Guo X, Cai M, Lin W. Side effects of long-term oral anti-seizure drugs on thyroid hormones in patients with epilepsy: a systematic review and network meta-analysis. *Neurol Sci.* 2022 Sep;43(9):5217-5227. PMID: 35644830

Schweiger BM, Lao AJ, Tavyev J. A case series of patients with central hypothyroidism from oxcarbazepine therapy. *J Child Neurol.* 2021;36(3):237-242. PMID: 33030389

18 ANSWER: D) Presence of macroprolactin

Hyperprolactinemia is commonly encountered in clinical practice, and it can be physiologic (ie, from pregnancy/lactation, stress, exercise, or nipple stimulation) or due to other causes such as medications, traumatic injury to the pituitary, pituitary disease, and systemic disorders. In evaluating and managing hyperprolactinemia, clinicians must be aware of the problems that can occur when evaluating circulating prolactin concentrations with currently available laboratory testing methodologies. An ideal prolactin assay would detect only its biologically active monomeric 23 kDa form. However, immunoassays for prolactin can also detect macroprolactin (Answer D), a biologically inactive form of prolactin, typically complexed to immunoglobulin, that can be 100 kDa or larger. Polyethylene glycol (PEG) precipitation leads to complexing of these bound forms of prolactin; when the fraction of PEG-precipitated prolactin is 60% or more of the total, the specimen is considered positive. In this vignette, PEG-precipitated prolactin was 65% of the total, and monomeric prolactin was normal.

Macroprolactinemia is a relatively common phenomenon, occurring in up to 18.9% of individuals with hyperprolactinemia according to one global meta-analysis. Given this high prevalence, some investigators advocate that all individuals with hyperprolactinemia be screened for macroprolactinemia before proceeding to the next diagnostic and management steps. Distinguishing macroprolactinemia from "true" hyperprolactinemia on the basis of clinical symptoms alone can be challenging. Others advocate having a low threshold to assess for macroprolactin and recommend testing all patients who have few or no symptoms of prolactin excess but have a prolactin concentration above the upper limit of normal but less than 250 ng/mL (<10.87 nmol/L).

Prolactin immunoassays can also underestimate the amount of "true" hyperprolactinemia when the amount of monomeric prolactin to be detected far exceeds the linear detection capacity of the assay, the so-called hook effect (Answer B). In particular, when the extent of clinical symptoms and/or the size of the tumor is substantial, but the prolactin concentration is less than 250 ng/mL (<10.87 nmol/L), considering the possibility of the hook effect by assessing the extent of true hyperprolactinemia with serial dilutions is essential. On clinical follow-up, this patient had no symptoms of prolactin excess and normal findings on pituitary MRI, so the hook effect is unlikely.

The normal pituitary MRI findings and lack of any symptoms of excess prolactin also make a prolactin-secreting neuroendocrine tumor (Answer E) and pituitary stalk disruption (Answer C) much less likely than the presence of macroprolactin. Testing for macroprolactin early in the course of evaluation for hyperprolactinemia could obviate the need for MRI in some cases (eg, when there are no symptoms suggestive of hyperprolactinemia).

Although biotin ingestion (Answer A) can affect hormonal assays that use biotinylation in their design (particularly some thyroid function tests), prolactin measurement is not typically affected, even if the patient's nutritional supplements include biotin.

Educational Objective

Identify potential pitfalls in the interpretation of prolactin assays.

Reference(s)

Casanueva FF, Molitch ME, Schlechte JA, et al. Guidelines of the Pituitary Society for the diagnosis and management of prolactinomas. *Clin Endocrinol (Oxf).* 2006;65(2):265-273. PMID: 16886971

Che Soh NAA, Yaacob NM, Omar J, et al. Global prevalence of macroprolactinemia among patients with hyperprolactinemia: a systematic review and meta-analysis. *Int J Environ Res Public Health.* 2020;17(21):8199. PMID: 33171973

Fahie-Wilson MN, McKenna TJ, Ahlquist JA, Smith TP. Macroprolactin and the Pituitary Society guidelines for the diagnosis and management of prolactinomas. *Clin Endocrinol (Oxf).* 2007;67(4):638-639. PMID: 17590168

Hauache OM, Rocha AJ, Maia ACM Jr, Maciel RMB, Vieira JGH. Screening for macroprolactinaemia and pituitary imaging studies. *Clin Endocrinol (Oxf).* 2002;57(3):327-331. PMID: 12201824

Melmed S, Casanueva FF, Hoffman AR, et al; Endocrine Society. Diagnosis and treatment of hyperprolactinemia: an Endocrine Society clinical practice guideline. *J Clin Endocrinol Metab.* 2011;96(2):273-288. PMID: 21296991

19 ANSWER: E) Phentermine/topiramate

The combination phentermine/topiramate extended-release capsule (Answer E) is approved for long-term weight management in pediatric patients who are 12 years and older who have a BMI in the 95th percentile or greater for age and sex. It suppresses appetite through mechanisms that are not fully understood. Phentermine is approved as short-term monotherapy (≤12 weeks) for weight control in individuals who are 16 years or older. Since it is an amphetamine analogue, it is a controlled, class IV substance. It is thought to enhance norepinephrine, dopamine, and epinephrine release in the central nervous system. Topiramate was first approved for the treatment of epilepsy and migraine prophylaxis. Its use for the treatment of obesity was pursued after weight loss was noted among patients with epilepsy who were taking the drug. Its mechanism of action in the central nervous system is not well-understood, but it may have effects on thermogenesis. Potential adverse effects of phentermine include dry mouth, increases in blood pressure and heart rate, palpitations, dizziness, tremor, insomnia, and restlessness. Topiramate can cause hypokalemia, metabolic acidosis, anhidrosis, nephrolithiasis, and dysgeusia (altered or impaired sense of taste), which the patient in the vignette is experiencing. Dysgeusia is often dosage-dependent. With combination therapy, there is a synergistic effect regarding weight loss, and lower dosages can be used than when these agents are prescribed independently. Depression, anxiety, sleep disorders, and suicidal ideation have been described and should be monitored for closely; the medication should be discontinued if suicidal ideation or behavior is encountered. The extended-release capsule is taken once daily in the morning, and the dosage can be gradually titrated depending on tolerability and whether the patient achieves desired weight loss. If ineffective, the medication must be slowly weaned to avoid risk of seizures with abrupt discontinuation.

Orlistat (Answer D) does not work at the level of the central nervous system, unlike several other antiobesity medications. Its mechanism of action involves inhibiting pancreatic and gastrointestinal lipases, which block triglyceride hydrolysis and fatty acid absorption by the intestinal endothelium. Approximately one-third of fatty acid absorption is blocked, which decreases the number of calories consumed. Orlistat is FDA-approved for pediatric patients who are 12 years and older. There is an over-the-counter version of orlistat (60 mg capsules), which is not as potent as prescribed orlistat (120 mg capsules). Orlistat does not affect patient appetite. While it is often well-tolerated, due to its mechanism of action, patients can experience frequent stooling, flatus, fecal incontinence, and steatorrhea. Use of a fiber-containing supplement, such as psyllium, may help decrease gastrointestinal adverse effects. Orlistat also prevents lipid-soluble vitamins from being absorbed, so those using it long-term should take supplemental vitamins A, D, E, and K.

Liraglutide (Answer A) is a GLP-1 receptor agonist that is approved for long-term weight management in adolescents with obesity who are 12 years and older. It is 97% identical to human GLP-1, but it has a much longer half-life (13 hours) compared with the half-life of human GLP-1 (minutes). Its mechanism of action is complex. It helps with glucose regulation by suppressing glucagon release in the pancreas and enhancing insulin secretion from pancreatic β cells. It also acts on GLP-1 receptors in the hypothalamus to suppress appetite and promote weight loss. Liraglutide also functions to slow gastric transit, thus enhancing satiety. The most common adverse effects are gastrointestinal-related. Nausea, vomiting, diarrhea, and dyspepsia are frequently reported, but they may be lessened by slow dosage titration. There have been concerns for risk of acute pancreatitis, although this is not common. Additionally, a higher incidence of thyroid C-cell cancer has been observed with liraglutide in rodent studies, so it is contraindicated in individuals with a personal or family history of medullary thyroid cancer or multiple endocrine neoplasia type 2.

Naltrexone/bupropion extended-release (Answer C) is approved for long-term weight management in individuals older than 18 years. Bupropion is a norepinephrine and dopamine reuptake inhibitor that, in addition to other actions, suppresses appetite and enhances energy expenditure. Naltrexone also inhibits appetite through blocking β-endorphin action, and it acts synergistically in combination with bupropion. Nausea is a very common adverse effect and can be severe, thus the dosage should be slowly titrated. Constipation, dizziness, dry mouth, insomnia, and headaches have also been reported. Risk of seizures, as well as concern for depression and suicidal ideation, must also be discussed.

Metformin (Answer B) is not an approved medication for the treatment of obesity in pediatric or adult patients. However, it is approved in children 12 years and older for the treatment of type 2 diabetes. Metformin has multiple sites of action. In the liver, it inhibits the mitochondrial respiratory chain, leading to activation of AMPK and lowering cyclic AMP, resulting in reduced gluconeogenesis and lipogenesis. At the level of the gut, it increases GLP-1 secretion, increases glucose use, and may also alter the microbiome. The most common adverse effects are gastrointestinal-related such as nausea, vomiting, diarrhea, and abdominal pain. While dysgeusia has been described with metformin therapy, it is less common than other gastrointestinal-related adverse effects. Rarely, lactic acidosis has been described.

Educational Objective

Identify common adverse effects associated with agents used in pharmacotherapy for weight loss.

Reference(s)

Son JW, Kim S. Comprehensive review of current and upcoming anti-obesity drugs. *Diabetes Metab J.* 2020;44(6):802-818. PMID: 33389955

Tak YJ, Lee SY. Long-term efficacy and safety of anti-obesity treatment: where do we stand? *Curr Obes Rep.* 2021;10(1):14-30. PMID: 33410104

20 ANSWER: E) Pathogenic variant in the *SHOX* gene

The *SHOX* gene (short stature homeobox-containing gene) is located in the pseudoautosomal region of the X and Y chromosomes. Pathogenic variants in the *SHOX* gene (Answer E) lead to short stature with a range of phenotypes. Heterozygous variants can lead to idiopathic short stature or Leri-Weill dyschondrosteosis, while biallelic recessive variants cause Langer mesomelic dysplasia, a rare, severe form of the disorder. The photograph of the mother's arms in this vignette demonstrates the classic Madelung deformity that can be found in individuals with short stature due to SHOX deficiency. SHOX deficiency causes disproportionate shortening of the extremities, resulting in an elevated sitting-height ratio. In a study by Malaquias et al of patients with SHOX deficiency, a sitting-height ratio above +2 SDS is present in 88% of children and in 96% of adults. Madelung deformity is a characteristic feature found in some individuals with SHOX deficiency. Pathogenic variants in *SHOX* can be de novo or inherited in a dominant fashion, as in this case (the mother is affected). SHOX deficiency is an approved indication for GH therapy.

A sitting-height ratio above +2 SDS is present in 48% of children with Turner syndrome (Answer A) in whom short stature is also often attributed to SHOX deficiency. However, Turner syndrome is not inherited in an autosomal dominant manner.

Individuals with pathogenic variants in *NPR2* (Answer D) or *ACAN* (Answer B) can present with either proportionate or disproportionate short stature, but they would not be expected to have Madelung deformity.

Pathogenic variants in *FGFR3* (Answer C) typically cause either achondroplasia or hypochondroplasia, which would lead to an elevated sitting-height ratio and disproportionate short stature, but again, without Madelung deformity.

Pathogenic variants in *NPR2, ACAN,* and *FGFR3* can also follow a dominant pattern of inheritance for short stature.

This case highlights the importance of measuring body proportions in the evaluation of patients with short stature. Normative charts exist for sitting-height ratio in the US population. It is important to note that body proportions do vary by racial background and the appropriate chart must be used when interpreting body proportions. This case also points to the low yield of traditional biochemical testing in patients with idiopathic short stature and normal growth velocity.

**Note: image in the stem reprinted from Makanji H.* OrthoBullets. *Madelung's deformity. Accessed December 7, 2023. https://www.orthobullets.com/hand/6070/madelungs-deformity*

Educational Objective

Explain the importance of measuring body proportions, including sitting height, and how this can suggest an underlying skeletal dysplasia such as a *SHOX* pathogenic variant.

Reference(s)

Blum WF, Crowe BJ, Quigley CA, et al; SHOX Study Group. Growth hormone is effective in treatment of short stature associated with short stature homeobox-containing gene deficiency: Two-year results of a randomized, controlled, multicenter trial. *J Clin Endocrinol Metab.* 2007;92(1):219-228. PMID: 17047016

Dantas NCB, Funari MFA, Vasques GA, et al. Adult height of patients with SHOX haploinsufficiency with or without GH therapy: a real-world single-center study. *Horm Res Paediatr.* 2022;95(3):264-274. PMID: 35390795

Hawkes CP, Mostoufi-Moab S, McCormack SE, Grimberg A, Zemel BS. Sitting height to standing height ratio reference charts for children in the United States. *J Pediatr.* 2020;226:221-227.e15. PMID: 32579888

Malaquias AC, Scalco RC, Fontenele EG, et al. The sitting height/height ratio for age in healthy and short individuals and its potential role in selecting short children for SHOX analysis. *Horm Res Paediatr.* 2013;80(6):449-456. PMID: 24296787

21 ANSWER: B) Monitor serum calcium every month

Inhibition of receptor activator of nuclear factor kappa-B ligand (RANKL) has been used as adjuvant treatment for aneurysmal bone cysts and other osteoclast-rich tumors to reduce tumor burden and aid in surgical resection. Denosumab is a fully human monoclonal antibody reversible inhibitor of RANKL. In the animal model, osteoclasts exposed to RANKL inhibition undergo fission into dormant "osteomorphs" that rapidly re-fuse into active osteoclasts upon treatment withdrawal. In human use, robust increases in bone resorption markers to above pretreatment levels have been observed upon cessation of denosumab. Adults who abruptly discontinue denosumab experience rapid loss of bone mineral density and an increase in vertebral fractures. Children have much higher rates of bone turnover and more time for skeletal mineralization than adults. Thus, when denosumab treatment is discontinued, hypercalcemia occurs more frequently (in up to 45% of pediatric patients vs in <1% of adults). The usual onset of hypercalcemia is between 1 and 7 months after treatment cessation. Current guidance is to monitor serum calcium, urinary calcium, and PTH levels at least monthly for this entire duration (Answer B), recognizing that the onset of hypercalcemia can be abrupt and severe. It is important to counsel patients and families about this phenomenon and to educate them about the signs and symptoms of hypercalcemia.

Dense metaphyseal bands are frequently seen in pediatric patients treated with high-dosage denosumab, which may explain hypocalcemia that occurs during active treatment and then the severe hypercalcemia noted after treatment as this mineral is released from these bands. However, there is no known correlation between hypocalcemia during treatment and risk of hypercalcemia upon treatment cessation. Obtaining lower-extremity x-rays again in 6 months (Answer E) may show an interval improvement in the sclerotic appearance of the metaphysis, which would be expected to continue to resolve as the child grows. However, this would not change clinical management.

Vertebral compression fractures have been described in adult patients 3 to 24 months after cessation of denosumab, again due to the rebound phenomenon of bone resorption. Many such fractures are asymptomatic and thus would only be detected on dedicated spinal imaging. However, this phenomenon has yet to be described in children. Therefore, spine x-rays (Answer C) are not the most important tool to monitor for adverse effects of denosumab treatment in children.

Adults are recommended to receive a dose of zoledronic acid 6 months after stopping denosumab (Answer A). While various regimens have been proposed to taper denosumab therapy and/or give bisphosphonate infusions at the end of treatment capitalizing on the different mechanism of action to reduce osteoclast activity, there is no preferred regimen in children. Some experts advise giving zoledronic acid 4 weeks and 8 weeks after the last denosumab dose because of the more rapid bone turnover in pediatrics. Rebound hypercalcemia can occur despite a single dose of zoledronic acid, especially given right at denosumab treatment cessation. As rebound hypercalcemia remains a risk even with this patient having received a dose of zoledronic acid, recommending no additional monitoring (Answer D) would be inappropriate.

Educational Objective

Identify and monitor for potential adverse effects of denosumab in children.

Reference(s)

Boyce AM. Denosumab: an emerging therapy in pediatric bone disorders. *Curr Osteoporos Rep.* 2017;15(4):283-292. PMID: 28643220

Horiuchi K, Kobayashi E, Mizuno T, Susa M, Chiba K. Hypercalcemia following discontinuation of denosumab therapy: a systematic review. *Bone Rep.* 2021;15:101148. PMID: 34825020

Vanderniet JA, Szymczuk V, Hogler W, et al. Managment of RANKL-mediated disorders with denosumab in children and adolescents: a global expert guidance document. *J Clin Endocrinol Metab.* 2024;109(5):1371-1382. PMID: 38041865

22 ANSWER: B) Moderate, active thyroid eye disease

Hyperthyroidism caused by Graves disease may be treated with the antithyroid drug methimazole, radioactive iodine (RAI), or thyroidectomy. Each of these treatment approaches has risks and benefits, and the choice of treatment should be determined based on individual patient characteristics and preferences.

In children with Graves hyperthyroidism, met!himazole is generally considered the first-line treatment because it has a low risk of severe adverse effects, does not result in permanent hypothyroidism, and allows the possibility that the patient may achieve disease remission. The likelihood of remission has been estimated at 25% after 2 years of initial methimazole treatment, and the probability of remission increases with longer duration of initial treatment, with a maximum remission rate of 45% to 90% after long-term treatment (8-10 years). For this reason, an initial period of methimazole treatment is often recommended for at least 2 years to assess for possible remission. Nevertheless, a patient may choose to undergo definitive therapy at any time, and not completing an initial 2-year trial of methimazole (Answer A) is not a contraindication to RAI therapy.

RAI therapy has risks and contraindications that must be considered before it is recommended to a patient. Definite contraindications to RAI therapy include:

1. **Active thyroid eye disease that is moderate or severe (Answer B).** Thyroid eye disease (TED, formerly termed Graves orbitopathy) is classified in terms of its activity of orbital inflammation (active or inactive) and the severity of clinical findings (mild, moderate, or severe). In individuals with active TED, RAI therapy is associated with a risk of worsening orbitopathy; therefore, RAI therapy is contraindicated in patients with active TED that is moderate or severe. Patients with TED that is active but mild may receive RAI, but usually with pretreatment using systemic glucocorticoids to reduce the risk of worsening orbitopathy. Inactive TED is unaffected by RAI therapy. Evaluation by an ophthalmologist is important to determine disease activity and severity prior to consideration of RAI therapy in patients with TED.
2. **Pregnancy or lactation**. Due to the risk of radiation exposure to the fetus or newborn, patients capable of pregnancy must be counseled about the need to avoid pregnancy during and at least 6 months following RAI therapy. In addition, a pregnancy test must be performed and a negative result confirmed within 48 hours prior to RAI therapy in any patient potentially capable of pregnancy. However, lack of reliable contraceptive use (Answer E) is not an absolute contraindication to RAI therapy as long as the patient is counseled about this risk and agrees to avoid pregnancy for at least 6 months following therapy.
3. **Diagnosis or suspicion of thyroid cancer**. If a thyroid nodule is present, RAI therapy should not be performed until the nodule can be evaluated and determined not to be thyroid cancer. The patient in this vignette has no thyroid nodules but rather tiny (<5 mm) cysts (Answer C), which may be present in up to 45% to 50% of normal adolescents, are not suspicious for thyroid cancer, and require no additional evaluation.
4. **Inability to comply with RAI safety guidelines**. After RAI, patients must comply with temporary radiation safety guidelines to avoid unnecessary radiation exposure to others. Specific guidelines vary by institution and by state but generally include avoidance of close contact, particularly with young children and pregnant individuals.

Larger thyroid size (Answer D) is associated with an increased risk that RAI therapy will be unsuccessful in inducing permanent hypothyroidism. In patients with a goiter 80 mL or more, the risk of RAI treatment failure is significant and treatment with antithyroid drugs or thyroidectomy may be favored. However, large thyroid size is not an absolute contraindication to RAI therapy and would not preclude RAI treatment in the patient in this vignette.

Educational Objective

Select patients with Graves disease for whom radioactive iodine therapy would be appropriate.

Reference(s)

Ross DS, Burch HB, Cooper DS, et al. 2016 American Thyroid Association guidelines for diagnosis and management of hyperthyroidism and other causes of thyrotoxicosis. *Thyroid.* 2016;26(10):1343-1421. PMID: 27521067

Shimura H, Sobue T, Takahashi H, et al; Thyroid Examination Unit of the Radiation Medical Center for the Fukushima Health Management Survey Group. Findings of thyroid ultrasound examination within 3 years after the Fukushima nuclear power plant accident: the Fukushima Health Management Survey. *J Clin Endocrinol Metab.* 2018;103(3):861-869. PMID: 29253182

23 ANSWER: D) Primary pigmented nodular adrenal disease

In this vignette describing ACTH-independent Cushing syndrome, several components increase the likelihood of primary pigmented nodular adrenal disease (PPNAD) (Answer D). The original dexamethasone test proposed by Liddle combined a low-dose dexamethasone test with a high-dose dexamethasone test to discriminate between pituitary and other causes of Cushing syndrome. The paradoxical rise of urinary free cortisol during the Liddle test has been reported to differentiate PPNAD from other forms of adrenocortical nodular disease. There is also the family history of a first-degree relative having a testicular lump removed, which should prompt suspicion of a large-cell calcifying Sertoli-cell tumor. Taken together, Carney complex should be suspected, which is why PPNAD is the most likely of the options. Classic Carney complex is diagnosed when a patient exhibits 2 of the diagnostic criteria or 1 diagnostic criterion and 1 supplemental criterion (*see table*).

Table. Carney Complex Diagnostic Criteria

Major criteria	Supplementary criteria	Suggestive features, not diagnostic
Spotty skin pigmentation with typical distribution (lips, conjunctiva and inner or outer canthi, vaginal and penile mucosa) **Myxoma*** (cutaneous and mucosal) **Cardiac myxoma*** **Breast myxomatosis*** or fat-suppressed MRI findings suggestive of this diagnosis **Primary pigmented nodular adrenocortical disease*** or paradoxical positive response of urinary glucocorticosteroid excretion to dexamethasone administration during Liddle test **Acromegaly** as a result of GH-producing adenoma* **Large-cell calcifying Sertoli-cell tumor*** or characteristic calcification on testicular ultrasonography **Thyroid carcinoma*** or multiple hypoechoic nodules on thyroid ultrasonography in a child younger than 18 years **Psammomatous melanotic schwannomas*** **Blue nevus, epithelioid blue nevus*** **Breast ductal adenoma*** **Osteochondromyxoma***	**Affected first-degree relative** Inactivating pathogenic variant in **PRKAR1A**	**Intense freckling** (without darkly pigmented spots or typical distribution) **Blue nevus** common type (if multiple) **Café-au-lait macules** or other "birthmarks" **Elevated IGF-1 concentrations**, abnormal glucose tolerance test, or paradoxical GH response to thyrotropin-releasing hormone testing in the absence of clinical acromegaly **Cardiomyopathy** **Pilonidal sinus** **History of Cushing syndrome**, acromegaly, or sudden death in extended family **Multiple skin tags** or other skin lesions; lipomas **Colonic polyps** usually in association with acromegaly **Hyperprolactinemia** usually mild and almost always combined with clinical or subclinical acromegaly **Single, benign thyroid nodule** in a child younger than age 18 years; multiple thyroid nodules in an individual older than age 18 years (detected on ultrasonography) **Family history of carcinoma** of the thyroid, colon, pancreas, and ovary; other multiple benign or malignant tumors

Adapted from Stratakis CA & Raygada M. Carney complex. 2003 Feb 5 (updated Aug 16, 2018). In Adam MP et al, eds. Gene Reviews. University of Washington, Seattle; 1993-2023. Available at: https://www.ncbi.nlm.nih.gov/books/NBK1286/.

*Denotes after histologic confirmation.

In this child, the presence of café-au-lait spots adds to the suspicion of Carney complex, although it is not diagnostic. Adrenal carcinoma (Answer A), bilateral macronodular disease (Answer B), isolated micronodular adrenocortical disease (Answer C), and sporadic nodular adrenocortical disease (Answer E) do not have these features. The summarizes the new World Health Organization classification of adrenocortical nodular diseases and refers to Answers B through E. PPNAD is characterized by multiple pigmented adrenal cortical micronodules (<10 mm, often 2 to 5 mm) throughout the adrenal cortex. The histologic classification can guide or be associated with specific germline variants. Although imaging (CT or MRI) may help define the type of adrenocortical nodular disease, this can be difficult. Whether nodules are visualized on imaging depends on their size. Imaging also determines whether overall adrenal size is enlarged. In individuals with PPNAD, imaging findings may be reported as normal or have the classic appearance of a "string of beads" because of multiple small nodules in an otherwise atrophic adrenal cortex.

Figure. The New World Health Organization Classification of Adrenocortical Nodular Disease

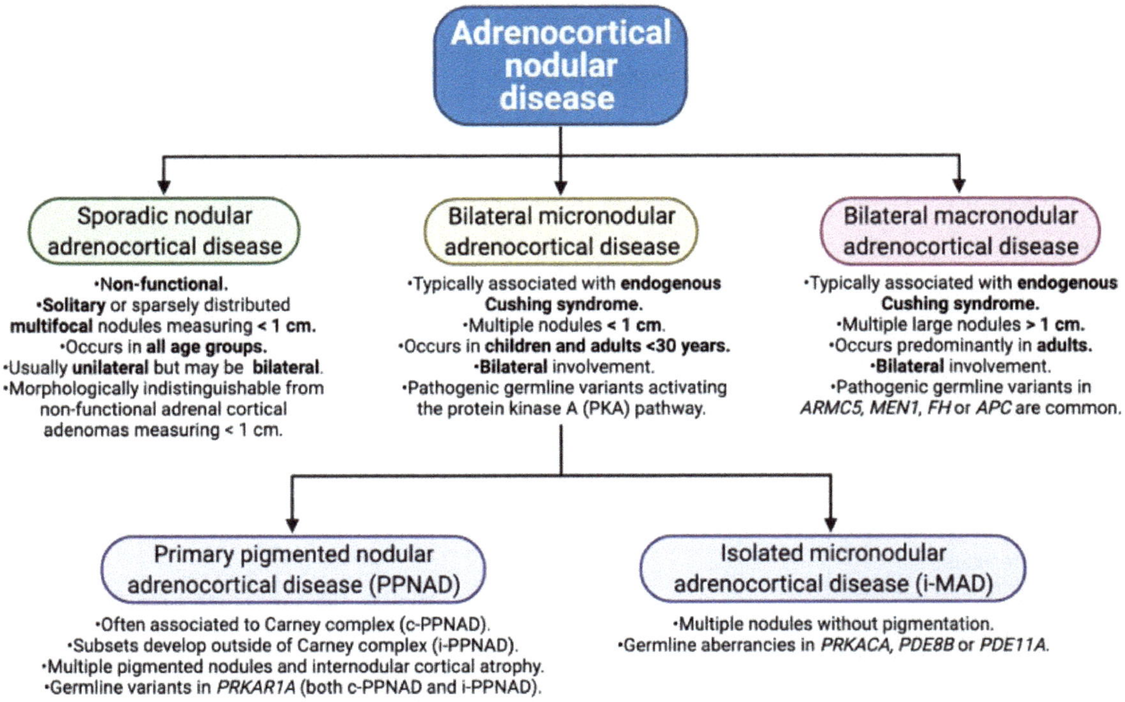

Fig. 1 The new WHO classification of adrenocortical nodular disease (Created with BioRender.com)

Educational Objective

Diagnose primary pigmented nodular adrenocortical disease leading to ACTH-independent Cushing syndrome and explain the histopathology.

Reference(s)

Correa R, Salpea P, Stratakis CA. Carney complex: an update. *Eur J Endocrinol.* 2015;173(4):M85-M97. PMID: 26130139

Mete O, Erickson LA, Juhlin CC, et al. Overview of the 2022 WHO classification of adrenal cortical tumors. *Endocr Pathol.* 2022;33(1):155-196. PMID: 35288842

Stratakis CA, Kirschner LS, Carney JA. Clinical and molecular features of the Carney complex: diagnostic criteria and recommendations for patient evaluation. *J Clin Endocrinol Metab.* 2001;86(9):4041-4046. PMID: 11549623

Stratakis CA, Raygada M. Carney complex. 2003 Feb 5 (updated Aug 16, 2018). In: Adamp MP, Mirzaa GM, Pagon RA, et al, eds. Gene Reviews. University of Washington, Seattle; 1993-2023. Available at: https://www.ncbi.nlm.nih.gov/books/NBK1286/.

Stratakis CA, Sarlis N, Kirschner LS, et al. Paradoxical response to dexamethasone in the diagnosis of primary pigmented nodular adrenocortical disease. *Ann Intern Med.* 1999;131(8):585-591. PMID: 10523219

24 ANSWER: E) Orthopedics consultation

X-linked hypophosphatemia or X-linked hypophosphatemic rickets (XLH) is a genetic disorder due to pathogenic variants in the *PHEX* gene resulting in elevated FGF-23, which causes renal phosphate wasting and reduced 1α-hydroxylation of 25-hydroxyvitamin D. Many patients are diagnosed early in life because of a family history of this X-linked dominant disorder. However, the diagnosis of de novo cases can be delayed because some leg bowing is often considered physiologic in toddlers. In fact, the patient in this vignette was seen by an orthopedist at age 2 and 3 years and radiographs at that time demonstrated femoral and tibial bowing, but metaphyseal fraying was overlooked. It was not until concerns of hip and knee pain prompted repeat imaging that a concern for metabolic bone disease was raised (*see images*).

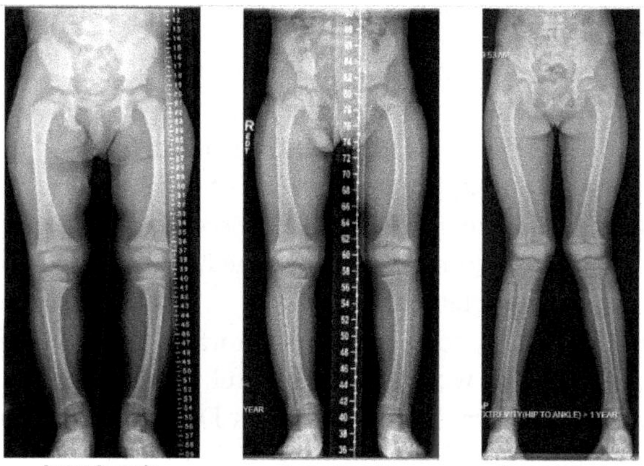

Standing lower-extremity x-rays depict the progression of the genu valgum deformity described in the vignette.

Treatment of XLH can improve rickets deformity and linear growth when initiated early (<1 year of age). Historical data show that patients treated with conventional therapy improve linear growth by approximately 1 standard deviation. In patients treated with burosumab, an anti–FGF-23 monoclonal antibody, modest improvements in growth velocity compared with conventional therapy are noted at 64 weeks. Children who continue on burosumab for 160 weeks show improvement in height Z-score (+0.35 SD) from baseline. GH therapy improves growth velocity in prepubertal children with XLH on conventional therapy, but long-term follow-up does not show sustained improvements in final adult height. Thus, GH therapy (Answer A) is not routinely recommended in the treatment of patients with XLH even if height predictions are suboptimal. In patients treated with burosumab, signs of rickets improve radiographically by 10 months. Obtaining another set of x-rays in 6 months (Answer D) is too soon to change the treatment course, but expert consensus recommends follow-up x-rays every 1 to 2 years in those with persistent deformity. Even with well-managed disease, approximately 40% of patients still require orthopedic intervention to correct bowing deformities. Surgical intervention is often indicated in those with rapidly progressive deformity after 7 years of age or persistent intermalleolar distance of 10 cm or more after 10 years of age, with the specific intervention depending on remaining growth potential. This patient has significant genu valgum deformity with pain. While symptoms may improve with treatment, consultation with orthopedics (Answer E) is the best next step.

Conventional therapy is associated with nephrocalcinosis due to the increased risk for hypercalciuria with calcitriol dosing. While targeted treatment with burosumab should minimize this risk, it is unknown whether patients are still at risk for nephrocalcinosis. Thus, periodic assessments with kidney ultrasonography (Answer C) every 1 to 2 years is still recommended. As nephrocalcinosis is a treatment complication, kidney ultrasonography at initiation of therapy is not necessary.

Head CT (Answer B) is recommended to assess for craniosynostosis in patients with XLH who are younger than 5 years and have an abnormal head shape. In older patients who have persistent headaches, brain MRI should be considered because of the risk of Chiari I malformation. While this patient has an abnormal head shape, her age and lack of neurologic concerns make imaging unnecessary now.

Educational Objective

Describe the expected outcomes with treatment of X-linked hypophosphatemia.

Reference(s)

Dahir K, Roberts MS, Krolczyk S, Simmons JH. X-linked hypophosphatemia: a new era in management. *J Endocr Soc.* 2020;4(12):bvaa151. PMID: 33204932

Haffner D, Emma F, Eastwood DM, et al. Clinical practice recommendations for the diagnosis and management of X-linked hypophosphataemia. *Nat Rev Nephrol.* 2019;15(7):435-455. PMID: 31068690

Imel EA, Glorieux FH, Whyte MP, et al. Burosumab versus conventional therapy in children with X-linked hypophosphataemia: a randomised, active-controlled, open-label, phase 3 trial. *Lancet.* 2019;393(10189):2416-2427. PMID: 31104833

Linglart A, Imel EA, Whyte MP, et al. Sustained efficacy and safety of burosumab, a monoclonal antibody to FGF23, in children with X-linked hypophosphatemia. *J Clin Endocrinol Metab.* 2022;107(3):813-824. PMID: 34636899

Rothenbuhler A, Schnabel D, Hogler W, Linglart A. Diagnosis, treatment-monitoring and follow-up of children and adolescents with X-linked hypophosphatemia (XLH). *Metabolism.* 2020;103S:153892. PMID: 30928313

25 **ANSWER: D) Perform karyotype analysis**

This patient has been short for more than 10 years. Her thyroid function is only mildly abnormal based on the laboratory values. Thus, her short stature cannot be explained by hypothyroidism, so assessing thyroid antibodies (Answer A) would not identify the cause of her short stature.

She does not have any clinical signs or symptoms suggestive of celiac disease, and the celiac screen was negative. Thus, there is no need to schedule an upper gastrointestinal endoscopy (Answer E).

A bone age x-ray (Answer B) could help confirm whether she has achieved final adult height, but it is not essential in identifying the cause of her short stature.

She has completed puberty and her IGF-1 concentration is normal. Thus, GH deficiency is unlikely and scheduling a GH-stimulation test (Answer C) would not be helpful.

Ruling out Turner syndrome with karyotype analysis (Answer D) is important in girls with unexplained short stature that is well below midparental target height. A diagnosis of Turner syndrome is not automatically excluded if a patient has onset, progression, and completion of spontaneous puberty. In fact, about 15% of girls with Turner syndrome start puberty normally and complete spontaneous puberty with regular menstrual cycles. Only about 50% of girls with Turner syndrome do not have spontaneous puberty and need pubertal induction therapy. The remaining patients have either arrested puberty or delayed puberty. Thus, Turner syndrome should be in the differential diagnosis of all girls with unexplained short stature despite normal pubertal onset, progression, and completion.

Educational Objective

Rule out Turner syndrome in a girl with short stature, even if she has completed spontaneous puberty and is having regular menstrual cycles.

Reference(s)

Hong YH, Shin YL. Turner syndrome masquerading as normal early puberty. *Ann Pediatr Endocrinol Metab.* 2014;19(4):225-228. PMID: 25654070

Pasquino AM, Passeri F, Pucarelli I, Segni M, Municchi G. Spontaneous pubertal development in Turner's syndrome. Italian Study Group for Turner's Syndrome. *J Clin Endocrinol Metab.* 1997;82(6):1810-1813. PMID: 9177387

Yuan X, Zhu Z. Turner syndrome with rapidly progressive puberty: a case report and literature review. *J Int Med Res.* 2020;48(5):300060519896914. PMID: 32357117

26 **ANSWER: A) Elevated BMI**

Both overweight and obesity are associated with earlier timing of thelarche and puberty in girls. Multiple studies indicate that elevated BMI (Answer A) is the single strongest predictor of earlier age of thelarche. Mechanisms are still poorly understood but may involve elevated leptin and adipokine levels, insulin resistance leading to increased adrenal androgen production, and increased aromatase activity in adipose tissue. Given this patient's history, elevated BMI is likely the most significant factor in her precocious puberty.

Although obesity may have a role in the development of central precocious puberty, particularly in girls, obesity does not significantly decrease the risk of central nervous system pathology in central precocious puberty. Thus, criteria for performing central nervous system imaging should not depend on BMI. The diagnostic evaluation remains essentially the same as it would in the absence of obesity. However, while basal LH concentrations do not seem to differ, girls with obesity and Tanner stage 2 to 3 breast development may have a lower peak LH value on stimulation testing.

The patient's mother reported an age of menarche that is earlier than average but still within the normal range, and there was no other family history of precocious puberty to suggest an underlying genetic predisposition (Answer B).

While some have suggested a higher rate of precocious puberty in children with autism spectrum disorder (Answer C), there are no reliable data to support this connection.

Nonclassic congenital adrenal hyperplasia (Answer E) can cause secondary central precocious puberty, but her history of thelarche preceding pubarche is not consistent with this etiology.

This patient's mild TSH elevation (Answer D) is most likely a consequence of elevated BMI rather than a cause of weight gain. One cross-sectional study in girls who underwent a GnRH-stimulation test showed that serum TSH concentration was higher in the central precocious puberty group than in the group without central precocious puberty. While the incidence of TSH elevation was higher in the central precocious puberty group, both groups had mean TSH levels in the normal range, and the central precocious puberty group actually had a lower mean BMI than the group without central precocious puberty. Far less frequently, prolonged, severe TSH elevation (ie, TSH >100 mIU/L) can occasionally cause early-onset of central puberty in girls, possibly due to cross-reactivity of TSH with FSH receptors. The patient in this vignette does not have a highly elevated TSH value, and there is inadequate evidence to suggest that mild TSH elevation associated with obesity increases the risk of precocious puberty.

Educational Objective

Explain how the presence of obesity influences the evaluation for precocious puberty.

Reference(s)

Tenedero CB, Oei K, Palmert MR. An approach to the evaluation and management of the obese child with early puberty. *J Endocr Soc.* 2021;6(1):bvab173. PMID: 34909516

27 ANSWER: C) Refer to a thyroid surgeon for consideration of hemithyroidectomy

Thyroid nodules in children have a higher risk of malignancy (20%-25%) than do thyroid nodules in adults (5%-15%), but most thyroid nodules in pediatric patients are benign. The goal of thyroid nodule evaluation is to identify thyroid nodules at significant risk of being thyroid cancer for proper management while avoiding unnecessary treatment of benign nodules.

For nonautonomous thyroid nodules, ultrasonography is the imaging modality of choice to assess for features associated with increased risk of thyroid cancer, including solid composition, hypoechogenicity, taller-than-wide shape in transverse view, irregular or invasive margins, calcifications, or abnormal lymph nodes. For nodules with suspicious characteristics, ultrasound-guided FNA is recommended to assess the risk of thyroid cancer.

Thyroid nodule FNA cytology should be interpreted using a standardized system, the most widely accepted of which is the Bethesda System for Reporting Thyroid Cytopathology. This system classifies thyroid cytology into 6 categories: nondiagnostic, benign, atypia of undetermined significance (AUS), follicular neoplasm, suspicious for malignancy, and malignant. Each category is associated with a specific risk of thyroid cancer that guides subsequent nodule management.

In both children and adults, the risk of malignancy in a thyroid nodule with benign cytology is very low (1%-3%). Therefore, most cytologically benign nodules in children do not require resection but should be observed by ultrasonography in 12 months. Repeat ultrasound in 3 months (Answer E) is unlikely to alter management and is generally not recommended. However, surgical resection (Answer C) should be considered for cytologically benign nodules larger than 4 cm in diameter because the false-negative rate of benign cytology is higher in these large nodules (~15%). In this vignette, hemithyroidectomy is the appropriate surgery in the absence of any reason to consider more extensive surgery (eg, contralateral nodules).

For certain thyroid nodules with nondiagnostic or AUS cytology that are associated with an intermediate risk of malignancy, repeated FNA in 3 to 6 months (Answer D) is an option to help clarify thyroid cancer risk and direct management. Another FNA generally is not necessary or recommended for nodules with benign cytology.

Thyroid scintigraphy is recommended for the evaluation of thyroid nodules suspected of being autonomous nodules. In a patient with a thyroid nodule, a low TSH concentration should raise suspicion for an autonomous nodule, and scintigraphy should be obtained to confirm this diagnosis. Thyroid scintigraphy (Answer B) is not indicated in the evaluation of thyroid nodules in a patient with a normal or elevated TSH concentration.

Levothyroxine therapy (Answer A) has been used in the management of benign thyroid nodules, with the rationale that suppressing TSH secretion may reduce nodule size and associated symptoms. Although levothyroxine may reduce nodule size in some patients, long-term TSH suppression is associated with increased risks to bone density and cardiovascular health. Therefore, levothyroxine therapy generally is not recommended for benign thyroid nodules in children and would not be considered for an asymptomatic benign nodule.

Educational Objective

Manage large (>4 cm) cytologically benign thyroid nodules in children.

Reference(s)

Ali SZ, Baloch ZW, Cochand-Priollet B, Schmitt FC, Vielh P, VanderLaan PA. The 2023 Bethesda System for Reporting Thyroid Cytopathology. *Thyroid.* 2023;33(9):1039-1044. PMID: 37427847

Cherella CE, Feldman HA, Hollowell M, et al. Natural history and outcomes of cytologically benign thyroid nodules in children. *J Clin Endocrinol Metab.* 2018;103(9):3557-3565. PMID: 29982665

Francis GL, Waguespack SG, Bauer AJ, et al; American Thyroid Association Guidelines Task Force. Management guidelines for children with thyroid nodules and differentiated thyroid cancer. *Thyroid.* 2015;25(7):716-759. PMID: 25900731

Ly S, Frates MC, Benson CB, et al. Features and outcome of autonomous thyroid nodules in children: 31 consecutive patients seen at a single center. *J Clin Endocrinol Metab.* 2016;101(10):3856-3862. PMID: 27501280

28 ANSWER: C) *GNAS*

The baby in this vignette has presented with neonatal Cushing syndrome. She also has biochemical evidence of hyperthyroidism and a large birthmark. The most likely diagnosis is therefore McCune-Albright syndrome (MAS). MAS is characterized by skeletal lesions, skin hyperpigmentation, and hyperfunctioning endocrinopathies. In general, MAS is diagnosed clinically with the presence of 2 of these 3 findings. Estimated prevalence is between 1 in 100,000 and 1 in 1,000,000. The genetic defect occurs due to postzygotic gain-of-function variants in the *GNAS* gene (Answer C), which encodes the α-subunit of the G_s protein involved in G protein–coupled receptor signaling (*see figure*). MAS occurs sporadically and vertical transmission has never been reported. *GNAS* pathogenic variants disrupt the intrinsic GTPase activity of $G_s\alpha$, leading to persistent stimulation of adenylyl cyclase and production of cyclic AMP. MAS is a mosaic disease with a broad clinical spectrum, ranging from an incidental x-ray finding to severe disease such as neonatal Cushing syndrome and hyperthyroidism as in this vignette. Other activating endocrinopathies include GH excess, and precocious puberty. The genomic diagnosis is most reliable from affected tissue (eg, skin biopsy of an affected area). Detecting a *GNAS* variant in DNA extracted from a blood peripheral blood sample is possible, although it is often negative, and the absence of a variant in blood does not exclude the diagnosis. Newer genomic amplification techniques have been suggested to increase the likelihood of determining the genetic etiology. Spontaneous resolution of neonatal Cushing syndrome in MAS is possible and has been reported.

Figure. Molecular Defect and Phenotype in McCune-Albright Syndrome

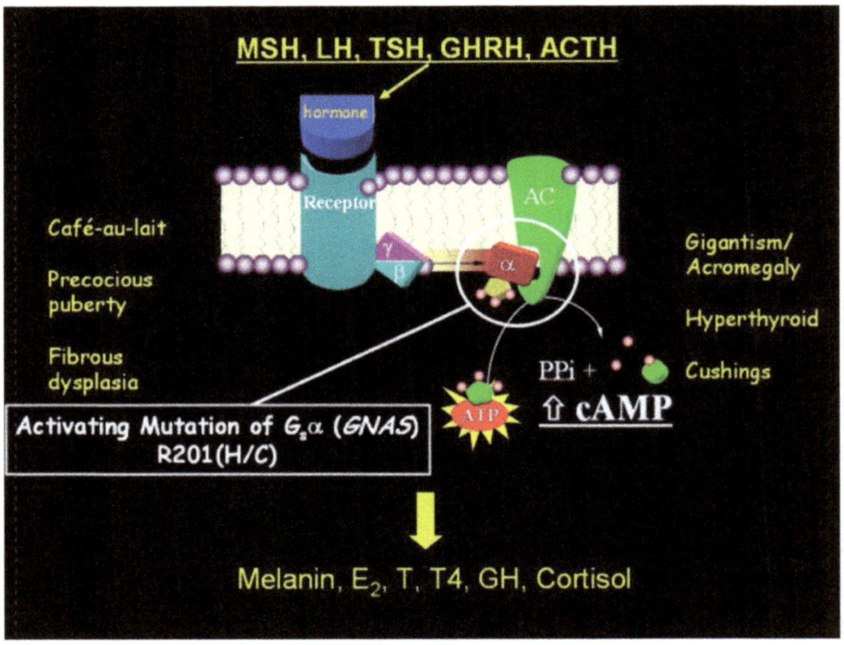

The hormones MSH (melanocyte-stimulating hormone), LH (luteinizing hormone), TSH (thyroid-stimulating hormone), GHRH (growth hormone–stimulating hormone), and ACTH (adrenocortical-stimulating hormone) all signal through the G protein (alpha, beta, gamma subunits) pathway. In McCune-Albright syndrome, the alpha subunit is modified in such a way as to induce constitutive activation of adenylate cyclase, and thus produce high levels of intracellular cAMP. This results in increased production of melanin, estradiol (E2), testosterone (T), thyroxine (T_4), growth hormone (GH), and cortisol. Dysregulated production of these hormones results in café-au-lait spots, precocious puberty, fibrous dysplasia, acromegaly, hyperthyroidism, and Cushing disease, depending on the tissue harboring the somatic mutation. Reprinted from Dumitrescu CE & Collins MT. Orphanet J Rare Dis, 2008; 3: 12. © The Authors. Published by BioMed Central Ltd., a part of Springer Nature.

The *DICER1* gene (Answer B) encodes the DICER1 protein, which is a small RNA processing endoribonuclease that cleaves precursor microRNAs (miRNA) into mature miRNAs. Germline pathogenic variants in the *DICER1* gene cause pleuropulmonary blastoma familial tumor and dysplasia syndrome. In affected patients, aggressive congenital pituitary blastomas lead to neonatal Cushing disease. Unlike the scenario in this vignette, Cushing disease associated with this syndrome would be ACTH-dependent.

Adrenocortical tumors represent most cases of neonatal Cushing syndrome, and pathogenic variants in the *TP53* gene (Answer E) are the most common cause of adrenocortical tumors, which can be observed in Li-Fraumeni syndrome. In light of the additional clinical features in this patient, variants in the *TP53* gene are unlikely.

The *PRKAR1A* gene (Answer D) encodes the regulatory subunit R1a of the protein kinase A leading to primary pigmented nodular adrenocortical disease (PPNAD) associated with Carney complex. PPNAD has not been described in children younger than 1 year.

The *AIP* gene (Answer A) encodes the aryl hydrocarbon receptor interacting protein, and germline variants are associated with pituitary adenomas. The most commonly occurring pituitary adenomas are GH-secreting adenomas (somatotropinoma), followed by prolactin-secreting adenomas (prolactinomas), GH and prolactin cosecreting adenomas (somatomammotropinomas), and nonfunctioning pituitary adenomas. Rarely, TSH-secreting adenomas are observed. *AIP* germline variants are not a cause of neonatal Cushing syndrome.

Educational Objective

Explain the genetics and pathophysiology of McCune-Albright syndrome.

Reference(s)

Dumitrescu CE, Collins MT. McCune-Albright syndrome. *Orphanet J Rare Dis.* 2008;3:12. PMID: 18489744

Elli FM, de Sanctis L, Bergallo M, et al. Improved molecular diagnosis of McCune-Albright syndrome and bone fibrous dysplasia by digital PCR. *Front Genet.* 2019;10:862. PMID: 31620168

Roszko KL, Guthrie L, Li X, Collins MT, de Castro LF, Boyce AM. Identification of GNAS variants in circulating cell-free DNA from patients with fibrous dysplasia/McCune Albright syndrome. *J Bone Miner Res.* 2023;38(3):443-450. PMID: 36593655

Salpea P, Stratakis CA. Carney complex and McCune Albright syndrome: an overview of clinical manifestations and human molecular genetics. *Mol Cell Endocrinol.* 2014;386(1-2):85-91. PMID: 24012770

Tatsi C, Stratakis CA. Neonatal Cushing syndrome: a rare but potentially devastating disease. *Clin Perinatol.* 2018; 45(1):103-118. PMID: 29406000

29 ANSWER: E) Start oral hydrocortisone and stop using diaper rash cream

This baby boy has classic features of iatrogenic Cushing syndrome from topical steroid use. Clobetasol is estimated to have a potency 600 times higher than that of hydrocortisone. Topical use of clobetasol has been reported to be the cause of iatrogenic Cushing syndrome in multiple case reports. Other topical steroid products such as triamcinolone cream, dexamethasone nasal drops (for conditions such as pyriform aperture stenosis), and dexamethasone ophthalmic drops (for conditions such as congenital glaucoma) also result in iatrogenic Cushing syndrome over time. In patients who have frank cushingoid features due to prolonged exposure to exogenous steroids, their hypothalamic-pituitary-adrenal axis is most likely suppressed. Thus, stopping the exogenous steroid abruptly could result in adrenal insufficiency. Initiating oral hydrocortisone replacement therapy and stopping the topical steroid (Answer E), with subsequent weaning of hydrocortisone treatment, is warranted in these situations.

There is a clear underlying etiology for this patient's mildly elevated fingerstick glucose value and slightly elevated hemoglobin A_{1c} value. Thus, there is no need for hospital admission (Answer A).

However, the patient has several ongoing medical problems, so waiting for results of genetic testing for neonatal diabetes (Answer C) or testing for diabetes-related antibodies (Answer B) would only result in a delayed diagnosis.

Brain MRI (Answer D) is not helpful in diagnosing iatrogenic Cushing disease.

Educational Objective

Identify exogenous topical steroid as the cause of iatrogenic Cushing syndrome and develop a management plan.

Reference(s)

Decani S, Federighi V, Baruzzi E, Sardella A, Lodi G. Iatrogenic Cushing's syndrome and topical steroid therapy: case series and review of the literature. *J Dermatolog Treat.* 2014;25(6):495-500. PMID: 23210698

Fukuhara D, Takiura T, Keino H, Okada AA, Yan K. Iatrogenic Cushing's syndrome due to topical ocular glucocorticoid treatment. *Pediatrics.* 2017;139(2):e20161233. PMID: 28104732

Joshi RR, Maresh A. Iatrogenic Cushing's syndrome and adrenal insufficiency in infants on intranasal dexamethasone drops for nasal obstruction - case series and literature review. *Int J Pediatr Otorhinolaryngol.* 2018;105:123-126. PMID: 29447799

Matejek N, Hoos J, Holterhus PM, Bettendorf M, Choukair D. Topical glucocorticoid application causing iatrogenic Cushing's syndrome followed by secondary adrenal insufficiency in infants: two case reports. *J Med Case Rep.* 2022;16(1):455. PMID: 36476353

30 ANSWER: D) Low FSH, low LH, low testosterone

The patient in this vignette has PCSK1 (proprotein convertase subtilisin/kexin type 1) deficiency. The *PCSK1* gene encodes prohormone convertase 1/3 (PC1/3) and was one of the first genes linked to monogenic early-onset obesity. PC1/3 (*PCSK1*) is predominantly expressed in neural and endocrine tissues. In the brain, PC1/3 expression is particularly prominent in the hypothalamus, but it is also present in other areas as well. PC1/3 is crucial for processing several neuropeptides and peptide hormones such as pro-opiomelanocortin, proinsulin, and proglucagon. Therefore, patients with PCSK1 deficiency most often present with early-onset obesity, hyperphagia, and a wide range of endocrinopathies. A hallmark of the condition is early and severe malabsorptive diarrhea in the postnatal period that often requires prolonged use of parenteral nutrition. Persistent diarrhea and malabsorption continue throughout life, potentially explaining why patients with PCSK1 deficiency may not exhibit the same degree of obesity as other individuals with monogenic forms.

One of the endocrinopathies that has been described in patients with PCSK1 deficiency is hypogonadotropic hypogonadism. Low levels of gonadotropins would be expected and this would result in low levels of sex steroids, in this case testosterone (Answer D). Micropenis has been described in some male patients in infancy.

In one series, at least one-third of patients with PCSK1 deficiency were found to be GH deficient; therefore, for many patients, a low IGF-1 concentration may be observed, rather than elevated IGF-1 (Answer B).

While not all individuals with PCSK1 deficiency have hypocortisolism, those who do have central adrenal insufficiency, not primary adrenal insufficiency (Answer A), where one would expect to see a markedly elevated ACTH concentration in the setting of low cortisol.

Central hypothyroidism has also been described in a number of patients with PCSK1 deficiency in whom free T_4 is low, coupled with an inappropriate TSH response, rather than a picture more consistent with primary hypothyroidism (Answer C).

Insulin is produced by pancreatic β cells from PC1/3- and PC2-mediated cleavage of proinsulin. Patients with PCSK1 deficiency therefore have markedly elevated proinsulin, not low levels (Answer E). Proinsulin has only a fraction of the activity of insulin, but in these patients, it is compensated for by secretion of significant amounts. Proinsulin has a half-life that is 4 to 6 times longer than that of insulin, which probably explains the postprandial hypoglycemia that has been reported in some patients.

Educational Objective

Describe the spectrum of the clinical phenotype observed in individuals with *PCSK1* pathogenic variants.

Reference(s)

Pépin L, Colin E, Tessarech M, et al. A new case of PCSK1 pathogenic variant with congenital proprotein convertase 1/3 deficiency and literature review. *J Clin Endocrinol Metab.* 2019;104(4):985-993. PMID: 30383237

Ramos-Molina B, Martin MG, Lindberg I. PCSK1 variants and human obesity. *Prog Mol Biol Transl Sci.* 2016;140:47-74. PMID: 27288825

Stijnen P, Ramos-Molina B, O'Rahilly S, Creemers JW. PCSK1 mutations and human endocrinopathies: from obesity to gastrointestinal disorders. *Endocr Rev.* 2016;37(4):347-371. PMID: 27187081

31 ANSWER: A) Activation of the TSH receptor

This infant has hyperthyroidism. He was born with intrauterine growth restriction with relative microcephaly, potentially due to craniosynostosis, which is a complication of thyrotoxicosis. In his case, hyperthyroidism is not due to the transplacental passage of TRAb because these antibodies were tested and were negative both during the pregnancy and in neonatal life. This infant most likely has activation of the TSH receptor (Answer A). Based on the maternal history of early-onset hyperthyroidism, lack of disease remission, lack of TRAb, and development of multiple nodules as a young adult, his mother probably has the same condition. She was misdiagnosed as having Graves disease instead of the much rarer condition of nonautoimmune hyperthyroidism due to an activating pathogenic variant in the TSH receptor gene.

Nonautoimmune hyperthyroidism due to activating variants in the TSH receptor gene can occur as an autosomal dominant condition (as described in this vignette) or sporadically (de novo variants). In the inherited form, the phenotype varies markedly, even among family members, and manifestations range from severe disease in utero with fetal hyperthyroidism and goiter to childhood- or adult-onset hyperthyroidism. The development of multinodular goiter in young adulthood is commonly described in this condition. Patients with the sporadic form tend to have a more severe phenotype. Hyperthyroidism associated with this condition can be treated initially with β-adrenergic blockade for symptom control and methimazole. However, long-term remission is not expected and definitive therapy is required with either radioactive iodine or surgery.

This condition can be confused with Graves disease, which is much more common. However, the diagnosis should be considered in anyone with a family history of hyperthyroidism or in anyone with hyperthyroidism without TRAb. Since this condition is not immune-mediated, it is not associated with thyroid eye disease. The diagnosis is confirmed when a variant in the TSH receptor gene is detected. Multiple pathogenic variants have been described in the literature. Because TPO antibodies are common in the population, the presence of these antibodies in the mother does not confirm an autoimmune cause of her prior hyperthyroidism.

Transplacental passage of maternal TPO antibodies (Answer E) is an incorrect explanation for this patient's goiter and hyperthyroidism. Autoantibodies do cross the placenta, but even if maternal TPO antibodies are present in the fetal circulation, they do not have any functional effect. Only TRAb affect thyroid function. Stimulatory antibodies result in hyperthyroidism, while blocking antibodies result in hypothyroidism.

Iodine deficiency (Answer B) during pregnancy can result in a goiter in the fetus and infant, but it should result in hypothyroidism rather than hyperthyroidism. This infant was born in the United States where iodine deficiency is not common. The mother was also taking a prenatal vitamin, thus ensuring adequate iodine intake.

Iodine excess (Answer C) in pregnancy can result in the development of a fetal goiter, but it would lead to fetal and neonatal hypothyroidism rather than hyperthyroidism. This mother is taking a health store thyroid supplement; all supplements should be reviewed with patients because iodine excess is possible through supplementation with nonregulated products.

A defect in iodide organification (Answer D) generally results in goiter development, but the lack of iodide organification causes hypothyroidism, not hyperthyroidism. TPO, dual oxidase (DUOX), and dual oxidase maturation factor 2 (DUOXA2) are all involved in iodide organification. Pathogenic variants in the *TPO* gene are the most commonly described variants in patients with dyshormonogenesis. Pathogenic variants in this gene typically result in the presence of a goiter, although rare cases of thyroid hypoplasia have also been described. Dyshormonogenesis due to *TPO* pathogenic variants is associated with hypothyroidism and is typically inherited in an autosomal recessive pattern.

Educational Objective

Identify nonautoimmune hyperthyroidism due to activating variants in the TSH receptor gene as a potential cause of neonatal goiter.

Reference(s)

Overcash RT, Marc-Aurele KL, Hull AD, Ramos GA. Maternal iodine exposure: a case of fetal goiter and neonatal hearing loss. Pediatrics. 2016;137(4):e20153722. PMID: 27006474

Stephenson A, Punjwani Z, Eszlinger M, Sawicka B, Bossowski A, Paschke R. Report of a family with three generations of undiagnosed familial nonautoimmune hyperthyroidism. Endocrinol Diabetes Metab Case Rep. 2021;2021:21-0019. PMID: 34866058

32 ANSWER: C) Repeat GH-stimulation testing after priming with β-estradiol

This patient is a prepubertal girl with obesity and poor growth who has a family history of constitutional pubertal delay. Patients with obesity may have slightly elevated TSH and normal T_4 concentrations. Thus, hyperthyrotropinemia is most likely a consequence of obesity and is reversible after weight loss without levothyroxine treatment (Answer E).

Although this patient is being monitored because of slow growth and obesity, she does not have any other clinical factors suggestive of Cushing syndrome and her growth velocity is acceptable for her prepubertal status. Thus, she does not need to be tested for Cushing syndrome (Answer A).

Although her total IgA value is low, it is not undetectable (<7 mg/dL) as is seen in patients with IgA deficiency. Hence, the negative tTG IgA antibodies can be used as a reliable screen to exclude celiac disease. Referral to gastroenterology (Answer B) is not necessary.

GH therapy (Answer D) should not be initiated, because a diagnosis of GH deficiency has not been conclusively established. She has no signs of puberty at age 11 years and 9 months and there is a strong family history of delayed puberty in her parents. Thus, she could have constitutional delay of puberty and growth.

To reduce the frequency of false-positive results in GH-stimulation testing, current guidelines recommend a 2-day course of 2 mg (1 mg for body weight) 17β-estradiol (Answer C) in prepubertal boys older than 11 years and in prepubertal girls older than 10 years on the evening preceding the test. Alternatively, a single testosterone dose of 50 to 100 mg given a week before the GH-provocative testing can be used as sex-steroid priming in eligible boys. Obesity blunts an individual's response to GH-provocative tests. Thus, lower cutoffs for peak GH values are recommended to diagnose GH deficiency in adults with or without obesity. However, the lack of consensus on such recommendations does not support adjusting GH peak cutoff values in children with obesity who undergo GH-provocative testing.

Educational Objective

Explain the limitations of diagnostic tests used in the evaluation of poor growth in children.

Reference(s)

Grimberg A, DiVall SA, Polychronakos C, et al; Drug and Therapeutics Committee and Ethics Committee of the Pediatric Endocrine Society. Guidelines for growth hormone and insulin-like growth factor-I treatment in children and adolescents: growth hormone deficiency, idiopathic short stature, and primary insulin-like growth factor-I deficiency. *Horm Res Paediatr.* 2016;86(6):361-397. PMID: 27884013

Kamoun C, Hawkes CP, Grimberg A. Provocative growth hormone testing in children: how did we get here and where do we go now? *J Pediatr Endocrinol Metab.* 2021;34(6):679-696. PMID: 33838090

Reinehr T, de Sousa G, Andler W. Hyperthyrotropinemia in obese children is reversible after weight loss and is not related to lipids. *J Clin Endocrinol Metab.* 2006;91(8):3088-3091. PMID: 16684827

Yau M, Rapaport R. Growth hormone stimulation testing: to test or not to test? That is one of the questions. *Front Endocrinol (Lausanne).* 2022;13:902364. PMID: 35757429

33 ANSWER: D) *HNF1B*

This vignette depicts the strong association between diabetes and kidney pathology. Maturity-onset diabetes of the young (MODY) type 5 due to *HNF1B* pathogenic variants (Answer D) have been reported in patients with kidney cysts and other kidney developmental disorders, early-onset diabetes, pancreatic atrophy, abnormal liver function tests, and genital tract abnormalities. Extrapancreatic involvement can be quickly recognized with the most consistent feature of cystic kidney disease. The kidney disease described is very heterogeneous but is always due to aberrant kidney development and includes kidney cysts, familial hypoplastic glomerulocystic kidney disease, and kidney malformations (eg, single kidney or horseshoe kidney).

GCK pathogenic variants (Answer B), characterized by limited phenotypic heterogeneity with hemoglobin A_{1c} values not exceeding 7.5% (60 mmol/mol), carry the nomenclature of MODY type 2. *GCK* encodes glucokinase, an enzyme catalyzing glucose phosphorylation at glycolysis initiation; therefore, GCK serves as a pancreatic β-cell glucose sensor. Genetic defects change the glucose-stimulated insulin secretion threshold without any other associated pathology.

HNF1A (Answer C) and HNF4A (Answer E) correspond to MODY type 3 and type 1, respectively. Pathogenic variants in these genes are the most common cause of MODY in the United States. HNF1A and HNF4A variants should be considered given the autosomal dominant inheritance pattern depicted in the vignette. However, kidney pathology is not an associated feature of *HNF1A* or *HNF4A* pathogenic variants.

MODY type 8 is caused by pathogenic variants in the gene encoding carboxyl ester lipase (*CEL*) (Answer A). *CEL* is highly expressed in pancreatic acinar cells and encodes one of the major lipases secreted in pancreatic enzymes. These variants lead to insulin-dependent diabetes in association with pancreatic exocrine dysfunction and atrophic pancreas with lipomatosis and cysts, but not kidney involvement.

Table. Genes Associated With MODY Types

MODY type	Gene
MODY 1	*HNF4A*
MODY 2	*GCK*
MODY 3	*HNF1A*
MODY 4	*PDX1*
MODY 5	*TCF2*
MODY 6	*NEUROD1*
MODY 7	*KLF11*
MODY 8	*CEL*
MODY 9	*PAX4*
MODY 10	*INS*
MODY 11	*BLK*
MODY 13	*KCNJ11*
MODY 14	*APPL1*

Adapted from Taylor R, Knight Johnson A, del Gaudio D. *Maturity Onset Diabetes of the Young Overview*. 2018 May 24. In Adam MP et al, eds. Gene Reviews. University of Washington, Seattle; 1993-2023.

Educational Objective

Explain the clinical correlation of *HNF1B* pathogenic variants associated with maturity-onset diabetes of the young type 5 and a family history of kidney disease.

Reference(s)

Edghill EL, Bingham C, Ellard S, Hattersley AT. Mutations in hepatocyte nuclear factor-1b and their related phenotypes. *J Med Genet.* 2006;43(1):84-90. PMID: 15930087

El Jellas K, Dušátková P, Haldorsen IS, et al. Two new mutations in the CEL gene causing diabetes and hereditary pancreatitis: how to correctly identify MODY8 cases. *J Clin Endocrinol Metab.* 2022;107(4):e1455-e1466. PMID: 34850019

Warncke K, Kummer S, Raile K, et al. Frequency and characteristics of MODY 1 (HNF4A mutation) and MODY 5 (HNF1B mutation): analysis from the DPV database. *J Clin Endocrinol Metab.* 2019;104(3):845-855. PMID: 30535056

34 ANSWER: B) Heparin

This patient has several risk factors that could lead to metabolic bone disease. Prematurity (Answer D) can cause osteopenia due to the inability to mimic the high rates of calcium deposition that occur during the third trimester. Some studies report birth before 32 weeks' gestation as a risk factor, whereas others use 28 weeks' gestation. Birthweight less than 1500 g is associated with prematurity, but this may also be an independent risk factor for metabolic bone disease of prematurity. Parenteral nutrition (Answer C) is also a risk factor because the amount of calcium and phosphorus is limited. Total parenteral nutrition use for more than 14 days is considered a risk factor for metabolic bone disease. This patient was not significantly premature and was able to be transitioned off parenteral nutrition quickly; thus, these risk factors do not explain the fractures at 3 months of age.

While systemic glucocorticoid exposure is a significant risk factor for skeletal fragility, a short course of dexamethasone (Answer A) would also not be expected to cause skeletal fragility at this age.

Ranitidine (Answer E) is a H2 blocker used to treat acid reflux. While proton-pump inhibitors have been associated with decreased calcium absorption and impaired bone health, H2 blockers have not been associated with skeletal fragility.

Anticoagulants (Answer B) have been associated with fractures in adult patients. Warfarin affects bone health by increasing the risk for vitamin K deficiency, a necessary cofactor for osteoclast function. Unfractionated heparin inhibits osteoprotegerin activity, thereby allowing RANKL to promote osteoclast-mediated bone resorption. Long-term use of heparin has also been shown to impair osteoblast activity. Adult patients who have been on heparin for 3 months or longer have decreased bone density and increased risk for vertebral fractures. Ongoing exposure of heparin is the most significant risk factor that would explain the long bone fractures and vertebral fractures in this patient.

Educational Objective

Identify risk factors of metabolic bone disease of prematurity and medications that can impair bone quality in infants.

Reference(s)

Li B, Lu D, Chen Y, Zhao M, Zuo L. Unfractionated heparin promotes osteoclast formation in vitro by inhibiting osteoprotegerin activity. *Int J Mol Sci.* 2016;17(4):613. PMID: 27110777

Kehinde F, Marinescu A, Turchi R. Catch it before it breaks!: managing metabolic bone disease of prematurity. *Curr Opin Pediatr.* 2021;33(6):676-683. PMID: 34734916

Signorelli SS, Scuto S, Marino E, Giusti M, Xourafa A, Gaudio A. Anticoagulants and osteoporosis. *Int J Mol Sci.* 2019;20(21):5275. PMID: 31652944

35 **ANSWER: B) Dexmedetomidine-induced arginine vasopressin deficiency**

Multiple medications used in sedation and anesthesia have been implicated in the development of diabetes insipidus (arginine vasopressin [AVP] deficiency), as has been recently reviewed. Of the cases reviewed, dexmedetomidine was the most common culprit. Typically, as in this case, AVP deficiency develops intraoperatively, responds to vasopressin and free water repletion, and resolves within 1 day. Dexmedetomidine, an $\alpha 2$ adrenergic agonist, causes diabetes insipidus, inhibiting both AVP release and also AVP action (AVP deficiency, as well as AVP resistance). Other medications used in the operating room and intensive care unit, including sevoflurane and ketamine, have also been implicated. Thus, clinicians should remain vigilant for these and other medication-related causes of transient diabetes insipidus (AVP deficiency/resistance) (Answer B).

Although this patient does not have cancer, individuals with cancer treated with novel targeted anticancer agents (eg, nivolumab, a PD-1 inhibitor) can develop AVP deficiency related to drug-induced hypophysitis. Other immune checkpoint inhibitors can also cause this. In some individuals with cancer, either the primary tumor—if it affects the hypothalamus/pituitary—and/or pituitary metastases can cause AVP deficiency, adding complexity to the diagnostic evaluation.

Undertreated hypothyroidism (Answer E) would be expected to lead to impaired free water clearance and physiology characteristic of syndrome of inappropriate antidiuretic hormone secretion (ie, oliguria and hyponatremia, not polyuria and hypernatremia, as in this vignette). Also, the degree of subclinical hypothyroidism is mild.

While dopamine (Answer C) can increase urine output via several mechanisms, including affecting renal perfusion and natriuresis, it would not typically produce hypernatremia, especially to this extent.

Cerebral salt-wasting (Answer A) would typically produce hyponatremia, and the hypernatremia suggests that she has lost free water out of proportion to salt.

Finally, while hypercalcemia (Answer D) can lead to an inability to concentrate urine, her serum calcium concentration is just above normal, which is more likely to reflect a consequence rather than a cause of dehydration.

Educational Objective

Identify medications as potential causes of arginine vasopressin deficiency or resistance (diabetes insipidus).

Reference(s)

Barnabei A, Strigari L, Corsello A, et al. Grading central diabetes insipidus induced by immune checkpoint inhibitors: a challenging task. *Front Endocrinol (Lausanne).* 2022;13:840971. PMID: 35388297

Fosci M, Pigliaru F, Salcuni AS, et al. Diabetes insipidus secondary to nivolumab-induced neurohypophysitis and pituitary metastasis. *Endocrinol Diabetes Metab Case Rep.* 2021;20-0123. PMID: 33522491

Kraus MB, Leuzinger K, Reynolds E, et al. Diabetes insipidus related to sedation in the intensive care unit: a review of the literature. *J Crit Care.* 2023;75:154233. PMID: 36738631

Rouch AJ, Kudo LH. Alpha 2-adrenergic-mediated inhibition of water and urea permeability in the rat IMCD. *Am J Physiol.* 1996;271(1 Pt 2):F150-F157. PMID: 8760256

Villela NR, do Nascimento Junior P, de Carvalho LR, Teixeira A. Effects of dexmedetomidine on renal system and on vasopressin plasma levels. Experimental study in dogs. *Rev Bras Anestesiol.* 2005;55(4):429-40. PMID: 19468631

36 ANSWER: D) Smith-Lemli-Opitz syndrome

Smith-Lemli-Opitz syndrome is caused by pathogenic variants in the *DHCR7* gene, which encodes 7-dehydrocholesterol reductase. More than 200 causative variants have been identified. The phenotypic spectrum is broad and can include distinctive facial features, cardiac defects, microcephaly, intellectual disability, growth restriction, and hypotonia. Syndactyly of toes 2 and 3 is the most common clinical finding. The degree of genital atypia is variable; in males, the phenotype ranges from isolated hypospadias to female-appearing external genitalia. Adrenal insufficiency is more likely in severely affected individuals. It is unclear to what extent features are due to cholesterol deficiency vs elevated dehydrocholesterol and other byproducts. Findings of atypical genitalia with microcephaly and low muscle tone in this patient are consistent with Smith-Lemli-Opitz syndrome (Answer D), which can be confirmed with an elevated 7-dehydrocholesterol concentration. Infants with Smith-Lemli-Opitz syndrome would be expected to have normal age-appropriate gonadotropin and sex steroid concentrations as exhibited by this patient's normal LH, FSH, testosterone, and dihydrotestosterone.

The other answer choices are all syndromes associated with genital abnormalities or atypia but have other features that are not consistent with the patient in this vignette. *NR0B1* (*DAX1*) (Answer C) encodes a nuclear receptor that is expressed in the adrenal glands, hypothalamus, pituitary gonadotrophs, and gonads and acts by inhibiting the transcriptional activity of other nuclear receptors such as SF-1. Duplication of the region of the X chromosome that contains *NR0B1* results in overexpression, impairing function of other nuclear transcription factors required for normal sexual differentiation in males. However, *NR0B1* variants are not associated with other features such as microcephaly or hypotonia.

WAGR syndrome (Answer E), Denys-Drash syndrome (Answer A), and Frasier syndrome (Answer B) are all caused by pathogenic variants in the *WT1* gene and are associated with an increased risk of Wilms tumor and atypical genitalia in males. WAGR syndrome is caused by deletions of the short arm of chromosome 11 involving the *WT1* and *PAX6* genes. In addition to Wilms tumor and abnormalities of the genitourinary tract, affected individuals can also have aniridia and other ocular defects (eg, cataracts, glaucoma) related to loss of *PAX6* gene function, developmental and intellectual delays, and obesity when the *BDNF* gene is also deleted.

Denys-Drash syndrome (Answer A) is characterized by impaired gonadal development resulting in variable degrees of genital atypia (primarily in males) without other dysmorphic features. Gonadotropins are expected to be elevated in the first weeks of life due to primary hypogonadism. The other key distinguishing feature is diffuse glomerulosclerosis that develops within the first few months of life.

Frasier syndrome (Answer B) is characterized by varying degrees of genital atypia in males, kidney failure due to focal segmental glomerulosclerosis, streak gonads, and high risk of gonadoblastoma. As with Denys-Drash syndrome, LH and FSH levels are expected to be elevated in the neonatal surge. There are no other associated dysmorphic features, and affected females usually have typical genitalia and gonads.

Educational Objective

Differentiate clinical and genetic features of individuals with 46,XY differences of sex development.

Reference(s)

Bianconi SE, Cross JL, Wassif CA, Porter FD. Pathogenesis, epidemiology, diagnosis and clinical aspects of Smith-Lemli-Opitz syndrome. *Expert Opin Orphan Drugs.* 2015;3(3):267-280. PMID: 25734025

Mendonca BB, Domenice S, Arnhold IJP, Costa EME. 46,XY disorders of sex development (DSD). *Clin Endocrinol (Oxf).* 2009;70(2):173-187. PMID: 18811725

37 ANSWER: B) Exenatide

Incretins are hormones produced by the gastrointestinal tract that promote insulin secretion in a glucose-dependent manner. The 2 main human incretins are GLP-1 and GIP (glucose-dependent insulinotropic peptide). Levels of both rise quickly after a meal but then are rapidly inactivated. GLP-1 is secreted from L cells in the distal small intestine. In addition to the actions at the level of the β cell, GLP-1 also helps to bolster satiety, inhibit glucose-dependent glucagon secretion, and reduce hepatic glucose production. While GLP-1 acts at numerous sites in the body, one of the major glucose-lowering effects is through the stimulation of insulin release after food intake. However, GLP-1 reduces blood glucose only when glucose concentrations are elevated above fasting levels, which is the case postprandially. As the postprandial blood glucose levels fall in response to GLP-1, GLP-1 action is self-terminating. In addition to promoting insulin secretion in a glucose-dependent fashion, GLP-1 also suppresses glucagon secretion by α cells. Exenatide (Answer B), a synthetic form of exendin-4, is an incretin mimetic that is administered subcutaneously. It is a high-affinity agonist at the GLP-1 receptor but is fairly resistant to the actions of DPP-4 in comparison to native GLP-1. DPP-4 is an enzyme that is responsible for the breakdown of the incretins GLP-1 and GIP. In addition to beneficial effects on glycemic control, GLP-1 receptor agonists also inhibit gastric emptying, suppress appetite, and, through their actions, promote weight loss. Since GLP-1 receptor agonists have minimal impact on insulin secretion in the absence of hyperglycemia, the risk for hypoglycemia is minimal.

Sitagliptin (Answer E) is a DPP-4 inhibitor. DPP-4 inhibitors suppress more than 90% of DPP-4 activity and therefore extend the half-life of endogenous GLP-1, which is normally very brief (only 1 to 2 min). DPP-4 inhibitors are administered orally and depend on native GLP-1 production being intact. They are typically weight-neutral, unlike GLP-1 receptor agonists, most likely because they do not provide supraphysiological stimulation of the GLP-1 receptor, so they would not aid in the goal of weight loss.

Sulfonylureas such as glyburide (Answer C) bind to and block the ATP-sensitive potassium channels on pancreatic β cells. As a result, potassium efflux decreases and the cell membrane depolarizes. This depolarization causes the opening of calcium channels, leading to increased calcium entering the β cell. This process stimulates insulin secretion from pancreatic β cells and ultimately leads to decreased glucose levels. Unlike GLP-1 receptor therapies, insulin release from sulfonylurea therapy is not glucose-dependent, so hypoglycemia is a risk. Weight gain is also a concern with this medication class because of the glucose-independent promotion of insulin secretion. Glyburide is a long-acting sulfonylurea that is available as an oral tablet, usually administered once daily, and it is currently only approved for use in adults with type 2 diabetes.

Empagliflozin (Answer A) is an SGLT-2 inhibitor that acts by increasing the excretion of glucose in the urine. SGLT-2 is a protein located in the renal proximal convoluted tubules that reabsorb filtered glucose from the tubular lumen. SGLT-2 inhibitors block this action in the kidneys, leading to increased glucose excretion and lowering of blood glucose. Because sodium and glucose are co-transported by SGLT-2, SGLT-2 inhibitors also inhibit sodium reabsorption with a resultant increase in distal tubular sodium load. While the exact mechanisms are still being elucidated, SGLT-2 inhibitors offer protective cardiac and renal effects due to these alterations in glucose and sodium reabsorption.

Metformin (Answer D) belongs to a class of medications called biguanides. While metformin has been available for the treatment of type 2 diabetes for many decades, its exact mechanism of action has been incompletely understood. It has an inhibitory effect on liver glucose production (gluconeogenesis), which is one of the main ways that it lowers blood glucose. However, it also enhances peripheral glucose uptake, enhances insulin sensitivity, and decreases the absorption of glucose from the gastrointestinal tract. More recently, metformin has been shown to have incretin-sensitizing effects as well. Metformin is administered orally.

Educational Objective

Explain how GLP-1 helps regulate glucose homeostasis.

Reference(s)

Brunton S. GLP-1 receptor agonists vs DPP-4 inhibitors for type 2 diabetes: is one approach more successful or preferable than the other? *Int J Clin Pract.* 2014;68(5):557-567. PMID: 24499291

Drucker DJ. Mechanisms of action and therapeutic application of glucagon-like peptide-1. *Cell Metab.* 2018;27(4):740-756. PMID: 29617641

Nadkarni P, Chepurny OG, Holz GG. Regulation of glucose homeostasis by GLP-1. *Prog Mol Biol Transl Sci.* 2014;121:23-65. PMID: 24373234

38 **ANSWER: D) Perform genetic testing for pathogenic variants in the *NSD1* gene**

This patient has features of Sotos syndrome. The classic triad of Sotos syndrome—characteristic facial features, learning disability, and overgrowth—is present in at least 90% of affected individuals. Sotos syndrome is due to pathogenic variants or deletions in the *NSD1* gene (Answer D). The important thing to note in this case is the presence of overgrowth and macrocephaly since birth, which should raise high suspicion for a genetic overgrowth syndrome. Characteristic facial features in persons with Sotos syndrome include a broad, prominent forehead with dolichocephaly; sparse frontotemporal hair, downslanting palpebral fissures; and a long narrow face. Children with Sotos syndrome characteristically have intellectual impairment, although the degree of impairment can vary significantly. Autism spectrum disorders are also more common than in the general population. In terms of overgrowth, affected children are large at birth with macrocephaly and often have rapid growth through childhood. However, adult height may be in the normal range. Bone age is characteristically advanced.

Sotos syndrome belongs to a class of genetic overgrowth syndromes. Other syndromes in the differential diagnosis include Weaver syndrome, Cohen-Gibson syndrome, Beckwith-Wiedemann syndrome, Simpson-Golabi-Behmel syndrome, Bannayan-Riley-Ruvalcaba syndrome, and fragile X syndrome. Some overgrowth syndromes are associated with increased risk of certain malignancies. Performing kidney ultrasonography (Answer E) alludes to the increased risk of Wilms tumor, which is seen in Beckwith-Wiedemann syndrome. However, this patient does not have other features of this syndrome such as body asymmetry, neonatal hypoglycemia, omphalocele, or macroglossia.

Measurement of IGF-1 (Answer B) is important as a screen for GH excess when one is concerned about pituitary gigantism. However, this would not present with macrocephaly and increased height since birth.

Measuring LH and testosterone (Answer C) is useful to assess for central precocious puberty. This 9-year-old patient has a testicular volume of 4 mL, which is within the normal range, and his growth pattern is not suggestive of central precocious puberty.

Considering adrenal androgen excess (Answer A) is important given the possibility of late-onset congenital adrenal hyperplasia in patients with advanced bone age and tall stature, but this patient has numerous other features pointing to a genetic overgrowth syndrome.

Educational Objective

Identify the characteristic clinical features of Sotos syndrome as a cause of tall stature and developmental delay.

Reference(s)

Albuquerque EVA, Scalco RC, Jorge AAL. Management of endocrine disease: diagnostic and therapeutic approach of tall stature. *Eur J Endocrinol.* 2017;176(6):R339-R353. PMID: 28274950

39

ANSWER: D) *FAM20C* (Raine syndrome)

The craniofacial findings and radiographic features of dense metaphyseal bands in long bones and osteosclerosis of the base of the skull make Raine syndrome the most likely diagnosis in this patient. Raine syndrome is due to homozygous pathogenic variants in the *FAM20C* gene (Answer D), which encodes a protein involved in the phosphorylation of several enzymes, including osteopontin, dentin matrix protein, and bone sialoprotein. The complex interactions of these enzymes and their products result in regulation of bone mineralization, as well as inhibition of extraskeletal calcification. Normal activity of *FAM20C* increases dentin matrix protein and decreases FGF-23 activity. Pathogenic variants, specifically missense variants or variants in the N-terminal portion of *FAM20C*, can lead to hypophosphatemia, renal phosphate wasting, dental anomalies similar to those of amelogenesis imperfecta, intracerebral calcifications, and osteosclerosis of long bones. Craniofacial features (midface hypoplasia, ocular proptosis, and intracerebral calcifications) can be detected in utero. Historically, Raine syndrome was thought to be a lethal condition with a life expectancy of only a few weeks due to pulmonary hypoplasia. However, more recent reports indicate that nearly half of patients survive into the second decade of life.

In contrast to other disorders associated with hypophosphatemia and elevated FGF-23, rickets is not a typical feature of Raine syndrome. Instead, the findings of generalized sclerosis (as depicted in the x-rays) and brain calcifications lead to classification as a form of osteosclerotic dysplasia. Treatment with calcitriol and multiple daily doses of phosphate salts is generally not indicated in Raine syndrome.

Biallelic loss-of-function variants in *ENPP1* (Answer C) can result in generalized arterial calcification of infancy and/or autosomal recessive hypophosphatemic rickets type 2. Generalized arterial calcification of infancy is fatal in nearly 50% of affected persons due to extensive and severe arterial calcifications in utero leading to multiorgan dysfunction and myocardial infarction.

Autosomal recessive hypophosphatemic rickets type 1 is due to pathogenic variants in *DMP1* (Answer B), and affected patients present similarly to those with autosomal recessive hypophosphatemic rickets type 2. In this vignette, the patient's intracranial calcifications and metaphyseal osteosclerosis are not consistent with *DMP1* pathogenic variants.

Patients with *SLC34A3* pathogenic variants (Answer E) have impaired function of the NaPi-IIc renal phosphate cotransporter leading to hereditary hypophosphatemic rickets with hypercalciuria. As the name implies, urinary calcium is high at diagnosis, which distinguishes it from other genetic hypophosphatemic disorders. In this condition, FGF-23 is not elevated, thus 1,25-dihydroxyvitamin D is usually elevated and PTH is frequently low or normal.

In Dent disease, pathogenic variants in *CNCL5* (Answer A) are inherited in an X-linked recessive manner and cause renal phosphate wasting, hypercalciuria, and proteinuria in male individuals.

Educational Objective

Differentiate among hypophosphatemic disorders based on phenotypic features.

Reference(s)

Carpenter TO. The expanding family of hypophosphatemic syndromes. *J Bone Miner Metab.* 2012;30(1):1-9. PMID: 22167381

Mameli C, Zichichi G, Mahmood N, et al. Natural history of non-lethal Raine syndrome during childhood. *Orphanet J Rare Dis.* 2020;15(1):93. PMID: 32299476

Palma-Lara I, Perez-Ramirez M, Alonso-Themann PG, et al. FAM20C overview: classic and novel targets, pathogenic variants and Raine syndrome phenotypes. *Int J Mol Sci.* 2021;22(15):8039. PMID: 34360805

40

ANSWER: A) *FOXE1*

The infant in the vignette has congenital primary hypothyroidism without a goiter and also has several other anomalies, including cleft palate and bilateral choanal atresia. Thyroid dysgenesis is the most common cause of congenital hypothyroidism, and the cause is unknown in most cases. The presence of congenital anomalies in addition to congenital hypothyroidism warrants an evaluation for a genetic cause. This infant has Bamforth-Lazarus syndrome due to homozygous pathogenic variants in the *FOXE1* gene (Answer A). The forkhead box protein E1 (*FOXE1*) gene is also known as thyroid transcription factor 2 (formerly *TTF-2*). As this syndrome is inherited in an autosomal recessive manner, there is frequently a history of consanguinity. The gene is expressed in the thyroid gland, oral cavity, and hair follicles. Homozygous variants in the gene cause thyroid dysgenesis, including athyreosis, along with spiky hair, cleft lip and/or palate, choanal atresia, and bifid uvula.

Pathogenic variants in the *TPO* gene (Answer E) cause dyshormonogenesis that results in primary hypothyroidism, as in this infant, but affected patients also typically have a goiter. Some rare cases of *TPO* pathogenic variants are associated with thyroid hypoplasia. The other congenital anomalies in this infant cannot be explained by *TPO* variants.

Pathogenic variants in the *NKX2-1* gene (Answer B) are responsible for the phenotype of brain-lung-thyroid syndrome. This condition is inherited in an autosomal dominant manner. Approximately one-half of those affected have the full phenotype with congenital primary hypothyroidism, respiratory distress syndrome, and choreoathetosis. The lung disease may manifest in infancy with severe respiratory distress syndrome due to surfactant deficiency at term or it may present later with recurrent pulmonary infections. The neurological disorder is characterized by abnormal choreoathetoid movements, hypotonia, and developmental delay. The phenotype is variable, even among affected individuals in the same family, and patients may manifest only hypothyroidism, lung disease, or neurological disease or any combination of features.

Pathogenic variants in the *PAX8* gene (Answer C) cause congenital primary hypothyroidism but not the other congenital anomalies seen in this patient. The protein encoded by *PAX8* is a transcription factor that regulates the expression of thyroglobulin, TPO, and the sodium-iodide symporter (*SLC5A5* gene). The thyroid gland may be normal in size or hypoplastic. Some affected patients have a partial organification defect, and this is likely because *TPO* and *SLC5A5* gene transcription is dependent on *PAX8*. Primary hypothyroidism associated with *PAX8* is inherited in an autosomal dominant fashion. The thyroid phenotype is variable, even among affected individuals in the same family. Some present with severe congenital hypothyroidism, others develop compensated hypothyroidism, and others remain euthyroid. *PAX8* is also expressed in the urogenital tract, and a few families have been described who have hypothyroidism and urogenital abnormalities (incomplete horseshoe kidney, undescended testicles, hydrocele, ureterocele), although these findings are rare.

The *POU1F1* gene (Answer D) encodes a transcription factor predominantly involved in pituitary development. Pathogenic variants in this gene can result in hypothyroidism, but the hypothyroidism would be central, not the primary hypothyroidism seen in this patient. The other congenital anomalies observed in this patient are not associated with hypopituitarism or variants in *POU1F1*.

Educational Objective

Identify *FOXE1* pathogenic variants as a rare cause of thyroid dysgenesis.

Reference(s)

Castanet M, Polak M. Spectrum of human FOXE1/TTF2 mutations. *Horm Res Paediatr.* 2010;73(6):423-429. PMID: 20453517

Kostopoulou E, Miliordos K, Spiliotis B. Genetics of primary congenital hypothyroidism-a review. *Hormones (Athens).* 2021;20(2):225-236. PMID: 33400193

41 **ANSWER: A) BMI percentile**

Disturbed eating behaviors include dieting for weight control and unhealthy weight-management behaviors, such as skipping meals, binging, or purging (more common in pre-teen and teenage girls with type 1 diabetes than in their peers without diabetes). Twenty to thirty percent of adolescent girls with type 1 diabetes display disturbed eating behaviors and are at risk for developing eating disorders. The problem in boys seems less prevalent but is still troublesome, with 5% to 10% reporting substantially disturbed eating behaviors. Adolescents with type 1 diabetes learn to manipulate body weight by insulin restriction or omission, and this behavior is reported in 35% to 40% of this cohort, especially in girls. Combined with other unhealthy behaviors, insulin manipulation may lead to higher hemoglobin A_{1c} values and premature diabetes complications. Study findings indicate that higher BMI percentile (Answer A) in adolescents may lead to significant body dissatisfaction and disturbed eating behaviors.

Diabetes distress reflects an emotional burden of daily diabetes management that can lead to depressive symptoms. There is a strong correlation between depression and disturbed eating behaviors. Furthermore, low self-esteem indicates a higher risk for depression and anxiety, difficulty coping with diabetes management, and suboptimal glycemic control. Puberty is a complex period marked by various physiological and psychological changes, and for individuals managing type 1 diabetes, this phase can introduce additional challenges. Studies have suggested that early or precocious puberty might be linked to an increased risk of disordered eating behaviors in adolescents with type 1 diabetes. The hormonal changes during puberty, coupled with the demands of managing diabetes, may contribute to heightened stress and body image concerns. Such factors could potentially influence the development of eating disorders or problematic eating behaviors in these individuals.

Studies do not show a significant association between duration of diabetes (Answer B) or the severity of its initial presentation, such as the history of diabetic ketoacidosis at the time of diagnosis (Answer D), and the occurrence of diabetes distress or disordered eating behaviors.

Fear of hypoglycemia (Answer C) is a complex psychological state fueled by diabetes-related fears and non–diabetes-related anxiety. Patients with fear of hypoglycemia may manipulate insulin doses and have irrational eating behaviors, yet they do not have a disturbed eating pattern as described in this vignette.

Refusal of a patient with type 1 diabetes to try an insulin pump (Answer E), on its own, would not directly increase the risk for disordered eating. The decision to decline an insulin pump could stem from various reasons, including fear, discomfort with technology, body image concerns, or a desire for more autonomy in diabetes management. It might reflect a broader issue related to the individual's relationship with their diabetes care regimen and how they perceive or cope with the demands of managing the condition.

Educational Objective

Identify patterns of and risk factors for disturbed eating in patients with type 1 diabetes.

Reference(s)

Colton P, Olmsted M, Daneman D, Rydall A, Rodin G. Disturbed eating behavior and eating disorders in pre-teen and early teenage girls with type 1 diabetes. *Diabetes Care.* 2004;27(7):1654-1659. PMID: 15220242

Colton PA, Olmsted MP, Daneman D, Rydall AC, Rodin GM. Natural history and predictors of disturbed eating behaviour in girls with type 1 diabetes. *Diabet Med.* 2007;24(4):424-429. PMID: 17298588

Luyckx K, Verschueren M, Palmeroni N, Goethals ER, Weets I, Claes L. Disturbed eating behaviors in adolescents and emerging adults with type 1 diabetes: a one-year prospective study. *Diabetes Care.* 2019;42(9):1637-1644. PMID: 31217162

42 ANSWER: B) GH resistance

Patients with anorexia nervosa can have poor growth due to caloric restriction. Several endocrine abnormalities affect growth in patients with anorexia nervosa, including GH resistance (Answer B), hypercortisolemia, hypogonadism due to loss of LH pulsatility, and low thyroid hormone and TSH concentrations.

Although growth improves once caloric intake is increased and sustained in children with anorexia nervosa, the catchup growth is not complete, making it unlikely for them to reach their genetic potential for adult height. Thus, this patient does not have normal growth (Answer E).

Her low normal TSH value and low free T_4 value are most likely the result of inadequate caloric intake, not hypopituitarism (Answer C) or hypothyroidism (Answer D).

She has normal pubertal development with normal height and BMI prior to the diagnosis of anorexia nervosa. Thus, her poor growth cannot be attributed to constitutional pubertal delay (Answer A).

Educational Objective

Identify anorexia nervosa as a cause of impaired linear growth and explain that catch-up growth is not complete after weight gain.

Reference(s)

Léger J, Fjellestad-Paulsen A, Bargiacchi A, Pages J, Chevenne D, Alison M, Alberti C, Guilmin-Crepon S. One year of GH treatment for growth failure in children with anorexia nervosa: a randomized placebo-controlled trial. *J Clin Endocrinol Metab.* 2021;106(7):e2535-e2546. PMID: 33772303

Misra M, Klibanski A. Endocrine consequences of anorexia nervosa. *Lancet Diabetes Endocrinol.* 2014;2(7):581-592. PMID: 24731664

Misra M, Miller KK, Bjornson J, et al. Alterations in growth hormone secretory dynamics in adolescent girls with anorexia nervosa and effects on bone metabolism. *J Clin Endocrinol Metab.* 2003;88(12):5615-5623. PMID: 14671143

Modan-Moses D, Yaroslavsky A, Pinhas-Hamiel O, et al. Prospective longitudinal assessment of linear growth and adult height in female adolescents with anorexia nervosa. *J Clin Endocrinol Metab.* 2021;106(1):e1-e10. PMID: 32816013

43 ANSWER: B) Lack of discussion initiated by her primary care physician about bariatric surgery

Although approximately 4.5 million adolescents in the United States are categorized as having severe obesity, the percentage of individuals who ultimately undergo metabolic and bariatric surgery (MBS) remains very low. This is concerning because data from the Teen-Longitudinal Assessment of Bariatric Surgery (TEEN-LABS) study and others have shown the positive benefits of MBS, both in terms of weight status, as well as improvement in comorbid conditions. Despite documented benefits of MBS, significant barriers remain for access to MBS, particularly in adolescent populations.

Campbell et al found that one of the significant barriers to MBS in adolescents is related to lack of knowledge about the procedure and lack of discussion initiated by medical providers regarding MBS (Answer B). National survey data suggest that providers are often reluctant to discuss MBS with patients and/or consider referral for MBS because of a variety of factors, including lack of knowledge regarding the efficacy and safety of the procedure, concerns about how MBS might affect linear growth (which has not been demonstrated), or personal weight bias (including skepticism that obesity is a chronic medical condition).

Adolescents from racial minority groups are more likely to have severe obesity and comorbid conditions but are less likely to undergo MBS than their White counterparts. Perez et al documented that Black and Hispanic adolescents are much less likely to undergo MBS than nonHispanic White adolescents. The authors also reported that being from a racial minority group and having Medicaid insurance further decreases the likelihood of having MBS, while the opposite is true for White adolescents. Although initial studies reported that postoperative outcomes did not appear to differ by race/ethnicity, more recent data have highlighted outcome disparities. Wood et al documented that nonHispanic Black patients have lower total body weight loss (32 kg vs 38.3 kg; $P < .001$) and lower percentage of excess weight loss (26% vs 29%; $P < .001$) compared with weight loss in nonHispanic White patients 1 year after MBS. Samaan et al also reported that Black patients lose significantly less weight compared with weight loss in White and Hispanic patients (thus, Answer C is incorrect). Additionally, recent data highlight that nonHispanic Black patients appear to experience higher rates of postoperative complications relative to complication rates in White patients.

While complications are possible with any surgical procedure, postoperative complications in young adults undergoing MBS are relatively infrequent (thus, Answer A is incorrect). Most reported complications (15%) are considered minor (eg, nausea, vomiting, and dehydration), and they typically occur in the immediate postoperative period. Major complications within 30 days of MBS were reported in 8% of TEEN-LABS participants, with 2.7% requiring reoperation before hospital discharge (similar to adult data). Postoperative micronutrient deficiencies are common and must be closely monitored.

While lifestyle counseling is important, data have shown that it alone is unlikely to lead to effective and sustained weight reduction compared with that achieved with MBS (thus, Answer D is incorrect). In the TEEN-LABS cohort, participants who underwent either Roux-en-Y gastric bypass or vertical sleeve gastrectomy had a mean weight reduction of 27%, as well as resolution of multiple comorbidities, including type 2 diabetes (95%), dyslipidemia (66%), and hypertension (74%) 3 years after surgery. Results from the AMOS cohort of adolescents undergoing Roux-en-Y gastric bypass demonstrated a mean weight loss of 81.1 lb (36.8 kg) at 5 years. This is in contrast to outcomes in adolescents enrolled in a lifestyle modification program who actually demonstrated a mean BMI increase of 3.3 kg/m^2. Indeed, more recent data highlight that "watchful waiting" may lead to further BMI increases, as well as an increase in the number of comorbid conditions.

Insurance coverage for MBS in adolescent patients also remains a significant barrier. A review from the TEEN-LABS research consortium documented that less than half (47%) of eligible surgical candidates received insurance approval upon initial request for authorization. Age less than 18 years was given as the most common reason for refusal. Obtaining insurance coverage would be more challenging if this patient were younger than 18 years (thus, Answer E is incorrect). In contrast, 85% of adults receive insurance approval for MBS with the first request.

Educational Objective

Describe some of the recognized barriers to bariatric surgery in the adolescent population.

Reference(s)

Armstrong SC, Bolling CF, Michalsky MP, Reichard KW; Section on Obesity, Section on Surgery. Pediatric metabolic and bariatric surgery: evidence, barriers, and best practices. *Pediatrics.* 2019;144(6):e20193223. PMID: 31656225

Campbell EG, Alasmar A, Lawrence R, et al. Barriers to metabolic bariatric surgery in adolescents: results of a qualitative study. *Surg Obes Relat Dis.* 2022;18(6):794-802. PMID: 35474008.

Perez NP, Westfal ML, Stapleton SM, et al. Beyond insurance: race-based disparities in the use of metabolic and bariatric surgery for the management of severe pediatric obesity. *Surg Obes Relat Dis.* 2020;16(3):414-419. PMID: 31917198

Samaan JS, Abboud Y, Yuan L, et al. Racial disparities in bariatric surgery postoperative weight loss and patient satisfaction. *Am J Surg.* 2022;223(5):969-974. PMID: 34583849

Wood MH, Carlin AM, Ghaferi AA, et al. Association of race with bariatric surgery outcomes. *JAMA Surg.* 2019;154(5):e190029. PMID: 30840063

44 ANSWER: E) Start a combined oral contraceptive pill

This patient presents with oligomenorrhea 3 years after menarche. Approximately 75% of girls develop a regular menstrual cycle within 1 year of menarche, with 5% more exhibiting regular cycles each of the next 3 years. As it can take up to 8 years to reach an adult ovulatory pattern, criteria for abnormal menstrual irregularity are different in adolescents than in adults. Oligomenorrhea is defined as fewer than 4 periods per year in postmenarcheal year 1, fewer than 6 periods per year in postmenarcheal year 2, fewer than 8 periods per year in postmenarcheal years 3 to 5, and fewer than 9 periods per year in adults.

Evaluation is indicated when menstrual dysfunction persists beyond 1 year, as is the case with the patient in this vignette, or when it is associated with other features such as hirsutism or galactorrhea. Assessment should include testing for chronic underlying disease (ie, complete blood cell count, erythrocyte sedimentation rate, comprehensive metabolic panel, and, when indicated, thyroid function testing, IGF-1, and assessment for celiac disease), sexual maturity (gonadotropins and estradiol), prolactin, and testosterone. Once underlying conditions (eg, prolactinoma, nonclassic congenital adrenal hyperplasia) have been ruled out, monophasic estrogen-progestin combined oral contraceptive pills (Answer E) should be prescribed for sexually mature girls. Benefits of treatment include improvement of endometrial hyperplasia and dysmenorrhea. Given the very infrequent menses in this case, reassurance and continued monitoring (Answer B) would not be the best choice.

In adolescents, polycystic ovaries on ultrasonography are a common and nonspecific finding. According to recent guidelines, there are no definitive criteria to define polycystic ovary morphology in adolescents. As such, pelvic ultrasonography (Answer C) at this point would not be helpful in determining the risk of polycystic ovary syndrome in this patient. Furthermore, her androgen concentrations are in the reference range, and thus she does not appear to be at risk of polycystic ovary syndrome now.

A progesterone withdrawal test (progestin challenge) (Answer A) can be used to assess adequacy of estrogenization; however, readily available sensitive assays to measure estradiol levels have generally rendered this test unnecessary. Cyclic progesterone therapy could, however, be used as an alternative to a hormonal contraceptive.

Obesity and insulin resistance are associated with dysmenorrhea and in this setting, lifestyle modification with counseling on diet and exercise (Answer D) can be helpful. However, the patient in this vignette has a normal BMI and no findings to suggest insulin resistance.

Educational Objective

Interpret laboratory test results in an adolescent with oligomenorrhea.

Reference(s)

Rosenfield RL. Clinical review: Adolescent anovulation: maturational mechanisms and implications. *J Clin Endocrinol Metab.* 2013;98(9):3572-3583. PMID: 23913942

Teede HJ, Tay CT, Laven JJE, et al. Recommendations from the 2023 international evidence-based guideline for the assessment and management of polycystic ovary syndrome. *J Clin Endocrinol Metab.* 2023;108(10):2447-2469. PMID: 37580314

45 ANSWER: B) Examine for hypermobility

Congenital adrenal hyperplasia (CAH) is caused by 21-hydroxylase deficiency in 95% of cases. The 21-hydroxylase enzyme is encoded by the *CYP21A2* gene and its highly homologous pseudogene, *CYP21A1P*. These genes are located on chromosome 6p21.3 within the class III major histocompatibility complex in a region referred to as *RCCX* copy number variation or module (*figure 1*). *RCCX* was named after the 4 genes located within: *STK19* (serine/threonine kinase 19; formerly **R**P), **C**4 (complement component 4), ***C**YP21* (steroid 21-hydroxylase), and *TN**X*** (tenascin-X).

Figure 1. Different Module Arrangement of Human RCCX

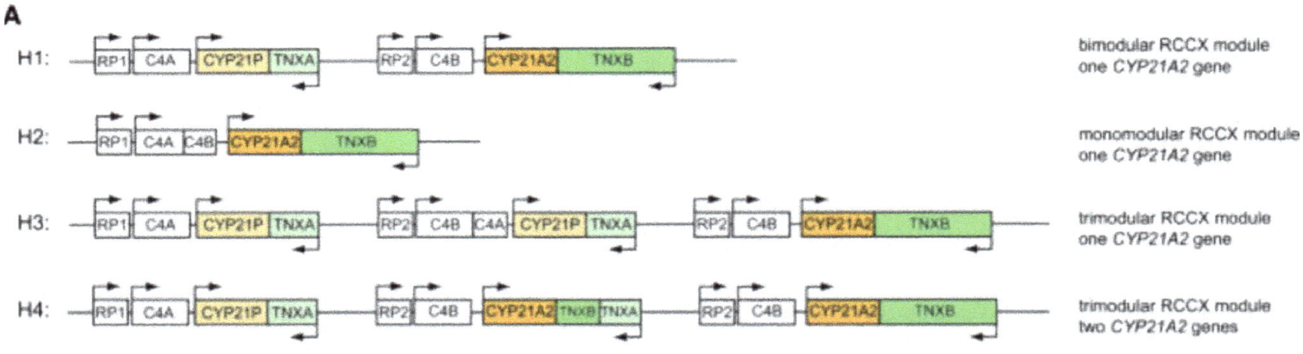

Reprinted from Fanis P et al. Front Endocrinol (Lausanne), 2023; 14: 1156616. © The Authors. Published by Frontiers Media S.A.

The *TNXB* gene encodes an extracellular matrix glycoprotein, tenascin-X. Pathogenic variants in *TNXB* cause Ehlers-Danlos syndrome. Deletions affecting both *CYP21A2* and *TNXB* result in a contiguous gene deletion syndrome known as CAH-X syndrome (*figure 2*). The first report of complete tenascin-X deficiency described a patient diagnosed with both CAH and Ehlers-Danlos syndrome. In one cohort of CAH, prevalence of CAH-X was reported to be 7%. Evaluation for Ehlers-Danlos syndrome should be performed in the presence of any suggestive features such as joint hypermobility (especially during childhood), chronic joint pain and multiple joint dislocations in adulthood, soft-tissue rheumatism, and other manifestations of tissue fragility. This is especially true for patients with CAH who have a *CYP21A2* deletion. Patients with known or suspected CAH-X syndrome should also have a cardiac evaluation to determine whether there are any structural abnormalities. The child in this vignette potentially has CAH-X; hence, the best mode of action is to examine for hypermobility (Answer B).

Figure 2. Genetic Changes in the CYP21A Locus and Clinical Presentation

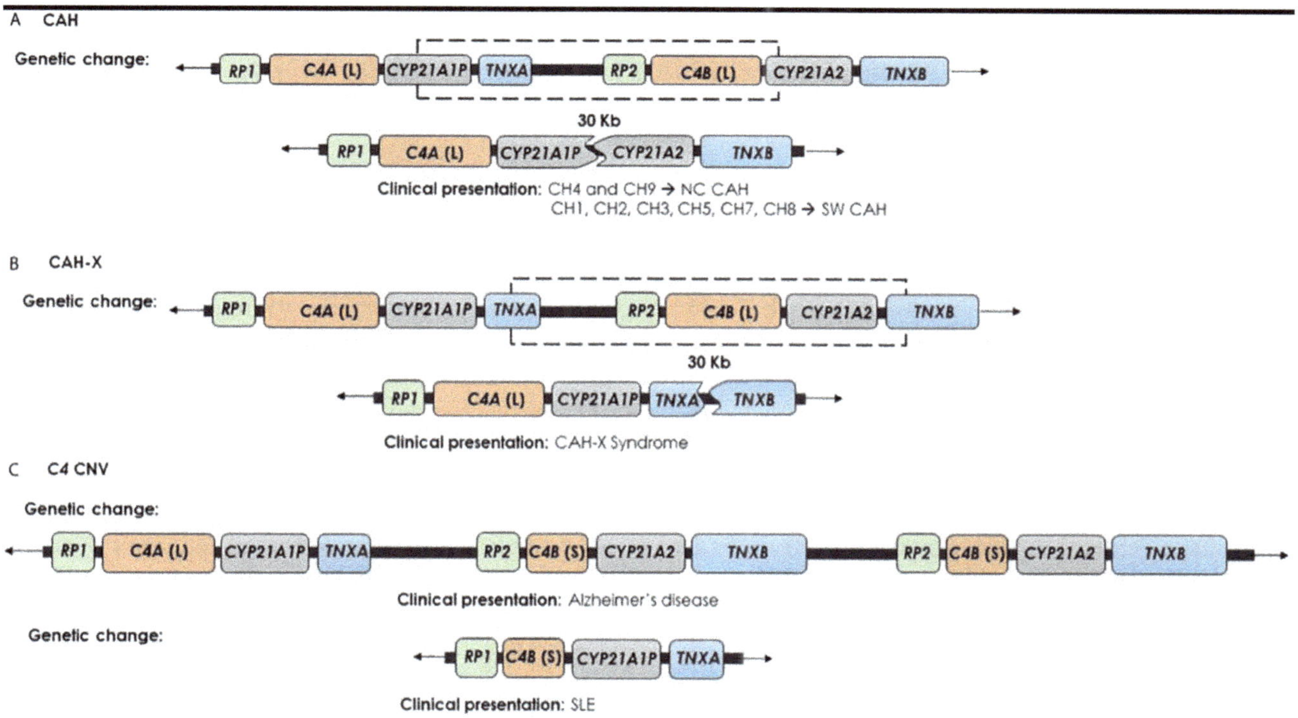

Panel A, Congenital adrenal hyperplasia (CAH) chimera (CYP21A1P/CYP21A2) is caused by recombination between CYP21A1P and CYP21A2 and causes the impairment of CYP21A2 and the deletion of C4B, but it leaves safe the *TNXB* gene. CH-1, CH-2, CH-3, CH-5, CH-6, CH-7, and CH-8 chimeras are involved in the severe SW form of CAH. In contrast, CH-4 and CH-9 chimeras are generally associated with a milder phenotype. *Panel B*, CAH-X chimera (*TNXA/TNXB*) is caused by recombination between *TNXA* and *TNXB* and results in complete deletion of the CYP21A2 gene, impairment of the *TNXB* gene, and deletion of C4B. This contiguous deletion is termed CAH-X, and it causes CAH-X syndrome. *Panel C*, Psychiatric and autoimmune diseases due to C4 CNV: high C4B copy number has been described as an Alzheimer disease risk factor, while C4A deficiency is related to systemic lupus erythematosus. Reprinted from Carrozza C et al. *Front Endocrinol (Lausanne)*, 2021; 12: 709758.

In individuals with Ehlers-Danlos syndrome, clotting factors, platelet aggregation, and bleeding time are usually normal. Prothrombin time and activated partial thromboplastin time are slightly prolonged in some patients. However, measuring prothrombin time (Answer C) would not be the best next step in this patient's management.

Assessing for rheumatoid factor (Answer A) would help pinpoint a diagnosis of rheumatoid arthritis, which is not suspected in this vignette.

Genetic testing for *VWF* gene variants (Answer D) would diagnose Von Willebrand disease, which is also not suspected in this vignette.

Reducing the hydrocortisone dosage (Answer E) is incorrect because a dosage within the recommended range of 10 to 15 mg/m^2 per day is unlikely cause of the symptom of bruising and would not be the cause of joint pain.

Educational Objective

Diagnose CAH-X syndrome.

Reference(s)

Burch GH, Gong Y, Liu W, et al. Tenascin-X deficiency is associated with Ehlers-Danlos syndrome. *Nat Genet.* 1997;17(1):104-108. PMID: 9288108

Lao Q, Merke DP. Molecular genetic testing of congenital adrenal hyperplasia due to 21-hydroxylase deficiency should include CAH-X chimeras. *Eur J Hum Genet.* 2021;29(7):1047-1048. PMID: 33824469

Merke DP, Chen W, Morissette R, et al. Tenascin-X haploinsufficiency associated with Ehlers-Danlos syndrome in patients with congenital adrenal hyperplasia. *J Clin Endocrinol Metab.* 2013;98(2):E379-E387. PMID: 23284009

46 **ANSWER: C) Measure serum free T_4 by equilibrium dialysis**

This patient's thyroid function tests show a persistent pattern of low (free) T_4 without appropriate TSH elevation. The differential diagnosis of this pattern includes central hypothyroidism, disorders of thyroid hormone binding, nonthyroidal illness, and medication effects. The latter 2 diagnoses are unlikely in this case given the history.

This male newborn has congenital deficiency of thyroxine-binding globulin (TBG), an X-linked condition that occurs in about 1 in 5000 infants and is 9 times more common in males than in females. When serum concentrations of TBG are low, the patient has a low concentration of total T_4 but normal circulating free T_4; therefore, patients with TBG deficiency have normal TSH concentrations, are euthyroid, and require no treatment. Thus, initiating levothyroxine (Answer A) is incorrect. However, states of markedly abnormal thyroid hormone binding may confound the measurement of free T_4 concentrations by many common direct immunoassays, which are designed for use in normal individuals with typical thyroid hormone binding. Therefore, free T_4 concentrations measured by standard free T_4 assays may be low in up to 10% of individuals with TBG deficiency. Measurement of free T_4 by a gold-standard assay technique such as equilibrium dialysis (Answer C) may confirm that free T_4 concentrations are normal, establishing the diagnosis of TBG deficiency rather than central hypothyroidism.

Central hypothyroidism must also be considered but is unlikely in this case. The patient has no clinical signs of hypothyroidism, although these signs may not be apparent in the first few weeks of life. In addition, most cases of congenital central hypothyroidism (65%-85%) are accompanied by additional pituitary hormone deficits. Evaluation of possible central hypothyroidism should include assessment for features such as hypoglycemia, hypotension, direct hyperbilirubinemia, microphallus, undescended testes, or polyuria. A cleft palate, other midline defects, or neurological features may suggest a structural brain lesion, and abnormal or roving eye movements may suggest optic nerve hypoplasia. The absence of any of these clinical findings in this patient makes central hypothyroidism much less likely, and cosyntropin-stimulation testing (Answer D) or MRI of the brain (Answer E) is less likely to yield a diagnosis than confirming the free T_4 concentration by equilibrium dialysis.

Familial dysalbuminemic hyperthyroxinemia is caused by a variant in the gene encoding albumin that increases the binding affinity of albumin for T_4, and in some cases for T_3. This abnormality leads to a pattern of high total T_4 concentrations with normal TSH, which may be mistaken for central hyperthyroidism (not the pattern observed in this patient). However, because free T_4 levels are normal, individuals with familial dysalbuminemic hyperthyroxinemia are euthyroid and no treatment is necessary. Serum albumin concentrations are not altered in this condition (Answer B), and although the albumin gene can be sequenced, this diagnosis is usually made clinically.

Educational Objective

Diagnose thyroxine-binding globulin deficiency.

Reference(s)

Connelly KJ, Pierce MJ, Hanna C, LaFranchi SH. Detecting congenital central hypothyroidism by newborn screening: difficulty in distinguishing from congenital thyroxine-binding globulin deficiency. *Horm Res Paediatr.* 2017;88(5):331-338. PMID: 28910808

Csako G, Zweig MH, Ruddel M, Glickman J, Kestner J. Direct and indirect techniques for free thyroxin compared in patients with nonthyroidal illness. III. Analysis of interference variables by stepwise regression. *Clin Chem.* 1990;36(4):645-650. PMID: 2136246

Lauffer P, Zwaveling-Soonawala N, Naafs JC, Boelen A, van Trotsenburg ASP. Diagnosis and management of central congenital hypothyroidism. *Front Endocrinol (Lausanne).* 2021;12:686317. PMID: 34566885

47 **ANSWER: E) Re-educate about the timely entry of all carbohydrates before meal consumption**

Management of type 1 diabetes has changed rapidly over the past 2 decades and is becoming increasingly dependent on technology. Several hybrid closed-loop systems are commercially available or in clinical trials, each with unique features to improve care for patients with type 1 diabetes. These systems incorporate continuous glucose monitoring values into an algorithm that adjusts the amount of insulin delivered. Current systems require the user to input carbohydrate intake for meals and glucose values for correction boluses while the system automates the basal insulin infusion to a target sensor glucose. Although these systems improve glycemic time in range, they still require input from the user and significant education to optimize glycemic control.

In this vignette, a 15-year-old patient is self-managing diabetes by keeping the system in automation 95% to 100% of the time, suggesting that he is well-versed in completing required checks to reach such high efficiency. A typical pitfall of the system is the automated increased rate of basal insulin delivery for any elevation detected by the glucose sensor, especially if the carbohydrate amounts are not entered on time (before consumption). For this reason, this patient is receiving an average of 60% of the daily total insulin as "basal," which is misleading because some of that insulin is delivered for correction due to elevated sensor glucose. Many patients enter the carbohydrate amount of the consumed meal or snack when they notice the elevation in the sensor glucose. Combination of insulin calculated for the programmed carbohydrate ratio and the insulin delivered attempting to "correct" sensor glucose to the target range causes stacking of insulin. This leads to hypoglycemia a few hours later when insulin action time is near complete. To avoid this risk, the patient should be educated about the importance of timely entry of carbohydrate amounts into the pump before consumption (Answer E). The improvement will not only help with the patient's concern regarding hypoglycemia but will also help minimize blood glucose excursions and therefore improve glycemic control (target time in range >70% and target hemoglobin A_{1c} <7.0% [<53 mmol/mol]).

Increasing the insulin amount for all meals (Answer B) without first improving the timing of carbohydrate entry would lead to more severe hypoglycemic episodes.

Activating "exercise/activity" mode (Answer A) raises target glucose levels to prevent potential hypoglycemia during physical activity/exercise. While activating the exercise/activity mode after a meal bolus could effectively mitigate the risk of hypoglycemia, it could become a cumbersome task to remember and complete after each meal. Moreover, this strategy would not address postprandial hyperglycemia or contribute to overall glycemic control. However, using the exercise/activity mode is an effective method to preempt the risk of hypoglycemia associated with exercise, especially when activated 90 to 120 minutes before commencing exercise.

Lowering the insulin amount calculated by the correction (insulin sensitivity) factor (Answer D) would help if the hypoglycemia were due to manual (or automated) correction bolus. In this vignette, there is no indication of a correction bolus administered either by the patient or by the pump that would lead to hypoglycemia. However, in some automated systems, a "correction bolus" is delivered for hyperglycemia by using (at least partially) insulin sensitivity.

Lowering the basal rate in the immediate postprandial period (Answer C) also does not have an impact because most automated systems determine the basal insulin infusion rate depending on the sensor glucose and target glucose set for that time.

Patients using hybrid closed-loop systems need to be aware that these automated systems do not eliminate the risk of severe hypoglycemia.

Educational Objective

Analyze data from an insulin pump download to optimize glycemic control in a patient using an automated hybrid closed-loop pump system.

Reference(s)

Buckingham BA, Forlenza GP, Criego AB, et al. Safety evaluation of the Omnipod® 5 automated insulin delivery system over three months of use in children with type 1 diabetes (T1D). *J Endocr Soc.* 2021;5(Suppl 1):A454.

Steenkamp DW, Piarulli A, Middelbeek RJW, Wolpert HA. Severe hypoglycaemia while using a hybrid closed-loop insulin pump system: a reminder of the continued importance of patient education for pre-emptive hypoglycaemia mitigation. *Diabet Med.* 2023;40(3):e14975. PMID: 36251520

48 **ANSWER: D) Pituitary hyperplasia**

In both children and adults with primary hypothyroidism (Answer D), TSH elevation from lack of feedback inhibition from thyroid hormone can be substantial, so much so that thyrotroph hyperplasia can lead to clinically apparent pituitary enlargement, as in this case. Associated complications, including mass effects, visual deficits, and deficiencies of other pituitary hormones, have also been described. Prolactin elevation also occurs because significantly increased thyrotropin-releasing hormone levels, as observed in untreated primary hypothyroidism, can stimulate lactotrophs and thyrotrophs. Thyroid hormone replacement typically leads to prompt decrease in pituitary size. Rarely, treatment of severe primary hypothyroidism can be accompanied by the development of pseudotumor cerebri syndrome and associated visual complications that add complexity. Follow-up imaging should be performed to exclude the very rare possibility of a co-occurrence between primary hypothyroidism and unrelated nonfunctional pituitary adenoma.

Overlooking the diagnostic possibility that primary hypothyroidism can cause pituitary hyperplasia can lead to unnecessary neurosurgical procedures. Thus, clinicians should be alert for this rare but well-described entity. A recent review summarized 110 reported cases of pituitary hyperplasia following primary hypothyroidism in pediatric patients. As expected, given the female predominance of autoimmune primary hypothyroidism (the most common cause), 74% of patients were female, and although most were school-aged, this phenomenon has been reported in children as young as 3 weeks of age. Affected children come to medical attention for growth attenuation (present in 78%), constipation (36%), and/or features of myxedema (18%). On average, it takes 7.2 months (range, 1-26 months) for pituitary hyperplasia and the associated abnormalities to resolve after treatment initiation. Clinicians may also be familiar with other potential endocrine manifestations of severe primary hypothyroidism, including galactorrhea and precocious puberty, often called Van Wyk Grumbach syndrome, in recognition of the 2 physicians who first described this entity in 1960.

Although prolactin elevation is common, hyperplasia of prolactin-producing pituitary cells in response to thyrotropin-releasing hormone, not a prolactin-producing adenoma, is the cause of hyperprolactinemia with TSH elevation. Macroprolactinomas (Answer B) can sometimes produce central hypothyroidism, in which case TSH is expected to be low. Also, a prolactinoma of this size would typically have higher concentrations of prolactin, and the lack of more substantial hyperprolactinemia was confirmed with serial dilution of the specimen (ie, no hook effect was present).

Although TSH-secreting pituitary adenomas (Answer E) have been described, these types of tumors would not be associated with undetectable free T_4. These tumors are also very rare, especially in children, and pituitary hyperplasia in response to primary hypothyroidism is the more likely cause. To distinguish the 2 etiologies (if the free T_4 is not clearly suggestive of hypothyroidism), a brief trial of high-dosage thyroid hormone and/or an acute T_3-suppression test could be pursued in appropriately selected patients.

Nonfunctioning pituitary macroadenomas (Answer C) are rare in children and might be expected to produce prolactin increase via pituitary stalk disruption, but this would not explain TSH elevation.

Craniopharyngiomas (Answer A) are brain tumors that affect the hypothalamus and pituitary in children. They often present with mass effect, including prolactin elevation from stalk disruption, and/or multiple pituitary hormone deficiencies, but they would not be expected to be associated with substantial TSH elevation. Instead, TSH would be low, normal, or mildly increased, as in central hypothyroidism.

Note: Image in the vignette is reprinted from Sarlis NJ, Brucker-Davis F, Doppman JL, Skarulis MC. MRI-demonstrable regression of a pituitary mass in a case of primary hypothyroidism after a week of acute thyroid hormone therapy. J Clin Endocrinol Metab. *1997;82(3):808-811.*

Educational Objective

Explain the relationship between pituitary hyperplasia and primary hypothyroidism.

Reference(s)

Bowers CY, Friesen HG, Folkers K. Further evidence that TRH is also a physiological regulator of PRL secretion in man. *Biochem Biophysical Res Commun.* 1973;51(3):512-521. PMID: 4634111

Passeri E, Tufano A, Locatelli M, Lania AG, Ambrosi B, Corbetta S. Large pituitary hyperplasia in severe primary hypothyroidism. *J Clin Endocrinol Metab.* 2011;96(1):22-23. PMID: 21209043

Sarlis NJ, Brucker-Davis F, Doppman JL, Skarulis MC. MRI-demonstrable regression of a pituitary mass in a case of primary hypothyroidism after a week of acute thyroid hormone therapy. *J Clin Endocrinol Metab.* 1997;82(3):808-811. PMID: 9062487

Sapkota S, Karn M, Sapkota S. Pituitary hyperplasia in childhood primary hypothyroidism: a review. *Childs Nerv Syst.* 2021;37(3):749-762. PMID: 33404718

Van Wyk JJ, Grumbach MM. Syndrome of precocious menstruation and galactorrhea in juvenile hypothyroidism: an example of hormonal overlap in pituitary feedback. *J Pediatrics.* 1960;57(3):416-435.

49 ANSWER: A) Disease state, active; disease severity, mild; recommendation, observation

This patient has Graves disease with hyperthyroidism and high thyroid-stimulating immunoglobulin. She also has evidence of thyroid eye disease. She is hyperthyroid at presentation, has mild eye symptoms, and is starting antithyroid medication. Improvement in eye symptoms is expected with control of hyperthyroidism. She should also be advised of the importance of avoiding cigarette smoking and passive smoke exposure.

Thyroid eye disease occurs most commonly in Graves disease but is occasionally seen in patients who are euthyroid or have immune-mediated hypothyroidism. Thyroid eye disease is observed almost exclusively in patients who have circulating thyrotropin-receptor antibodies. Both the TSH receptor and the IGF-1 receptor are important targets in the disease, and their stimulation on orbital fibroblasts results in inflammation, adipogenesis, and tissue remodeling. The disease is characterized by distinct phases: (1) an active phase when infiltration of orbital tissues, edema, and adipogenesis occur and (2) an inactive phase when fat infiltration and fibrosis are prominent. Thyroid eye disease is less common in children, and it is typically milder than in adults.

When evaluating a patient with thyroid eye disease, clinical activity and disease severity should be assessed independently. A commonly used clinical activity score assigns 1 point to each of the following 7 items:

- Spontaneous retrobulbar pain
- Pain on upward or lateral gaze
- Redness of the eyelids
- Redness of the conjunctiva
- Swelling of the eyelids
- Swelling of the conjunctiva (chemosis)
- Inflammation of the caruncle or plica

A score of 3 or higher or a subjective history of worsening of any thyroid eye disease symptoms suggests active disease.

Disease severity is classified into 3 categories:

- Mild: Disease features have only a minor impact on daily life.
- Moderate to severe: No sight-threatening disease but the effect on daily life is sufficient to warrant more aggressive therapy and the potential risks that treatment entails. These patients often have more significant lid lag and proptosis, diplopia, and marked inflammatory changes.
- Sight-threatening: The threat to vision can come from optic neuropathy, corneal abrasions, or subluxation of the globe.

This patient has active disease (clinical activity score = 4 for redness of conjunctiva, redness of eyelids, swelling of conjunctiva, and swelling of eyelids) of mild severity (the features have a minor impact on daily life) (Answer A).

Teprotumumab (Answer B and E) is a human IGF-1 receptor inhibitory monoclonal antibody and is FDA approved for the treatment of thyroid eye disease in patients who are 18 years and older. The medication is not approved in children due to concerns about growth. TSH-receptor antibodies interact with TSH receptors and IGF-1 receptors on orbital fibroblasts and promote inflammation. Studies have shown that teprotumumab decreases disease activity level, proptosis, and diplopia. The medication is given as an intravenous infusion in 8 doses, administered every 3 weeks. Adverse effects include muscle cramps, nausea, alopecia, fatigue, and hearing impairment (which may persist after completion of therapy). Although the medication is FDA approved, it is not recommended as first-line therapy for mild disease and is typically reserved for patients with active moderate to severe disease, especially in those with significant proptosis.

Orbital surgery (Answer C) is not recommended for this patient, at least right now. She has proptosis with normal vision and normal eye movements, which may improve with stabilization of her thyroid function. Proptosis that does not threaten sight can still have a clinically significant impact on quality of life, and surgery can be considered in such cases. However, in the absence of urgent surgical intervention for sight-threatening disease (eg, urgent decompression for dysthyroid optic neuropathy), surgery should only occur when a patient is euthyroid and during the inactive phase of the disease.

Observation for inactive mild disease (Answer D) is incorrect because this patient has active disease.

Educational Objective

Determine both disease activity and disease severity when assessing children with thyroid eye disease and explain how these designations guide treatment choices.

Reference(s)

Burch H, Perros P, Bednarczuk T, et al. Management of thyroid eye disease: a consensus statement by the American Thyroid Association and the European Thyroid Association. *Thyroid*. 2022;32(12):1439-1470. PMID: 36480280

Chua MR, Tomlinson LA, Binenbaum G, Katowitz WR. Pediatric thyroid eye disease: clinical characteristics and orbital decompression outcomes. *Ophthal Plast Reconstr Surg*. 2018;34(4S Suppl 1):S52-S55. PMID: 29985836

50 **ANSWER: C) GH deficiency**

This patient has a classic presentation of GH deficiency with a fall-off in height percentiles due to subnormal growth velocity and preserved weight gain. Her IGF-1 concentration is low. Although there is a grandparent with short stature, this progressive decline in height SD score is not consistent with familial short stature (Answer B). Additionally, the very low IGF-1 value and severity of growth deceleration make GH deficiency much more likely than constitutional delay (Answer A).

The patient has proportionate short stature, which makes a *SHOX* deletion (Answer D) unlikely.

While Turner syndrome (Answer E) is a consideration, the IGF-1 level should not be low in that setting.

This case scenario raises the very important point about delayed diagnosis of GH deficiency (Answer C) in girls and in minority patients. Large postmarketing databases of GH use show significant sex- and race-based disparities. Male patients and White patients are much more likely to be treated with GH than female patients and patients from racial and ethnic minority populations. These treatment disparities reflect differences in referrals, parental desires, and the diagnostic and therapeutic decisions of pediatric endocrinologists.

In addition to the large referral biases that lead to fewer female and minority patients being evaluated for short stature, recent studies also shed light on the likelihood of an endocrinologist ordering GH-stimulation tests, as well as initiating treatment based on the test results. A large retrospective study of 7425 children referred for growth evaluation examined the role of race. NonHispanic White patients were 1.4 times more likely than nonHispanic Black patients to undergo GH-stimulation testing. Once a GH-stimulation test was performed, patients with a GH peak less than 7.0 ng/mL (<7.0 µg/L) had similar GH therapy initiation rates regardless of race (~90% in all racial and ethnic groups). However, nonHispanic Black patients with GH peaks between 7 and 10 ng/mL (7-10 µg/L) were less likely than nonHispanic White patients to be treated with GH (53% vs 77%; *P* = .04).

In a separate study, male patients referred for short stature were more likely than female patients to have a GH-stimulation test performed. Female patients, on average, had lower height Z-scores than male patients at the time of evaluation. However, once a stimulation test was performed, the proportion of patients who received a GH prescription at a given peak GH value was similar regardless of sex.

Educational Objective

Discuss the racial-, ethnic-, and sex-based biases in the diagnostic and therapeutic approach to patients with short stature.

Reference(s)

Hawkes CP, Gunturi H, Dauber A, Hirschhorn JN, Grimberg A. Racial and ethnic disparities in the investigation and treatment of growth hormone deficiency. *J Pediatr.* 2021;236:238-245. PMID: 33901521

Kamoun C, Hawkes CP, Gunturi H, Dauber A, Hirschhorn JN, Grimberg A. Growth hormone stimulation testing patterns contribute to sex differences in pediatric growth hormone treatment. *Horm Res Paediatr.* 2021;94(9-10):353-363. PMID: 34662877

51 **ANSWER: A) Broadening of the medial tibial physis**

This adolescent has Blount disease, also known as tibia vara. Blount disease is a disorder of the growth plates around the knee in which there is asymmetric growth of the proximal tibia. The main radiographic finding is broadening of the medial tibial physis (Answer A), although other abnormalities are also observed, such as a wedge-shaped epiphysis, tibial shaft in the varus position, and femoral deformities. Blount disease has 2 clinical variants: an early-onset form of the condition, also called infantile Blount disease, and a late-onset or adolescent form, the latter of which occurs after age 10 years. Approximately 50% of cases in adolescents are bilateral. While the etiology appears multifactorial, excessive compressive forces lead to a relative lack of growth of the medial proximal tibial physis, which alters bone formation and causes progressive genu varum. Risk factors for adolescent Blount disease include severe obesity and Afro-Caribbean ethnicity. Blount disease can be diagnosed by obtaining long-leg anteroposterior radiographs of both legs. This condition should be suspected in patients with obesity who present with knee pain, particularly on the medial aspect. All patients with suspected Blount disease must be referred for orthopedic evaluation and management, which is typically surgical.

Swelling of the tibial tuberosity (Answer D) is seen with Osgood-Schlatter disease, which is a cause of frequent knee pain in adolescents. In patients with Osgood-Schlatter disease, there is inflammation, swelling, and pain in the area below the knee where the patellar tendon attaches to the tibia. It most often occurs during periods of rapid growth and is more common in children who are very physically active in sports. The symptoms are often worse with running/jumping. Typically, affected children describe knee pain and tenderness at the tibial tuberosity. An x-ray is not absolutely necessary to make the diagnosis.

Thickening of the proximal patellar tendon (Answer E) is seen with Sinding-Larsen-Johansson syndrome. Sinding-Larsen-Johansson is an injury to the growth plate of the knee, which typically affects children between the ages of 10 and 14 years. It is almost always due to overuse from playing sports. Sinding-Larsen-Johansson syndrome shares a lot of commonalities with Osgood-Schlatter disease; however, the location of the injury is different. In Sinding-Larsen-Johansson syndrome, the injury is to the top of the patellar tendon. In both conditions, rest and anti-inflammatory medications are typically the recommended treatment.

Lucencies in the articular epiphysis (Answer C) are seen in osteochondritis dissecans, which is a condition that affects the joints, most commonly the knee, in children and adolescents. In osteochondritis dissecans, a small segment of bone starts to separate due to a lack of blood supply. While the exact etiology is unknown, repeated trauma/stress to the joint from playing sports, for example, and possible genetic factors are thought to have a role. Symptoms include pain and swelling of the affected joint that is often made worse by activity, a feeling that the joint is "giving way" or "locking and catching," or decreased range of joint motion.

In patients with metaphyseal chondrodysplasia, radiographs show metaphyseal irregularities of the long bones, such as enlarged metaphyses and widened cupped physes (Answer B). Metaphyseal chondrodysplasia is an autosomal dominant skeletal dysplasia. Individuals with this condition typically exhibit short stature by age 2 years characterized by shortened limbs, genu varum, and a waddling gait.

Educational Objective

Diagnose Blount disease in adolescents and guide the appropriate diagnostic workup.

Reference(s)

de Pablos J, Arbeloa-Gutierrez L, Arenas-Miquelez A. Update on treatment of adolescent Blount disease. *Curr Opin Pediatr.* 2018;30(1):71-77. PMID: 29315109

Janoyer M. Blount disease. *Orthop Traumatol Surg Res.* 2019;105(1S):S111-S121. PMID: 29481866

52 ANSWER: B) Follow-up assessment and repeated hemoglobin A_{1c} measurement in 3 months

Prediabetes is an intermediate state between normal glucose homeostasis and type 2 diabetes. In the 2005-2006 National Health and Nutrition Examination Survey, the overall prevalence of prediabetes among adolescents in the United States was 16.1%. While individuals with prediabetes are asymptomatic, there is evidence of associations between prediabetes and early forms of nephropathy, neuropathy, diabetic retinopathy, and macrovascular disease.

The annualized incidence of type 2 diabetes in adults with prediabetes is between 7% and 10%, and it has been estimated that approximately 70% of adults with prediabetes eventually progress to diabetes. While youth-onset type 2 diabetes is more aggressive than in adults, children and adolescents with prediabetes may revert to normal glucose metabolism at higher rates than adults. GH and IGF-1 levels contribute to the normal physiologic decrease in insulin sensitivity that occurs in puberty. As these hormone levels decrease towards the end of puberty, insulin sensitivity improves, contributing to a higher rate of reversion to normoglycemia in late adolescence. Thus, different interventions are indicated. A US study of 526 adolescents with obesity and dysglycemia at baseline reported that 65% reverted to normoglycemia, 27% had persistent dysglycemia, and 8% progressed to type 2 diabetes. In a cohort of White Canadian children with prediabetes at baseline and a parental history of obesity, 73% of children aged 8 to 10 years and 53% of children aged 10 to 12 years reverted to normoglycemia by age 17 years.

While there is no consensus on how often testing should be performed in youth with prediabetes, it is reasonable to repeat testing in this patient in 3 months (or sooner if progression to diabetes is suspected) (Answer B). A comprehensive review by Magge et al in 2020 presented an algorithm that starts with lifestyle modifications and education on symptoms of diabetes with follow-up after 3 months to assess progress and hemoglobin A_{1c}. While the optimal strategy for identifying prediabetes is still a matter of debate, current American Diabetes Association and International Society for Pediatric and Adolescent Diabetes guidelines consider fasting plasma glucose, oral glucose tolerance testing, and hemoglobin A_{1c} all acceptable to diagnose prediabetes and diabetes in youth. Thus, oral glucose tolerance testing (Answer D) is not needed.

Lifestyle intervention via improved nutrition, increased physical activity, and decreased sedentary activity is the cornerstone to prediabetes management, targeting the most important modifiable risk factors for developing diabetes. While data on treatment of prediabetes in youth are limited, there is some evidence that intensive lifestyle modification can reduce BMI and improve insulin sensitivity.

Currently there are no FDA-approved pharmacologic agents for treatment of prediabetes in youth. Metformin (Answer C) has been shown to improve insulin sensitivity and modestly lower BMI in some studies, while other clinical trials failed to show an effect on progression to diabetes. As such, addition of metformin after 6 months of attempted lifestyle intervention may be helpful if hemoglobin A_{1c} remains above 6.0% (>42 mmol/mol) but there is no consensus on this treatment. Adding metformin at this patient's initial endocrine encounter would not be the best option because existing data do not show a convincing benefit in this scenario. Semaglutide (Answer E) is indicated as an adjunct to diet and exercise for chronic weight management in patients 12 years and older with a BMI at the 95th percentile or greater, but it is not FDA approved to treat prediabetes. While this patient may be able to lose some weight with semaglutide, he does not meet BMI or hemoglobin A_{1c} criteria for use of this medication.

While this patient's laboratory test results are consistent with mixed dyslipidemia, current American Heart Association guidelines recommend statin therapy for children and adolescents with an LDL-cholesterol concentration persistently greater than 190 mg/dL (>4.92 mmol/L) (or >160 mg/dL [>4.14 mmol/L] in the context of familial hypercholesterolemia) despite 3 to 6 months of lifestyle intervention. Although American Diabetes Association guidelines recommend statin therapy for those with diabetes if LDL cholesterol remains greater than 130 mg/dL (>3.37 mmol/L) after 6 months of dietary intervention, these criteria do not apply to those with prediabetes. Thus, treatment with atorvastatin (Answer A) is not indicated for this patient.

Educational Objective

Initiate management of prediabetes in children and adolescents.

Reference(s)

Galderisi A, Giannini C, Weiss R, et al. Trajectories of changes in glucose tolerance in a multiethnic cohort of obese youths: an observational prospective analysis. *Lancet Child Adolesc Health.* 2018; 2:726–735. PMID: 30236381

Harnois-Leblanc S, Van Hulst A, Ybarra M, et al. Natural history and determinants of dysglycemia in Canadian children with parental obesity from ages 8-10 to 15-17 years: The QUALITY cohort. *Pediatr Diabetes.* 2022;23(3):274-285. PMID: 35023257

Magge SN, Silverstein J, Elder D, Nadeau K, Hannon TS. Evaluation and treatment of prediabetes in youth. *J Pediatr.* 2020;219:11-22. PMID: 32143933

Ng HY, Chan LTW. Prediabetes in children and adolescents: an updated review. *World J Clin Pediatr.* 2023;12(5):263-272. PMID: 38178932

53 ANSWER: A) Calculation of sitting height-to-standing height ratio

In a child with unexplained short stature, assessment of proportionality is required before determining which investigations are required. Various approaches to identifying disproportionate short stature have been described, including measurement of arm span, sitting height, and upper-to-lower segment or sitting height-to-standing height ratios (Answer A). This assessment can be performed during the clinic visit and would thus be the appropriate next step in this case.

Assessing proportionality in children can be challenging, as body proportions change throughout childhood. At 1 year of age, sitting height represents almost two-thirds of body length. In adolescence, sitting height accounts for approximately 50% of body length. Sitting height represents a greater proportion of body size in non-Hispanic White children than in non-Hispanic Black children, indicating that ethnicity-specific reference data should be used when assessing whether a child's proportions are within the expected range.

When a skeletal dysplasia is suspected, a skeletal survey (Answer E) does not always identify an anomaly. In one retrospective review, approximately one-third of children with a skeletal dysplasia did not have the diagnosis made on skeletal survey. Thus, genetic testing may be indicated in the setting of clinical suspicion even when the skeletal survey is normal.

While celiac disease and GH deficiency are causes of short stature, testing for these conditions (Answers B and C) would not be the best next step before completing the anthropometric assessment.

Although this boy's parents have short stature, reassurance (Answer D) would not be correct without first performing a complete assessment, including assessment of proportionality.

Educational Objective

Evaluate for disproportionate short stature in a child.

Reference(s)

Dauber A, Rosenfeld RG, Hirschhorn JN. Genetic evaluation of short stature. *J Clin Endocrinol Metab.* 2014;99(9):3080-3092. PMID: 24915122

Fredriks AM, van Buuren S, van Heel WJ, Dijkman-Neerincx RH, Verloove-Vanhorick SP, Wit JM. Nationwide age references for sitting height, leg length, and sitting height/height ratio, and their diagnostic value for disproportionate growth disorders. *Arch Dis Child.* 2005;90(8):807-812. PMID: 15863466

Hawkes CP, Mostoufi-Moab S, McCormack SE, Grimberg A, Zemel BS. Sitting Height to standing height ratio reference charts for children in the United States. *J Pediatr.* 2020;226:221-227.e15. PMID: 32579888

Mazicioglu MM, Hatipoglu N, Ozturk A, Gun I, Ustunbas HB, Kurtoglu S. Age references for the arm span and stature of Turkish children and adolescents. *Ann Hum Biol.* 2009;36(3):308-319. PMID: 19274587

Veeramani AK, Higgins P, Butler S, et al. Diagnostic use of skeletal survey in suspected skeletal dysplasia. *J Clin Res Pediatr Endocrinol.* 2009;1(6):270-274. PMID: 21274308

54 **ANSWER: A) Measure serum 17-hydroxyprogesterone, testosterone, electrolytes, and plasma renin**
The most common cause of atypical genitalia in 46,XX newborns is congenital adrenal hyperplasia (CAH) due to 21-hydroxylase deficiency (21-OHD), and it should be part of the differential diagnosis and initial diagnostic workup of differences of sex development. A negative newborn screen for CAH does not exclude the diagnosis of classic CAH due to 21-OHD. Thus, reassuring the baby's family that she does not have CAH (Answer D) would be incorrect at this point. Newborn screening identifies infants who may have CAH, but the diagnosis is made after referral to a pediatric endocrinologist and initial confirmatory testing that includes measurement of 17-hydroxyprogesterone (17-OHP), electrolytes, and plasma renin (Answer A). Although electrolytes and plasma renin may be normal at birth, hyponatremia, hyperkalemia, and low blood glucose may be present by 8 days of life in affected newborns. In this case, testosterone should be included in the workup to evaluate whether increased testosterone production from either the adrenal glands or gonads may have led to clitoromegaly.

Although most females with classic CAH present with Prader stage 2 to 3 external genitalia, there are affected female newborns who present on a spectrum ranging from severe virilization and penile urethra (Prader stage V) to mild clitoromegaly (Prader stage I) or no clitoromegaly. Prader classification depicts the increasing degrees of virilization of the female internal and external genitalia (*see figure*). The different stages are defined as follows:

- Stage I: clitoral enlargement
- Stage II: clitoral enlargement, partial labioscrotal fusion, and a funnel-shaped urogenital sinus
- Stage III: increased phallus size with complete labioscrotal fusion forming a urogenital sinus at the base of the penis
- Stage IV: further increased phallus size and further elongated urogenital sinus
- Stage V: female with normal male-appearing penile urethra

Figure. Prader Classification

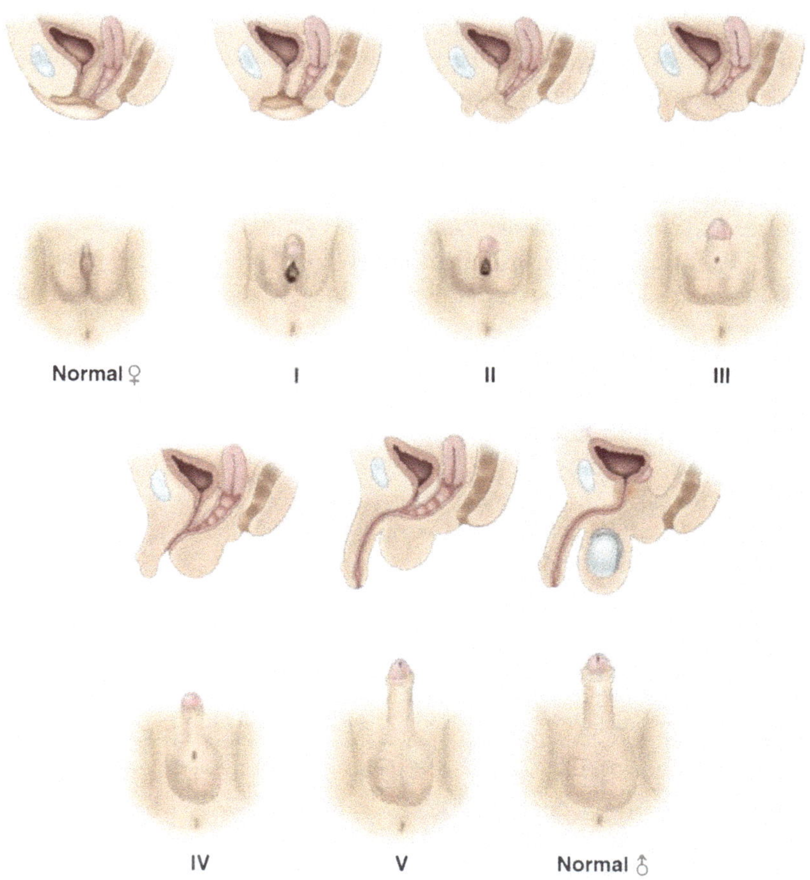

Reprinted with permission from Sarafoglou K, Hoffmann GF & Roth KS, eds. *Pediatric Endocrinology and Inborn Errors of Metabolism.* 2nd edition. New York, NY: McGraw-Hill Education; 2017. © The McGraw-Hill Companies, Inc.

State newborn screening programs use a fluoroimmunoassay to measure 17-OHP from a dried blood spot, which is typically collected on filter paper between 24 and 36 hours of life. There is a generally held belief that newborn screening can detect almost all cases of classic CAH and that this screening has 100% sensitivity. However, several studies have reported false-negative rates ranging from 2.5% to 30% with one-tier 17-OHP testing at 1 to 2 days of life. Several states that routinely test repeat specimens collected at approximately 2 weeks of age have reported missing as many as one-third of CAH cases on the first screen.

One explanation for false-negative CAH newborn screening results could be a delayed rise in 17-OHP due to the influence of intrauterine biological factors on the fetal hypothalamic-pituitary-adrenal (HPA) axis causing 17-OHP levels to be transiently lower at 24 to 48 hours of life when the blood spot sample is collected. During pregnancy, the fetus is protected from most maternal cortisol, as maternal cortisol cannot reach the fetus because it is oxidized to the inactive form of cortisone by the placental enzyme 11β-hydroxysteroid dehydrogenase (11β-HSD2). Pathogenic variants in the *HSD11B2* gene may alter enzyme activity, allowing a greater proportion of maternal cortisol to cross into the placenta and then enter fetal circulation. In a fetus affected with CAH, a decrease in 11β-HSD2 activity would allow higher amounts of maternal cortisol in fetal circulation, leading to decreased activity of the fetal HPA axis and transiently low 17-OHP levels 24 to 48 hours after birth when the blood sample is collected for newborn screening. Another potential cause of delayed rise of 17-OHP is increased glucocorticoid sensitivity of the fetal HPA axis to maternal cortisol that crosses into fetal circulation. Specific glucocorticoid receptor haplotypes have been associated with varying glucocorticoid sensitivity, including those that cause individuals to be more sensitive to glucocorticoids. Therefore, while first-tier fluoroimmunoassay or second-tier liquid chromatography–tandem mass spectrometry may accurately capture 17-OHP concentrations at 24 to 48 hours of life, these levels may not represent the presence or absence of disease in the newborn at the time of sample collection, as steroid assays cannot account for the inherent biological factors that influence HPA-axis activity and 17-OHP levels.

A high-dose cosyntropin-stimulation test (Answer B) should not be the first test, as an elevated random serum 17-OHP concentration greater than 10,000 ng/dL (>300 nmol/L) is diagnostic of classic CAH due to 21-OHD. However, female newborns with atypical genitalia and borderline elevations of 17-OHP should undergo a high-dose cosyntropin-stimulation test to differentiate between the intermediate 21-OHD form (nonclassic/simple virilizing), 11β-hydroxylase deficiency, 3β-hydroxysteroid dehydrogenase type II deficiency, and P450 oxidoreductase deficiency (PORD). PORD is an autosomal recessive disorder due to pathogenic variants in the *POR* gene, and it has a broad clinical phenotype that includes skeletal malformations resembling the Antley-Bixler syndrome phenotype.

Pelvic ultrasonography (Answer C) should follow hormonal evaluation, as it may not be sensitive in detecting a uterus and ovaries in the neonatal period.

Genetic counseling and a gene panel for differences of sex development (Answer E) should not be the initial evaluation in a neonate with mild clitoromegaly and otherwise normal external genitalia.

Educational Objective

Rule out the diagnosis of classic congenital adrenal hyperplasia in a female newborn with clitoromegaly despite a negative newborn screening result.

Reference(s)

Held PK, Bird IM, Heather NL. Newborn screening for congenital adrenal hyperplasia: review of factors affecting screening accuracy. *Int J Neonatal Screen.* 2020;6(3):67. PMID: 33117906

Sarafoglou K, Banks K, Gaviglio A, Hietala A, McCann M, Thomas W. Comparison of one-tier and two-tier newborn screening metrics for congenital adrenal hyperplasia. *Pediatrics.* 2012;130(5):e1261-e1268. PMID: 23071209

Sarafoglou K, Banks K, Kyllo J, Pittock S, Thomas W. Cases of congenital adrenal hyperplasia missed by newborn screening in Minnesota. *JAMA.* 2012;307(22):2371-2374. PMID: 22692165

Sarafoglou K, Gaviglio A, Wolf C, et al. Can incorporating molecular testing improve the accuracy of newborn screening for congenital adrenal hyperplasia? *J Clin Endocrinol Metab.* 2024. [Online ahead of print] PMID: 38701341

Yauch L, Mayhew A, Gomez-Lobo V, Shimy K, Sarafoglou K. Nonvirilized genitalia in 3 female newborns with the salt-wasting congenital adrenal hyperplasia phenotype. *J Endocr Soc.* 2021;5(1):bvaa169. PMID: 33294764

55 ANSWER: A) Calcitonin

This child has a thyroid nodule that requires evaluation to determine whether it is benign or malignant. Most thyroid malignancies in children are papillary carcinomas (~85%) and a minority are follicular carcinomas (~10%). Medullary thyroid carcinoma (MTC) is rare in children and is usually associated with multiple endocrine neoplasia (MEN) type 2, which is caused by pathogenic variants in the *RET* proto-oncogene. Certain *RET* variants causing MEN type 2A (specifically variants in codons 609, 611, 618, and 620) are also associated with Hirschsprung disease. In this adolescent, the family history and the findings of a thyroid nodule and ipsilateral lymphadenopathy raise the possibility of a hereditary *RET* variant causing MEN type 2A and MTC. Therefore, measurement of serum calcitonin (Answer A) is important in this case. In most children with MTC, serum calcitonin is elevated at diagnosis, often markedly so (>100 pg/mL [>29.2 pmol/L]). When MTC due to an inherited *RET* variant is discovered clinically (as in this vignette) rather than through family-based screening, lymph node metastases are already present at diagnosis in two-thirds of cases.

In general, the evaluation of a thyroid nodule begins with TSH measurement to determine whether the nodule is autonomous. Radioiodine uptake (Answer C) and scintigraphy should be performed in patients with a thyroid nodule who have a low TSH concentration, which suggests a possible autonomous thyroid nodule. Measuring radioiodine uptake is not indicated for thyroid nodule evaluation unless the TSH concentration is low. Similarly, measurement of free T_4 (Answer B) is not indicated in the evaluation of a thyroid nodule unless TSH is low or there are clinical signs of hyperthyroidism.

Measurement of thyroglobulin (Answer D) is an important component of postoperative staging and surveillance for differentiated (papillary or follicular) thyroid cancer. However, measuring serum thyroglobulin is not useful or indicated for the evaluation of thyroid nodules.

Measurement of TPO antibodies (Answer E) is a diagnostic test for autoimmune thyroid disease, which can be associated with goiter but does not cause an isolated thyroid nodule. Measurement of TPO antibodies is not standard in the evaluation of thyroid nodules.

Educational Objective

Recognize Hirschsprung disease as a condition associated with multiple endocrine neoplasia type 2A and guide the appropriate evaluation.

Reference(s)

Francis GL, Waguespack SG, Bauer AJ, et al; American Thyroid Association Guidelines Task Force. Management guidelines for children with thyroid nodules and differentiated thyroid cancer. *Thyroid.* 2015;25(7):716-759. PMID: 25900731

Hensley SG, Hu MI, Bassett RL, et al. Pediatric medullary thyroid carcinoma: clinical presentations and long-term outcomes in 144 patients over 6 decades. *J Clin Endocrinol Metab.* 2024;109(9):2256-2268. PMID: 38441533

Wells SA Jr, Asa SL, Dralle H, et al; American Thyroid Association Guidelines Task Force on Medullary Thyroid Carcinoma. Revised American Thyroid Association guidelines for the management of medullary thyroid carcinoma. *Thyroid.* 2015;25(6):567-610. PMID: 25810047

56 ANSWER: E) Random GH measurement

Unlike in older children, random GH concentrations tend to be elevated in neonates. Thus, random GH measurement (Answer E) can help identify infants with sufficient GH production. In a study by Mamilly et al, a random serum GH value of 4.5 ng/mL (4.5 µg/L) had 100% sensitivity and 83% specificity for identifying neonates with congenital GH deficiency.

GH does not have a significant role in regulating in utero growth. Length of infants with congenital GH deficiency can be within the normal range. Thus, short stature is not a specific finding of GH deficiency in neonates, and this infant's normal length does not rule out GH deficiency. IGF-1, however, has a prominent role in regulating in utero growth. Infants with IGF-1 deficiency or resistance would have attenuated prenatal growth, so measuring IGF-1 (Answer D) is not the best next step.

Although GH measurement is part of the "critical sample" when investigating hypoglycemia in children, studies in older children have demonstrated that low GH levels are poorly specific for disease. Up to 70% of children without GH deficiency have concentrations below 7.5 ng/mL (<7.5 µg/L) during hypoglycemia. Thus, low GH levels during hypoglycemia (Answer A) would not be sufficient to diagnose GH deficiency. While GH-stimulation testing (Answer B) may be required if random GH concentrations are not elevated, it would not be the best next step. Random GH measurement in this case may demonstrate a sufficient GH concentration and thus GH-stimulation testing could potentially be avoided.

IGFBP-1 (Answer C) levels are low during hypoglycemic episodes in infants with hyperinsulinism, but measurement of this binding protein does not have a role in the evaluation of possible GH deficiency.

Educational Objective

Identify the most specific findings of GH deficiency in newborns.

Reference(s)

Abuzzahab MJ, Schneider A, Goddard A, et al, Intrauterine Growth Retardation Study G. IGF-I receptor mutations resulting in intrauterine and postnatal growth retardation. *N Engl J Med.* 2003;349(23):2211-2222. PMID: 14657428

Hawkes CP, Grimberg A. Measuring growth hormone and insulin-like growth factor-I in infants: what is normal? *Pediatr Endocrinol Rev.* 2013;11(2):126-146. PMID: 24575549

Kelly A, Tang R, Becker S, Stanley CA. Poor specificity of low growth hormone and cortisol levels during fasting hypoglycemia for the diagnoses of growth hormone deficiency and adrenal insufficiency. *Pediatrics.* 2008;122(3):e522-e528. PMID: 18694902

Leger J, Noel M, Limal JM, Czernichow P. Growth factors and intrauterine growth retardation. II. Serum growth hormone, insulin-like growth factor (IGF) I, and IGF-binding protein 3 levels in children with intrauterine growth retardation compared with normal control subjects: prospective study from birth to two years of age. Study Group of IUGR. *Pediatr Res.* 1996;40(1):101-107. PMID: 8798254

Mamilly L, Pyle-Eilola AL, Chaudhari M, Henry RK. The utility of a random growth hormone level in determining neonatal growth hormone sufficiency. *Clin Endocrinol (Oxf).* 2021;94(3):392-398. PMID: 33140844

57 ANSWER: A) α-Subunit

Many individuals with pituitary adenomas come to attention because they experience characteristic clinical symptoms from excess secretion of pituitary hormones by the tumor. Lactotroph adenomas can cause hyperprolactinemia and associated galactorrhea and secondary hypogonadism. Somatotroph adenomas produce GH excess and associated gigantism (in individuals continuing to experience linear growth) or acromegaly (in those in whom linear growth has ceased).

In contrast, individuals with clinically nonfunctioning pituitary adenomas, which this patient has, often come to attention when imaging is done for an unrelated indication, or from mass effect (eg, headache from elevated intracranial pressure, vision loss from chiasmic compression). This patient had mild prolactin elevation, likely from pituitary stalk disruption (pathology did not show differentiated lactotrophs, and a prolactinoma of this size would be expected to produce much higher prolactin values), leading to galactorrhea. She also had evolving pituitary hormone deficits (central hypothyroidism) and visual deficits that may have produced symptoms over time.

Unlike individuals with excess secretion of pituitary hormones, monitoring for recurrence or growth of any residual nonfunctional pituitary adenoma typically requires serial imaging, which this patient should undergo. Prolactin elevation in this patient was most likely due to stalk disruption and/or possibly localized weak tumor prolactin production not observed on immunohistochemistry. Ongoing surveillance of prolactin could be potentially useful if any of these processes recurred.

Additionally, a subset of individuals with nonfunctional pituitary adenomas have elevated circulating levels of free α-subunit (Answer A) that can thus serve as a tumor biomarker over time. Free α-subunit, if elevated at diagnosis, can serve as a proxy measure of tumor burden. Preoperative measurement of α-subunit could be considered in individuals with a suspected nonfunctional pituitary adenoma and planned surgical resection. The common α-subunit can combine with each of 3 separate specific β-subunits to form LH, FSH, and TSH, respectively. These pituitary glycoprotein hormones are also sometimes produced by pituitary adenomas, but this patient had prepubertal gonadotropins and inappropriately normal TSH (ie, central hypothyroidism), and pathology was negative for TSH. Thus, TSH measurement (Answer E) is incorrect.

While some pituitary tumors also secrete GH and/or evolve to have this capacity, GH staining was negative and IGF-1 was within the reference range, thus α-subunit is the more likely meaningful biomarker. IGF-1 (Answer D) will be monitored, along with 8-AM cortisol (Answer B), to detect evolving evidence of multiple pituitary hormone deficiencies, but these measurements would be indirect measures of tumor recurrence.

While hCG (Answer C) can be a circulating marker of germ-cell tumors, the patient does not have this tumor type.

Educational Objective

Explain the relevance of α-subunit secretion in nonfunctional pituitary adenomas.

Reference(s)

Asa SL, Mete O, Perry A, Osamura RY. Overview of the 2022 WHO classification of pituitary tumors. *Endocr Pathol.* 2022;33(1):6-26. PMID: 35291028

Gupta S, Hoffman SE, Mehta NH, et al. Elevated risk of recurrence and retreatment for silent pituitary adenomas. *Pituitary.* 2024;27(2):204-212. PMID: 38345720

Oppenheim DS, Kana AR, Sangha JS, Klibanski A. Prevalence of alpha-subunit hypersecretion in patients with pituitary tumors: clinically nonfunctioning and somatotroph adenomas. *J Clin Endocrinol Metab.* 1990;70(4):859-864. PMID: 1690748

Shomali ME, Katznelson L. Medical therapy of gonadotropin-producing and nonfunctioning pituitary adenomas. *Pituitary.* 2002;5(2):89-98. PMID: 12675506

58 ANSWER: B) Reassure her that no thyroid intervention is needed; semaglutide can be prescribed if indicated

This patient has subclinical hypothyroidism and no evidence of thyroid autoimmunity based on thyroid autoantibody testing. Thyroid ultrasonography shows a mildly enlarged thyroid gland and loss of homogeneity with generalized hypoechogenicity. These laboratory and ultrasound findings are common in patients with obesity; therefore, no thyroid intervention is needed (Answer B). The mechanism is not entirely understood but is thought to be related to the proinflammatory state induced in patients with obesity. Multiple inflammatory cytokines have been shown to impair the sodium-iodide symporter system, resulting in a compensatory rise in TSH. In addition, inflammatory cytokines may cause vasodilation and increased permeability of thyroid vessels, resulting in thyroid parenchymal changes on ultrasonography. Studies in both adults and children with obesity show that these laboratory and ultrasound changes improve with weight loss. The appropriate intervention for this patient is to help support her in weight-loss measures. GLP-1 receptor agonists such as semaglutide are highly effective agents for treating obesity. Rodent studies suggest an association between use of GLP-1 receptor agonists and development of medullary thyroid cancer. This has resulted in a black box warning for these agents in patients at risk for medullary thyroid cancer. There is no proof of any association with other types of thyroid cancer. There is no reason to suspect that this patient is at increased risk of medullary thyroid cancer: she has no family history of thyroid cancer, she has a smooth thyroid gland on palpation, and no nodules were detected on ultrasonography. Thus, semaglutide is not contraindicated in her case.

Initiation of levothyroxine (Answer E) is not needed because this patient has a mildly elevated TSH value, normal free T_4 value, and no evidence of thyroid autoimmunity. Even if overt hypothyroidism were present, initiation of levothyroxine should not delay the start of a GLP-1 receptor agonist if its use is indicated.

When patients present with subclinical hypothyroidism, follow-up thyroid function tests (Answer D) are often recommended to check for restoration of normal thyroid function or progression to overt hypothyroidism. In this case, remeasuring TSH may be reasonable; however, there is no indication to measure thyroid autoantibodies again. If thyroid autoimmunity was not responsible for the lab change when first evaluated, there is no need to serially check antibody levels. In addition, thyroid hormone levels should not influence the decision to prescribe a GLP-1 receptor agonist.

Thyroid ultrasonography (Answer C) should be repeated in patients with suspicious thyroid nodules. This patient has thyroid parenchymal changes that mimic autoimmune thyroiditis. She has no evidence of autoimmune disease, but even if she did, there is no indication for serial thyroid ultrasonography in patients with thyroiditis. There is also no indication to routinely perform thyroid ultrasonography after treatment with a GLP-1 receptor agonist has been initiated.

Educational Objective

Recognize that abnormal thyroid function and alterations in the echotexture of the thyroid gland occur in the setting of obesity and explain the potential link between GLP-1 receptor agonists and thyroid cancer.

Reference(s)

Espinosa De Ycaza AE, Brito JP, McCoy RG, Shao H, Singh Ospina N. Glucagon-like peptide-1 receptor agonists and thyroid cancer: a narrative review. *Thyroid.* 2024;34(4):403-418. PMID: 38343381

Lass N, Barth A, Reinehr T. Thyroid volume and thyroid function parameters are independently associated with weight status in overweight children. *Horm Res Paediatr.* 2020;93(5):279-286. PMID: 33040066

Licenziati MR, Valerio G, Vetrani I, De Maria G, Liotta F, Radetti G. Altered thyroid function and structure in children and adolescents who are overweight and obese: reversal after weight loss. *J Clin Endocrinol Metab.* 2019;104(7):2757-2765. PMID: 30874808

Radetti G, Kleon W, Buzi F, et al. Thyroid function and structure are affected in childhood obesity. *J Clin Endocrinol Metab.* 2008;93(12):4749-4754. PMID: 18840640

Rotondi M, Cappelli C, Leporati P, et al. A hypoechoic pattern of the thyroid at ultrasound does not indicate autoimmune thyroid diseases in patients with morbid obesity. *Eur J Endocrinol.* 2010;163(1):105-109. PMID: 20453114

59 ANSWER: D) Perform MRI of her brain

This 15-year-old girl presents with primary amenorrhea 3 years after thelarche. While some girls may take up to 4 years to have menarche after thelarche, her pubertal breast development has stalled at early Tanner stage 3. Therefore, she needs evaluation to determine the cause of her primary amenorrhea. She has low estradiol, low IGF-1, and borderline-low free T_4, which—along with the clinical picture of stalled puberty—make the diagnosis of central hypogonadism/hypopituitarism likely. Furthermore, gonadotropins are not elevated, which rules out causes of primary ovarian insufficiency. Normal gonadotropins can be found in cases of central hypogonadotropic hypogonadism. Therefore, the most appropriate next step is to perform MRI of the brain and pituitary gland (Answer D) to look for structural abnormalities.

Offering reassurance (Answer B) is inappropriate. Primary amenorrhea is defined as the absence of menarche at age 15 years if there are secondary sexual characteristics or the absence of menarche at age 13 years if there is complete absence of secondary sexual characteristics such as breast development.

Congenital adrenal hyperplasia with a high 17-hydroxyprogesterone value (Answer A) may be associated with primary amenorrhea. However, this patient does not have advanced bone age, she has no signs of hyperandrogenism on physical examination, and her testosterone concentration is normal. Late-onset congenital adrenal hyperplasia is an unlikely diagnosis.

Congenital malformation of internal female organs (ie, absent uterus or cervix or cervical outlet obstruction) can be associated with primary amenorrhea, and this needs to be evaluated with pelvic ultrasonography, which the patient already had. There is no benefit of MRI (Answer E) in this scenario if findings on pelvic ultrasonography are normal.

This patient is also very short, and even though her karyotype is normal (46,XX), it is still possible she has Turner syndrome due to a small deletion on the X chromosome that general karyotyping cannot identify. However, results of fluorescence in situ hybridization microarray were normal. When there is strong suspicion of mosaic Turner syndrome, genetic testing might need to be repeated using cells from a different source (ie, skin fibroblasts). However, this patient has no signs of primary ovarian insufficiency and her clinical picture is more consistent with central hypogonadism. Genetic testing to identify causes of central hypogonadism may be helpful in the future.

She has a baseline cortisol concentration of 9.0 µg/dL (248.3 nmol/L), which can be a normal value at 8 AM. While she is at risk for adrenal insufficiency if central hypopituitarism is confirmed, and her cortisol value does not exclude central adrenal insufficiency, she currently has no clinical signs of adrenal insufficiency. She most likely needs to be evaluated with cosyntropin-stimulation testing (Answer C) to rule out central adrenal insufficiency, but it is not the most appropriate next step.

This patient might benefit from use of an oral contraceptive pill and eventually could need that for management of primary amenorrhea. However, it is best to complete the workup for an underlying etiology of amenorrhea before initiating treatment. Furthermore, a gradual increase in her breast development can be best achieved with increasing doses of estradiol patches and later add-on cyclical progesterone. Once she has fully matured breasts, she could switch to an oral contraceptive pill.

Educational Objective

Evaluate primary amenorrhea in a patient with sexual infantilism and other signs of secondary sexual maturation.

Reference(s)

Seppä S, Kuiri-Hänninen T, Holopainen E, Voutilainen R. Management of endocrine disease: diagnosis and management of primary amenorrhea and female delayed puberty. *Eur J Endocrinol.* 2021;184(6):R225-R242. PMID: 33687345

Stuenkel CA, Gompel A, Davis SR, Pinkerton JV, Lumsden MA, Santen RJ. Approach to the patient with new-onset secondary amenorrhea: is this primary ovarian insufficiency? *J Clin Endocrinol Metab.* 2022;107(3):825-835. PMID: 34693971

60 ANSWER: E) Sequencing the *IGF2* gene

This patient has the classic features of Russell-Silver syndrome, including being born small-for-gestational-age, postnatal short stature, relative macrocephaly, feeding difficulties, a prominent forehead, and a triangular-shaped face. The most common genetic etiology of Russell-Silver syndrome is hypomethylation of the imprinted region on chromosome 11p15. This hypomethylation leads to loss of paternal *IGF2* expression and gain of maternal *H19* expression, which causes growth restriction. However, methylation analysis of chromosome 11p15 was normal in this case.

Therefore, she has a less common cause of Russell-Silver syndrome, and the pedigree gives an important clue to the etiology. The patient has a paternal half-brother and paternal first cousin who are both affected. The patient's father, paternal uncle, and paternal grandparents are not affected. This pattern is consistent with inheritance of a pathogenic variant in an imprinted gene. Imprinted genes are those in which only 1 allele of the gene is expressed, and the copy that is expressed is based on whether it was inherited from the mother or the father. In this case, the patient has inherited a pathogenic variant in the *IGF2* gene (Answer E). *IGF2* is maternally imprinted, meaning that the maternal copy is silenced and only the paternal copy is expressed. In this case, the patient, her half-brother, and her first cousin all inherited the pathogenic variant from their fathers who were clinically unaffected. The patient's father and his brother must have inherited the same pathogenic variant from their mother, and due to the imprinting of the gene, they are clinically unaffected.

The second most common genetic cause of Russell-Silver syndrome is maternal uniparental disomy of chromosome 7 (Answer A). However, uniparental disomy is not an inherited condition and would not fit this pedigree.

Pathogenic variants in *IGF1* (Answer C) and *IGF1R* (Answer D) both present in children who are born small-for-gestational-age and have postnatal short stature. In both conditions, affected individuals usually have microcephaly, not relative macrocephaly. Neither condition is an imprinted disorder. Patients with pathogenic variants in the *IGF1R* gene tend to have IGF-1 levels in the upper half of the reference range or frankly elevated, although this is not uniformly the case.

Karyotype analysis (Answer B) would not identify abnormalities causing Russell-Silver syndrome, and abnormalities present in a karyotype would not be inherited in an imprinted fashion.

Educational Objective

Identify *IGF2* pathogenic variants as a rare cause of Russell-Silver syndrome and recognize an imprinted pattern of inheritance in a pedigree.

Reference(s)

Abi Habib W, Brioude F, Edouard T, et al. Genetic disruption of the oncogenic HMGA2-PLAG1-IGF2 pathway causes fetal growth restriction. *Genet Med.* 2018;20(2):250-258. PMID: 28796236

Begemann M, Zirn B, Santen G, et al. Paternally inherited IGF2 mutation and growth restriction. *N Engl J Med.* 2015;373(4):349-356. PMID: 26154720

Wakeling EL, Brioude F, Lokulo-Sodipe O, et al. Diagnosis and management of Silver-Russell syndrome: first international consensus statement. *Nat Rev Endocrinol.* 2017;13(2):105-124. PMID: 27585961

61 ANSWER: D) Start asfotase alfa

This patient has hypophosphatasia (HPP), as evidenced by his clinical presentation, undetectable alkaline phosphatase (ALP), and radiographic findings. HPP is a rare bone disease characterized by impaired bone mineralization due to the accumulation of inorganic pyrophosphate (PPi), a potent inhibitor of hydroxyapatite crystal formation. HPP is caused by pathogenic variants in the *ALPL* gene, which encodes the tissue-nonspecific alkaline phosphatase (TNSALP) enzyme. TNSALP normally hydrolyzes PPi, preventing its accumulation and allowing proper bone mineralization. *ALPL* pathogenic variants cause TNSALP deficiency, leading to PPi accumulation and defective skeletal and dental mineralization. Low serum ALP is the hallmark of HPP. There are 6 clinical forms of varying severity according to age of symptom onset (benign prenatal, perinatal, infantile, childhood, adult) or whether only teeth are affected (odontohypophosphatasia). Severe forms present with skeletal abnormalities, rickets, fractures, bone pain, skeletal deformities, failure to thrive, short stature, and hypotonia. This patient exhibits all these features, along with abnormal radiographs showing marked metaphyseal fraying and characteristic radiolucent "tongues" projecting from growth plates into metaphyses, most pronounced in the distal radius and ulna. Dental manifestations, especially premature primary tooth loss, are nearly universal due to defective cementum formation.

Infants and children with HPP often have normal or elevated calcium and phosphorus levels due to impaired bone mineralization and inability to incorporate calcium and phosphorus into hydroxyapatite. Hypercalcemia may necessitate low-calcium and/or low-phosphorus formula in infants. This patient has mildly elevated calcium and phosphorus concentrations. Vitamin D supplementation (Answer E) is not recommended in patients with HPP and hypercalcemia. Kidney ultrasonography should be performed to evaluate for nephrocalcinosis, which occurs in severe HPP. TNSALP deficiency leads to accumulation of PPi, which binds to calcium and forms insoluble calcium pyrophosphate crystals. These crystals cannot be broken down due to TNSALP deficiency, and they deposit in the kidneys, causing nephrocalcinosis. Hypercalcemia with hypercalciuria also contributes to the development of nephrocalcinosis.

Diagnostic criteria for HPP, as recently proposed by Rush et al, require either 2 major criteria or 1 major and 2 minor criteria. Low ALP for age and sex is an obligate diagnostic criterion. Major and minor diagnostic criteria are shown (*see table*).

Table. Proposed Diagnostic Criteria for the Diagnosis of Hypophosphatasia in Children and Adolescents

Obligate Criteria	
Low alkaline phosphatase for age and sex	
Major criteria	**Minor criteria**
ALPL gene variant(s)	Short stature
Elevation of TNSALP substrates	Delayed motor milestones
Early nontraumatic loss of primary teeth	Chronic musculoskeletal pain
Presence of rickets on radiograph	Impaired mobility
	Genu valgum/varum
	Craniosynostosis
	Nephrocalcinosis/nephrolithiasis
	Low muscle tone
	B_6-responsive seizures

Diagnosis of hypophosphatasia requires either 2 major criteria or 1 majorand 2 minor criteria. Adapted from Rush E et al. Osteoporos *Int*, 2024; 35(1): 1-10. © The Authors. Published by Springer Nature.

HPP can be diagnosed clinically in this patient based on the above diagnostic criteria. To confirm the diagnosis, additional laboratory studies could be obtained, including vitamin B_6 measurement and urinary phosphoethanolamine excretion, both of which are substrates and are expected to be elevated in HPP. Although the plasma pyridoxal 5′-phosphate concentration, the principal circulating form of vitamin B_6, is markedly elevated in HPP and is considered a biochemical hallmark of this condition, serum pyridoxic acid (Answer A), the degradation product of vitamin B_6 used to assess B_6 sufficiency, is typically normal or low in persons with HPP. Thus, measuring pyridoxic acid is nondiagnostic.

Genetic testing of the *ALPL* gene can confirm HPP, but it may not be necessary in straightforward cases such as this vignette. *ALPL* gene analysis in affected individuals and family members can clarify inheritance patterns, recurrence risks, and guide genetic counseling. It is important to note that a pathogenic variant in the *ALPL* gene is not always present and is not required for diagnosis.

Asfotase alfa (Answer D) is a human recombinant TNSALP enzyme replacement therapy approved in 2015 for patients with pediatric-onset HPP. Asfotase alfa has revolutionized outcomes for severe, previously fatal forms and improved patients' quality of life. Asfotase alfa therapy is indicated in this patient to provide the missing enzyme activity to hydrolyze accumulated PPi. By reducing PPi levels, asfotase alfa promotes proper bone mineralization and improves the skeletal and nonskeletal manifestations of HPP.

Bisphosphonate treatment (Answer C) is contraindicated in patients with HPP because it exacerbates the underlying pathophysiology by further inhibiting bone mineralization. Bisphosphonates are analogues of inorganic pyrophosphate, which is already elevated in HPP, leading to increased deposition of calcium pyrophosphate crystals in bone and other tissues. Patients with HPP may present with low bone mass and fractures resembling osteoporosis (as in this patient), but bisphosphonates worsen clinical outcomes and can increase the risk of atypical femoral fractures in these patients.

Osteogenesis imperfecta is a genetic bone disorder characterized by pathogenic variants in the *COL1A1* and *COL1A2* genes that affect the production or structure of type I collagen, a crucial component for bone strength. Persons with osteogenesis imperfecta typically present with multiple fractures but do not exhibit radiolucency in bone radiographs. Serum alkaline phosphatase levels in osteogenesis imperfecta are either normal or elevated. In this vignette, genetic testing for osteogenesis imperfecta (Answer B) would not be of diagnostic value.

**Image in the vignette reprinted from Bowden SA, Adler BH. Asfotase alfa treatment for one year in a 16 year-old male with severe childhood hypophosphatasia.* Osteoporos Int. *2018;29(2):511-515.*

Educational Objective

Identify the defining features, clinical manifestations, and diagnostic criteria of hypophosphatasia in children and recommend asfotase alfa enzyme replacement therapy.

Reference(s)

Bowden SA, Foster BL. Alkaline phosphatase replacement therapy for hypophosphatasia in development and practice. *Adv Exp Med Biol.* 2019;1148:279-322. PMID: 31482504

Khan AA, Brandi ML, Rush ET, et al. Hypophosphatasia diagnosis: current state of the art and proposed diagnostic criteria for children and adults. *Osteoporos Int.* 2024;35(3):431-438. PMID: 37982857

Rush E, Brandi ML, Khan A, et al. Proposed diagnostic criteria for the diagnosis of hypophosphatasia in children and adolescents: results from the HPP International Working Group. *Osteoporos Int.* 2024;35(1):1-10. PMID: 37982855

62 ANSWER: A) Ectopic posterior pituitary

This infant has congenital central hypothyroidism, which in most cases is a component of combined pituitary hormone deficiency (CPHD). The most common cause of CPHD is an isolated structural abnormality of the pituitary usually consisting of interrupted pituitary stalk, anterior pituitary hypoplasia, and/or ectopic posterior pituitary (pituitary stalk interruption syndrome [PSIS]). Among newborns diagnosed with central hypothyroidism, PSIS is the most common etiology, and ectopic posterior pituitary (Answer A) is the most likely finding to be observed in this patient.

Less commonly, CPHD is syndromic and is associated with other central nervous system and extracranial abnormalities affecting the eyes, ears, or facial structures (eg, palate, teeth); optic nerve hypoplasia (Answer C); or midline brain malformations such as absent corpus callosum or holoprosencephaly. Many such cases are caused by monogenic pathogenic variants in genes encoding a variety of transcription factors, and the associated abnormalities usually are identified on physical examination and/or imaging. Two rare monogenic causes of CPHD (*PROP1* and *POU1F1*) have normal pituitary findings on MRI (Answer B), but these are much less common than PSIS as a cause of congenital central hypothyroidism.

Congenital central hypothyroidism can be isolated (not part of CPHD) in up to 25% to 35% of cases, and in these patients, MRI findings are normal. Most cases of isolated congenital central hypothyroidism are monogenic. The most commonly involved genes are *IGSF1* (~50% of cases), *IRS4* (~15%), and *TBL1X* (~15%), which are all X-linked and therefore cause hypothyroidism in only males. Very rare variants occur in *TSHB* and *TRHR*, and about 10% of cases have no known genetic cause.

Pituitary blastoma (Answer D) is a very rare hypothalamic tumor that occurs in infants younger than 2 years. It typically presents with signs of intracranial mass effect or ACTH-dependent Cushing syndrome, not with pituitary hormone deficiencies. Pituitary blastomas generally are caused by pathogenic variants in *DICER1* and have a poor prognosis.

Thickening of the pituitary stalk (Answer E) can be observed in infiltrative disorders such as germinoma and Langerhans cell histiocytosis, and it can result in pituitary hormone deficits, most often arginine vasopressin deficiency and less commonly central hypothyroidism. These conditions are very unlikely to occur in a newborn.

Educational Objective

Identify pituitary stalk interruption syndrome as the most common cause of congenital central hypothyroidism.

Reference(s)

Lauffer P, Zwaveling-Soonawala N, Naafs JC, Boelen A, van Trotsenburg ASP. Diagnosis and management of central congenital hypothyroidism. *Front Endocrinol (Lausanne).* 2021;12:686317. PMID: 34566885

Liu APY, Kelsey MM, Sabbaghian N, et al. Clinical outcomes and complications of pituitary blastoma. *J Clin Endocrinol Metab.* 2021;106(2):351-363. PMID: 33236116

Moszczyńska E, Kunecka K, Baszyńska-Wilk M, et al. Pituitary stalk thickening: causes and consequences. The Children's Memorial Health Institute experience and literature review. *Front Endocrinol (Lausanne).* 2022;13:868558. PMID: 35669693

Naafs JC, Verkerk PH, Fliers E, van Trotsenburg ASP, Zwaveling-Soonawala N. Clinical and genetic characteristics of Dutch children with central congenital hypothyroidism, early detected by neonatal screening. *Eur J Endocrinol.* 2020;183(6):627-636. PMID: 33107432

63 ANSWER: A) Continue basal-bolus insulin

Individuals with monogenic diabetes are often misdiagnosed as having type 1 diabetes, particularly when they present in early childhood. Maturity-onset diabetes of the young (MODY) type 10 is caused by variants in the insulin gene (*INS*) and is referred to as either INS-NDM if presenting as neonatal diabetes or INS-MODY if presenting after 1 year of age. While INS-MODY is a rare cause of diabetes, one large-scale study showed that pathogenic *INS* variants were among the 3 most common causes of neonatal diabetes, along with activating pathogenic variants in *KCNJ11* and *ABCC8.* The *figure* demonstrates the penetrance of *INS* pathogenic variants in families where the proband was diagnosed in the first year of life.

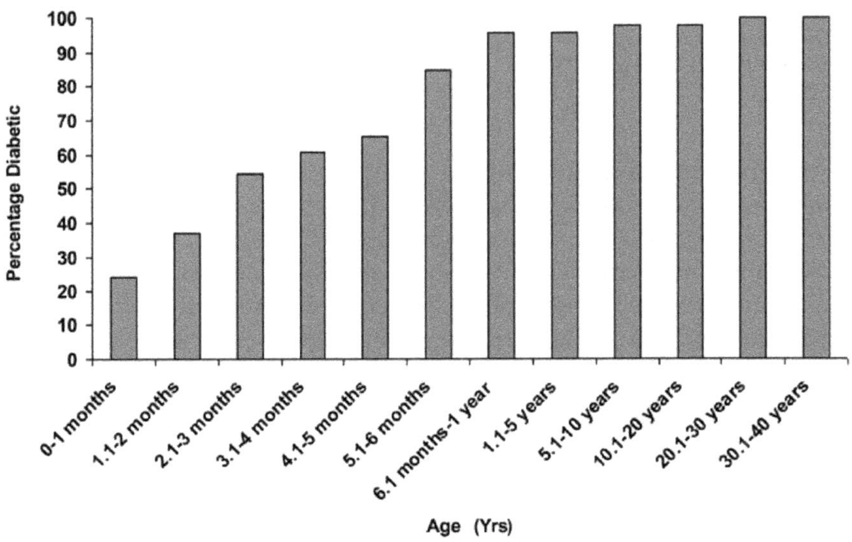

FIG. 3. Penetrance of *INS* gene mutations in 46 individuals from 35 families where the proband was diagnosed in the first year of life.
The percentage of patients with an *INS* mutation and diabetes at any given age is shown.

Pathogenic variants disrupt folding of the proinsulin molecule, resulting in the misfolded protein response in the endoplasmic reticulum, endoplasmic reticulum stress, and cell apoptosis. Depletion of β-cell mass results in hyperglycemia and symptoms of diabetes. MODY type 10 requires treatment with insulin, typically at full replacement dosages; thus, a basal-bolus insulin regimen (Answer A) is most appropriate.

In 46 patients with diabetes due to *INS* gene variants, 100% required insulin treatment at an average dosage of 0.7 (0.3-1.9) units/kg per day. Glycemic control was variable; the average hemoglobin A_{1c} value in the study population was 7.95% (63 mmol/mol) (range, 4.6%-13.8% [27-127 mmol/mol]) Because MODY type 10 is due to insulin deficiency caused by β-cell depletion, once symptomatic, patients require lifetime insulin treatment, so tapering insulin (Answer C) would not be appropriate. Treatment with basal insulin alone (Answer B) is unlikely to result in adequate glycemic control. Furthermore, there is some suggestion that minimizing hyperglycemia through early intensive insulin therapy may slow the progression of β-cell loss, resulting in better long-term outcomes.

The most common forms of monogenic diabetes are due to heterozygous variants in genes encoding transcription factors HNF1A and HNF4A and glucokinase, the pancreatic glucose sensor (MODY type 2). In many cases, *HNF1A*-MODY and *HNF4A*-MODY can be effectively treated with oral sulfonylureas (Answer D), which bypass the defect in glucose-stimulated insulin secretion in the intact β cell. Repaglinide (Answer E) is an oral agent in the meglitinide class that is used in the management of type 2 diabetes, and it has demonstrated efficacy in treating *HNF1A*-associated monogenic diabetes. However, these medications are not expected to be effective in MODY type 10 due to the mechanism of insulin deficiency.

Educational Objective

Recommend appropriate management of maturity-onset diabetes of the young type 10.

Reference(s)

Edghill EL, Flanagan SE, Patch AM, et al. Insulin mutation screening in 1,044 patients with diabetes: mutations in the INS gene are a common cause of neonatal diabetes but a rare cause of diabetes diagnosed in childhood or adulthood. *Diabetes.* 2008;57(4):1034-1042. PMID: 18162506

Riddle MC, Philipson LH, Rich SS, et al. Monogenic diabetes: from genetic insights to population-based precision in care. Reflections from a *Diabetes Care* editors' expert forum. *Diabetes Care.* 2020;43(12):3117-3128. PMID: 33560999

64 **ANSWER: D) Reduce synthetic clothing items**

Global plastic production has increased drastically since World War II, with more than 8300 megatons of plastic manufactured in that time. Single-use plastics represent 35% to 40% of current production and are the most rapidly growing segment of plastic manufacturing. Disposal of plastic waste is a major barrier, with rates of recovery and recycling below 10% globally. Twenty-two megatons of plastic waste are estimated to enter the environment each year.

Due to the ubiquitous use of plastic, there is widespread exposure to the chemicals found in plastics, not only for humans, but for all living creatures. As exposure has increased globally, it has become evident that plastics and plastics-containing chemicals are associated with a growing number of health effects, including risk for overweight/obesity. While the exact mechanisms are not fully understood, microplastics (MPs) have been shown to induce oxidative stress and may affect metabolism by promoting the growth of adipocytes. Additionally, several plastic additives act as endocrine-disrupting chemicals that can cause changes within developing cells and organs with increased risk of disease and disability in childhood and beyond. The antenatal period, as well as early childhood, are 2 periods in the human life cycle that appear to harbor increased susceptibility to plastics-related health effects.

Microplastics is a term used to denote plastic particles that are 1 μm to 5 mm in diameter. They can be classified into 2 categories: *primary MPs* and *secondary MPs.* Primary MPs are plastic particles manufactured to a small size, which are then added to consumer products (usually cosmetic and/or biomedical), as well as microfibers that shed from synthetic sources. Secondary MPs are created from the breakdown of larger plastic items, often plastic litter, after entering the environment. Humans are exposed to MPs in a multitude of ways, and once they enter the human body, MPs can travel through the circulation to all organ systems where accumulation is likely. It is estimated that an average human being ingests several milligrams of MPs daily.

Inhalation and ingestion are currently believed to be the main sources of MP exposure for humans. Recent studies have shown that inhaled indoor air is a prominent source of airborne MP exposure. Airborne MPs are directly inhaled by humans, and a major source of those airborne MPs is synthetic textiles. Polyester and other synthetic textiles such as acrylic, nylon, and rayon are known to "shed" tiny plastic microfibers, which are a type of MP, during manufacturing, use, washing, and disposal. Washing these textiles is the primary source of MP pollution. Thus, reducing synthetic clothing items (Answer D) is the best way to decrease this child's MP exposure.

While dietary ingestion of MPs is a prominent source of MP exposure in humans, certain foods and beverages are much more significant sources than others. Drinking water, particularly bottled water, is a major source of MP exposure, as well as other dietary items such as seafood (MPs are ingested by marine organisms), table salt (primarily produced from evaporation of seawater, which is contaminated from ocean plastic pollution), ultra-processed foods, and foods purchased in plastic packaging. While MPs are still found in produce, fresh whole foods typically contain fewer MPs than amounts in more processed options. Thus, limiting the amount of fresh produce this child consumes (Answer A) is not the best answer.

Both cotton and linen are natural fibers. Thus, if left untreated, neither is likely to shed MPs, so switching from cotton to linen sheets (Answer C) is incorrect.

Dermal contact (Answers B and E) is considered a less significant route of MP exposure for potential systemic uptake, since skin absorption is believed to be minimal for MPs larger than 10 to 100 nm in diameter. Therefore, while limiting use of topical body lotions and switching to a shampoo bar could result in less MP exposure, neither lotion nor shampoo is likely to be the most abundant source of MP exposure for this child.

Educational Objective

Describe the burden of microplastics exposure and how it may contribute to obesity risk.

Reference(s)

Harris L. 10 simple ways to avoid microplastics in your everyday life. EcoWatch. October 12, 2021. Accessed November 2024. https://www.ecowatch.com/avoid-microplastics-at-home-2655282616.html

Kannan K, Vimalkumar K. A review of human exposure to microplastics and insights into microplastics as obesogens. *Front Endocrinol (Lausanne).* 2021;12:724989. PMID: 34484127

Landrigan PJ, Raps H, Cropper M, et al. The Minderoo-Monaco Commission on Plastics and Human Health. *Ann Glob Health.* 2023;89(1):23. PMID: 36969097

Zuri G, Karanasiou A, Lacorte S. Microplastics: human exposure assessment through air, water, and food. *Environ Int.* 2023;179:108150. PMID: 37607425

65 ANSWER: E) Measurement of very long-chain fatty acids

X-linked adrenoleukodystrophy (X-ALD) is a rare genetic disorder due to pathogenic variants in the *ABCD1* gene, which encodes the synthesis of adrenoleukodystrophy protein (ALDP), a peroxisomal membrane protein that transports very long-chain fatty acids (VLCFAs) into peroxisomes. ALDP deficiency leads to accumulation of VLCFAs (≥C22) in the plasma, white matter, spinal cord, and adrenal cortex. It presents more severely in males and is often categorized into 3 main clinical phenotypes; cerebral adrenoleukodystrophy (CALD); adrenomyeloneuropathy (AMN); and/or primary adrenal insufficiency (PAI). CALD is characterized by progressive behavioral, cognitive, and neurologic deficits. Symptoms may develop during childhood (ages 4 to 8 years), adolescence (ages 11 to 21 years), or adulthood. Clinical symptoms of AMN include leg weakness, stiffness, and bladder and bowel dysfunction with typical age of onset of 20 to 30 years. The onset of PAI ranges from age 2 years to adulthood (most commonly by age 7.5 years). Heterozygous females are at increased risk of developing AMN and PAI with increasing age.

All boys with primary adrenal insufficiency, especially in the setting of behavioral problems and decline in school performance, should have measurement of VLCFA (Answer E) to rule out X-ALD. Children with X-ALD typically have absent circulating adrenocortical autoantibodies. Presenting X-ALD symptoms can be subtle and nonspecific and often mimic psychiatric or developmental disorders of childhood, especially attention-deficit/hyperactivity disorder. The presence of similar behavioral and academic difficulties in his older brother suggests that both boys are most likely affected with X-ALD. If results of VLCFA analysis are abnormal, *ABCD1* gene testing (Answer A) should follow to confirm the diagnosis.

High-dose cosyntropin-stimulation testing (Answer D) is not needed because the patient's baseline ACTH and cortisol levels indisputably indicate primary adrenal insufficiency.

AIRE gene testing (Answer B) for autoimmune polyglandular type 1 syndrome in a child with negative adrenal antibodies would be recommended only after other causes of primary adrenal insufficiency with negative antibodies have been ruled out.

Brain MRI (Answer C) is not a first-line test in the evaluation for X-ALD, but it would be relevant after X-ALD is diagnosed. The onset of cerebral involvement in childhood is typically between 2.5 and 10 years of age. MRI findings include extensive demyelination in the periventricular deep white matter and parietal and occipital regions. Disease progression is often associated with inflammatory white matter demyelination.

Educational Objective

Rule out X-linked adrenal leukodystrophy in all boys presenting with primary adrenal insufficiency and a decline in school performance, even in those with underlying autoimmune disease.

Reference(s)

Cappa M, Todisco T, Bizzarri C. X-linked adrenoleukodystrophy and primary adrenal insufficiency. *Front Endocrinol (Lausanne).* 2023;14:1309053. PMID: 38034003

Paparella R, Menghi M, Micangeli G, et al. Autoimmune polyendocrine syndromes in the pediatric age. *Children (Basel).* 2023;10(3):588. PMID: 36980146

66 ANSWER: B) Radioactive iodine

The patient has a high TRAb titer, and these antibodies cross the placenta. The presence of high TRAb levels, regardless of thyroid hormone levels, predicts risk of developing fetal and neonatal Graves disease. Typically, maternal TRAb levels greater than 5 times the upper normal limit are associated with significant risk of fetal or neonatal disease.

The decrease in TRAb after radioactive iodine therapy is slower than after treatment with medication or thyroidectomy. Therefore, the short-term risk of having a pregnancy complicated by fetal Graves disease is highest in a woman treated with radioactive iodine (Answer B). TRAb levels typically decrease to low levels by 6 to 12 months after thyroidectomy or methimazole treatment, while it may take up to 2 years to reach similar levels after radioactive iodine therapy. For pregnancy planning in the short term, both thyroidectomy and methimazole result in similar and prompt decreases in TRAb levels and have a low risk of fetal Graves disease (thus, Answers A, C, D, and E are incorrect). If pregnancy is not anticipated for several years, the risk of having an affected pregnancy is similar across treatment modalities.

Fetal hyperthyroidism is uncommon and affects less than 5% of babies of mothers with a history of Graves disease. However, if it occurs and is not recognized, the fetal outcome can be severe (cardiac failure, hydrops, craniosynostosis). Monitoring required in this patient's future pregnancies will depend on her clinical course and the selected treatment modality. Women who are hyperthyroid during pregnancy require treatment of the hyperthyroidism and monitoring for fetal Graves disease. Euthyroid women who have had definitive therapy (either thyroidectomy or radioactive iodine therapy) should have TRAb levels checked during the first trimester and, if positive, rechecked subsequently (at 18-22 weeks and 30-34 weeks). If TRAb antibodies are positive at a titer greater than 3 times the upper normal limit, increased fetal monitoring is required. However, measurement of TRAb is not necessary for women with an intact thyroid gland who are in remission after a course of medical management. These women should have thyroid function checked in the first trimester; normal thyroid function confirms the absence of clinically significant TRAb levels. Thyroid function tests should only be repeated if hyperthyroid symptoms occur.

Educational Objective

Describe the timing of TRAb changes after treatment of Graves disease and explain how this may affect choice of therapy.

Reference(s)

Kim J, Choi MS, Park J, et al. Changes in thyrotropin receptor antibody levels following total thyroidectomy or radioiodine therapy in patients with refractory Graves' disease. *Thyroid.* 2021;31(8):1264-1271. PMID: 33947272

Laurberg P, Wallin G, Tallstedt L, Abraham-Nordling M, Lundell G, Torring O. TSH-receptor autoimmunity in Graves' disease after therapy with anti-thyroid drugs, surgery, or radioiodine: a 5-year prospective randomized study *Eur J Endocrinol.* 2008;158(1):69-75. PMID: 18166819

Van Dijk MM, Smits IH, Fliers E, Bisschop PH. Maternal thyrotropin receptor antibody concentration and the risk of fetal and neonatal thyrotoxicosis: a systematic review. *Thyroid.* 2018;28(2):257-264. PMID: 29325496

67 ANSWER: A) Calcium and calcitriol

Metabolic bone disease of prematurity (MBDP), also known as osteopenia of prematurity, is characterized by undermineralization of the skeleton due to inadequate calcium and phosphate accretion prenatally and postnatally. Preterm infants have inadequate calcium and phosphorus reserves at birth due to premature delivery before the third trimester when most mineral accretion occurs in utero. The deficiency of these minerals leads to osteopenia, which increases the risk of rickets and fractures in severe cases. This infant has multiple risk factors for MBDP, including prematurity, low birth weight, total parenteral nutrition, necrotizing enterocolitis, diuretic use (by causing hypercalciuria and calcium depletion), caffeine (by inhibiting intestinal calcium absorption and promoting urinary excretion of calcium), and corticosteroid use (by increasing osteoclastic activity and reducing osteoblast proliferation) to treat chronic lung disease.

In preterm infants, phosphorus and/or calcium deficiency are often the key factors contributing to MBDP. Phosphorus deficiency leads to low levels of FGF-23, which normally inhibits renal phosphate reabsorption. This causes increased production of 1,25-dihydroxyvitamin D, resulting in increased intestinal absorption of both calcium and phosphorus and increased renal phosphorus reabsorption. In cases of calcium deficiency, elevated PTH levels activate 25-hydroxyvitamin D to 1,25-dihydroxyvitamin D, increasing intestinal absorption of calcium and phosphorus. Elevated PTH also increases bone resorption, which releases calcium and phosphorus, and enhances renal calcium reabsorption while increasing renal phosphorus excretion. The net effect is normal serum calcium, low serum phosphorus, and elevated alkaline phosphatase. All the above lead to decreased bone mineralization, resulting in MBDP. Importantly, hypophosphatemia is a universal feature of MBDP, occurring due to PTH-mediated renal phosphate excretion in calcium deficiency and reduced phosphate absorption in phosphate deficiency. Therefore, further testing with PTH and tubular reabsorption of phosphorus can help identify the primary etiology.

Calcium deficiency is often accompanied by elevated PTH levels due to secondary hyperparathyroidism. PTH serves as a sensitive biomarker of calcium deficiency. A high PTH concentration with low tubular reabsorption of phosphorus would suggest calcium deficiency, whereas a low or normal PTH concentration with high tubular reabsorption of phosphorus would indicate phosphorus deficiency. Phosphate supplementation should be initiated as first-line therapy for infants with phosphorus deficiency.

This infant has hypophosphatemia, eucalcemia, low tubular reabsorption of phosphorus, elevated alkaline phosphatase and PTH levels, and normal 25-hydroxyvitamin D concentration, suggestive of calcium deficiency. Calcium supplementation is required to normalize elevated PTH and thereby reduce resultant bone resorption and hypophosphatemia. Despite having hypophosphatemia, phosphate supplementation (Answers B, C, D, and E) without addressing underlying calcium deficiency should be avoided because it can precipitate hypocalcemia, resulting in worsening hyperparathyroidism, leading to exacerbation of MBDP. This can have severe consequences such as rickets and pathologic fractures.

Serum calcium is not a reliable marker of calcium adequacy because serum calcium is maintained at the expense of depletion of skeletal stores by secondary hyperparathyroidism.

In cases of severe calcium deficiency with significant secondary hyperparathyroidism (as in this patient), active vitamin D (calcitriol) supplementation (Answer A) is required in addition to calcium supplementation to help normalize hyperparathyroidism. Calcitriol can directly suppress PTH secretion at pharmacologic dosages, thereby reducing PTH-mediated bone resorption and phosphate wasting. Calcitriol can also help increase intestinal absorption of calcium and phosphorus when given with mineral supplementation. Typical calcitriol dosages are 0.05 to 0.1 mcg/kg per day, or up to 0.2 mcg/kg per day, in 1 or 2 divided doses, to improve enteral calcium and phosphorus absorption in infants with secondary hyperparathyroidism. Monitoring serum calcium, PTH, and the urinary calcium-to-creatinine ratio is required to adjust calcitriol dosing, as high dosages can cause hypercalcemia and hypercalciuria.

In some infants, metabolic abnormalities may persist despite initial treatment with calcium (persistent hypophosphatemia despite improved tubular reabsorption of phosphate and PTH) or phosphate (triggering or worsening secondary hyperparathyroidism), and combined calcium and phosphate treatment may be required. When prescribed together, calcium and phosphate should be administered at least 2 hours apart to avoid precipitation with poor absorption.

Nutritional consensus guidelines recommend providing preterm and low-birthweight infants with 120 to 200 mg/kg per day of calcium and 60 to 140 mg/kg per day of phosphorus through enteral feeds. For optimal absorption and retention, the enteral calcium-to-phosphate intake ratio should be maintained at 1.5:1 to 1.8:1 on a mg-to-mg basis. A higher calcium requirement is crucial because preterm infants have an estimated calcium absorption efficiency of 50% to 60% and phosphorus absorption efficiency of 80% to 90%. A calcium-to-phosphate ratio of 1:2 (Answer E) is incorrect.

** Image in the vignette reprinted from Boddu SK, Lankala R. Are we undertreating calcium deficiency in metabolic bone disease of prematurity? A case report and review.* Front Pediatr. *2022;10:991488.*

Educational Objective

Distinguish between calcium and phosphorus deficiency as 2 distinct etiologies of metabolic bone disease of prematurity using laboratory investigations and outline appropriate treatment strategies for each type.

Reference(s)

Chinoy A, Mughal MZ, Padidela R. Metabolic bone disease of prematurity: causes, recognition, prevention, treatment and long-term consequences. *Arch Dis Child Fetal Neonatal Ed.* 2019;104(5):F560-F566. PMID: 31079069

Grover M, Ashraf AP, Bowden SA, et al. Invited mini review metabolic bone disease of prematurity: overview and practice recommendations. *Horm Res Paediatr.* 2024 [Online ahead on print] PMID: 38211570

Rustico SE, Kelly A, Monk HM, Calabria AC. Calcitriol treatment in metabolic bone disease of prematurity with elevated parathyroid hormone: a preliminary study. *J Clin Transl Endocrinol.* 2015;2(1):14-20. PMID: 29159104

68 **ANSWER: D) Reassurance with no further testing**

The patient described in this vignette is demonstrating growth acceleration due to relatively early puberty. The timing of puberty affects growth velocity and the magnitude of the growth spurt seen in both boys and girls. Children with relatively early onset of puberty achieve a higher peak growth velocity than those with average or later puberty. This patient is currently in midpuberty as evidenced by his testicular volume. He is at the appropriate point in puberty for when a growth spurt should be occurring. A growth velocity of 10.5 cm/y is the 97th percentile for an early maturing male, so while this is on the higher side, it is still within the normal range for pubertal development (*see figure*). The increase in height percentiles is due to his growth accelerating earlier than that of average boys his age. The Centers for Disease Control growth charts are cross-sectional charts that represent the average population growth. A child with relatively early puberty will have a greater-than-average growth velocity and thus an increase in growth percentiles during a pubertal growth spurt. On the other end of the spectrum, a child with later puberty will have a slower-than-average growth velocity from ages 12 to 14 years, as well as a decrease in height percentiles at that time. This child and his parents can be reassured that no further testing is necessary (Answer D).

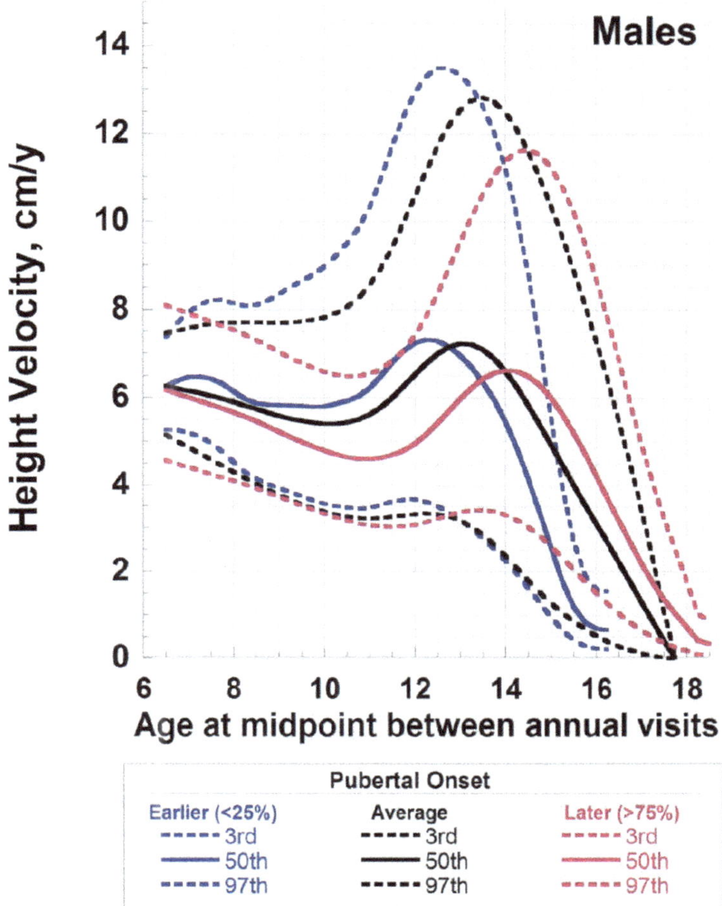

Reprinted from Kelly A et al. *J Clin Endocrinol Metab*, 2014; 99(6): 2104-2112. © The Endocrine Society.

The IGF-1 value is elevated based on this child's chronological age, but it would not be elevated when adjusted for Tanner stage. Therefore, there is no concern for GH excess, and a GH-suppression test (Answer B) is unnecessary. If a patient has an excessive growth rate inappropriate for the stage of puberty or if the IGF-1 is elevated above the normal range even adjusted for pubertal stage, then one must consider GH excess.

While hyperthyroidism can lead to growth acceleration, this patient had normal findings on thyroid examination and is not tachycardic, which makes hyperthyroidism unlikely. Thus, thyroid function testing (Answer E) is unnecessary.

With symmetric enlargement of both testes, this patient clearly has central puberty, and there is no need to measure gonadotropins and testosterone (Answer C) to confirm his pubertal status. A peripheral cause of early puberty would present with small testes or asymmetric enlargement due to a testicular mass. Boys with activating pathogenic variants in the LH receptor gene can present with bilateral testicular enlargement and sexual precocity, but the typical age of presentation is between 1 and 4 years.

Because there is no concern for GH excess or pathological precocious puberty, there is no need for brain MRI (Answer A).

Educational Objective

Explain the influence of pubertal timing on growth velocity in childhood.

Reference(s)

Kelly A, Winer KK, Kalkwarf H, et al. Age-based reference ranges for annual height velocity in US children. *J Clin Endocrinol Metab.* 2014;99(6):2104-2112. PMID: 24601728

Tanner JM, Davies PS. Clinical longitudinal standards for height and height velocity for North American children. *J Pediatr.* 1985;107(3):317-329. PMID: 3875704

69 ANSWER: A) Measure β-hCG

This child has precocious puberty that is not central in origin, given the low gonadotropins, high testosterone, and evidence of virilization on physical examination. All boys with precocious puberty should be evaluated for germ-cell tumors that secrete β-hCG. If β-hCG is elevated, the patient will eventually need brain MRI to exclude a germinoma. However, in that circumstance, he would also need a referral to oncology and a more extensive workup. As an immediate next step, β-hCG should be measured (Answer A). Germ-cell tumors are relatively rare in childhood, and they often present with very large tumors in both gonadal and extragonadal locations.

Seminomas and dysgerminomas are primitive germ-cell tumors that lack the ability for further differentiation. These tumors occur most commonly in the ovary, mediastinum, or central nervous system. Management consists of surgical resection for localized disease, chemotherapy for residual or metastatic disease, and neoadjuvant chemotherapy and delayed surgical excision for unresectable lesions. Most germ-cell tumors secrete either hCG or α-fetoprotein. hCG has a similar structure to that of LH, which is normally produced by the pituitary gland. Because of this, hCG can mimic LH's action and stimulate Leydig cells in the testes to produce testosterone and cause precocious puberty in boys.

Measuring LH again (Answer B) is unlikely to be helpful in this case given that the patient has no significant testicular enlargement. One would expect a boy with central precocious puberty and a testosterone concentration of 200 ng/dL (7.0 nmol/L) to have an LH concentration greater than 0.30 mIU/mL (>0.30 IU/L) and a testicular volume greater than 4 cc.

Although brain MRI (Answer C) is recommended for all boys with central precocious puberty to rule out central nervous system brain tumors that could cause increased LH, this patient does not have evidence of central precocious puberty.

Pathogenic variants in the kisspeptin 1 gene (*KISS1*) (Answer D) and the gene encoding its G protein–coupled receptor (*KISS1R*) have been implicated in the pathogenesis of some cases of central precocious puberty. Loss-of-function variants in *KISS1R* can cause hypogonadotropic hypogonadism. However, in these cases, one would expect the LH to be in the pubertal range, accompanied by larger testicular volume.

Familial male-limited precocious puberty can cause a form of GnRH-independent precocious puberty in boys and is due to activating pathogenic variants in the gene encoding the LH receptor (*LHCGR*) (Answer E). This condition is inherited in an autosomal dominant manner, but it can occur sporadically. It is unlikely this patient's father had an *LHCGR* pathogenic variant given that he reached normal height with no treatment. Boys with familial male-limited precocious puberty usually present at a much younger age, between 2 and 5 years. This diagnosis is less likely in a child who is already 8 years old.

Educational Objective

Guide the evaluation of precocious puberty in a boy.

Reference(s)

Bradley SH, Lawrence N, Steele C, Mohamed Z. Precocious puberty. *BMJ.* 2020;368:l6597. PMID: 31932347

Latronico AC, Brito VN, Carel J-C. Causes, diagnosis, and treatment of central precocious puberty. *Lancet Diabetes Endocrinol.* 2016;4(3):265-274. PMID: 26852255

Rescorla FJ. Pediatric germ cell tumors. *Semin Surg Oncol.* 1999;16(2):144-158. PMID: 9988869

70 **ANSWER: E) *THRA* (thyroid hormone receptor alpha)**

This child has a pathogenic variant in *THRA* (Answer E), which encodes thyroid hormone receptor alpha (TRα), leading to decreased thyroid hormone signaling in tissues that primarily express this thyroid hormone receptor, including the skeleton, heart, gastrointestinal tract, and brain. The resulting syndrome is called resistance to thyroid hormone alpha (RTHα), and common physical features include relatively slow growth with disproportionately short lower extremities, typical facial features as in this case, bradycardia, low blood pressure, severe constipation, and neurological findings such as delayed milestones, slow or dysarthric speech, slow or ataxic gait, and impaired gross and fine motor skills. Because hypothalamic-pituitary regulation of the thyroid axis is mediated primarily by thyroid hormone receptor beta, thyroid function testing in patients with RTHα may be normal or have only subtle abnormalities. The typical pattern is normal TSH, normal or low (free) T_4, and normal or high T_3, resulting in an abnormally low ratio of T_4 to T_3. Patients with RTHα frequently have mild normocytic anemia that may be related to an effect of thyroid hormone on hematopoiesis that is mediated by TRα. In some cases, treatment with levothyroxine improves growth, constipation, and some neurological features. Pathogenic variants in *THRA* are dominant and may be familial or occur de novo.

Variants in *ALB* (Answer A) that increase the affinity of albumin for T_4 cause familial dysalbuminemic hyperthyroxinemia. This is a benign condition characterized biochemically by elevated total T_4, normal free T_4, and normal TSH. T_3 concentrations are usually normal. Persons with familial dysalbuminemic hyperthyroxinemia are euthyroid and have no clinical findings.

Variants in *IGSF1* (Answer B) are the most common cause of isolated congenital central hypothyroidism. *IGSF1* is on the X chromosome, and pathogenic variants cause a syndrome of congenital central hypothyroidism and macroorchidism in males. Females usually are not affected, although about 10% may have mildly low free T_4 levels. Individuals with IGSF1 deficiency have central hypothyroidism (low free T_4 without proportionate TSH elevation) but do not have disproportionate growth, dysmorphism, or neurological findings.

SLC16A2 (Answer C) encodes the thyroid hormone transporter monocarboxylate transporter 8 (MCT8). Pathogenic variants in this gene cause Allan-Herndon-Dudley syndrome, a rare X-linked syndrome in which decreased transport of thyroid hormone in the central nervous system causes profound neurological sequelae, including severe hypotonia and developmental delay. Most affected boys are unable to sit or stand independently or to speak. The typical biochemical pattern of normal TSH, low (free) T_4, and elevated T_3 somewhat resembles that of RTHa, but the other clinical features should distinguish these disorders.

Variants in *TBL1X* (Answer D) are a rare cause of isolated congenital central hypothyroidism. This gene is on the X chromosome, and affected males have central hypothyroidism, as well as mild hearing deficits in some cases. However, affected individuals do not have disproportionate growth, dysmorphism, or neurological findings as observed in this vignette.

Educational Objective

Describe the clinical presentation of resistance to thyroid hormone alpha.

Reference(s)

Bochukova E, Schoenmakers N, Agostini M, et al. A mutation in the thyroid hormone receptor alpha gene. *N Engl J Med.* 2012;366(3):243-249. PMID: 22168587

Moran C, Chatterjee K. Resistance to thyroid hormone due to defective thyroid receptor alpha. *Best Pract Res Clin Endocrinol Metab.* 2015;29(4):647-657. PMID: 26303090

Persani L, Rodien P, Moran C, et al. 2024 European Thyroid Association Guidelines on diagnosis and management of genetic disorders of thyroid hormone transport, metabolism and action. *Eur Thyroid J.* 2024;13(4):e240125. PMID: 38963712

71 **ANSWER: A) Occasional mild hypoglycemia**

The SGLT-2 inhibitor empagliflozin was approved by the US FDA for use in patients with type 2 diabetes as young as 10 years based on findings from the DINAMO study, a multicenter, randomized, double-blinded, placebo-controlled trial of empagliflozin and linagliptin. There were no severe hypoglycemic events reported in the DINAMO study. However, there were significantly higher rates of hypoglycemia for those in the empagliflozin arm vs the placebo arm (23.1% vs 9.4% and a greater frequency of plasma glucose levels detected below 54 mg/dL (<3.0 mmol/L) (19.2% vs 7.5%) (Answer A).

The DINAMO study included individuals who were already being treated with metformin or insulin, and patients were eligible for enrollment if their hemoglobin A_{1c} values were between 6.5% and 10.5% (48 and

91 mmol/mol). Empagliflozin lowered hemoglobin A_{1c} by an average of 0.8% vs placebo at week 26, indicating that most adolescents should not expect a hemoglobin A_{1c} reduction greater than 1% (thus, Answer B is incorrect). In subgroup analysis, empagliflozin showed greater efficacy in participants with higher baseline hemoglobin A_{1c} and fasting plasma glucose.

SGLT-2 inhibitors have demonstrated efficacy in reducing weight and lowering blood pressure in adults. Several studies have demonstrated between 2% and 4% weight loss for adults, but this has not been demonstrated in adolescents (thus, Answer E is incorrect). In the DINAMO study, the adjusted mean change in body weight from baseline to week 26 was −0.75 kg and the adjusted mean change in systolic blood pressure vs placebo was −1.42 mm Hg, but neither difference achieved significance.

While nausea, vomiting, and diarrhea are a concern as a potential risk with GLP-1 receptor agonists, this has not been demonstrated in patients treated with SGLT-2 inhibitors (thus, Answer D is incorrect). Rates of gastrointestinal adverse effects in the DINAMO study were low and did not differ between empagliflozin and placebo groups.

SGLT-2 inhibitors work to lower blood glucose by reducing reabsorption of filtered glucose from the renal tubular lumen, which reduces the passive reabsorption of water within the collecting duct. This causes a transient increase in urine volume that generally normalizes within a week. Sustained polyuria has been observed in studies of adult patients with congestive heart failure treated with SGLT-2 inhibitors but not in other populations (thus, Answer C is incorrect).

SGLT-2 inhibitors appear to be safe and well-tolerated in adolescents with type 2 diabetes, with efficacy similar to that of GLP-1 receptor agonists. However, existing data do not indicate a benefit in terms of weight reduction. The American Diabetes Association Standards of Care in Diabetes 2024 recommendations include addition of a GLP-1 receptor agonist or SGLT-2 inhibitor in youth with type 2 diabetes who are not meeting hemoglobin A_{1c} goals with insulin and/or metformin.

Educational Objective

Guide appropriate use of SGLT-2 inhibitors in pediatric patients and advise patients on expected effects.

Reference(s)

American Diabetes Association Professional Practice Committee. 14. Children and adolescents: standards of care in diabetes-2024. *Diabetes Care.* 2024;47(Suppl 1):S258-S281. PMID: 38078582

Laffel LM, Danne T, Klingensmith GJ, et al. Efficacy and safety of the SGLT2 inhibitor empagliflozin versus placebo and the DPP-4 inhibitor linagliptin versus placebo in young people with type 2 diabetes (DINAMO): a multicentre, randomised, double-blind, parallel group, phase 3 trial. *Lancet Diabetes Endocrinol.* 2023;11(3):169-181. PMID: 36738751

72 ANSWER: E) Zinc measurement

Zinc has an essential role in GH biosynthesis and secretion, as well as in IGF-1 generation and responsiveness. Low IGF-1 and IGFBP-3 levels are seen in children with zinc deficiency (Answer E), and these levels improve with zinc replacement. Furthermore, in children with GH deficiency, GH responsiveness is reduced if there is coexisting zinc deficiency.

Clinical zinc deficiency can be seen with prolonged breastfeeding with delayed introduction of foods beyond 6 months. Premature infants are particularly at risk. Natural grains have low zinc concentrations, and dietary phytates reduce zinc absorption. Mild zinc deficiency is common and is likely underrecognized. In severe cases, deficiency can be associated with diarrhea, impaired immune function, hypogonadism, and the rash observed in this patient (acrodermatitis enteropathica).

Iron deficiency (Answer C) is associated with fatigue, pica, hair loss, and angular cheilitis.

Copper deficiency (Answer A) causes edema, brittle hair, and neurological abnormalities.

Although this boy's IGF-1 level is low, this can be seen in zinc deficiency. GH-stimulation testing (Answer B) would not identify the diagnosis in this case, as GH deficiency is not associated with this characteristic rash. Micronutrient deficiencies should always be considered in children presenting with faltering growth on a background of a restrictive diet.

Scurvy is caused by vitamin C deficiency (Answer D) and is characterized by ecchymoses, perifollicular hemorrhage, gingivitis, and arthralgia.

Note: Image in the vignette is reprinted from Zhao M, Shen C. Acrodermatitis enteropathica. N Engl J Med. *2023;389(19):1803.*

Educational Objective

Identify the role of mineral deficiencies in growth failure.

Reference(s)

Hamza RT, Hamed AI, Sallam MT. Effect of zinc supplementation on growth hormone-insulin growth factor axis in short Egyptian children with zinc deficiency. *Ital J Pediatr.* 2012;38:21. PMID: 22625223

Jen M, Yan AC. Syndromes associated with nutritional deficiency and excess. *Clin Dermatol.* 2010;28(6):669-685. PMID: 21034991

Miletta MC, Schoni MH, Kernland K, Mullis PE, Petkovic V. The role of zinc dynamics in growth hormone secretion. *Horm Res Paediatr.* 2013;80(6):381-389. PMID: 24296719

Petkovic V, Miletta MC, Mullis PE. From endoplasmic reticulum to secretory granules: role of zinc in the secretory pathway of growth hormone. *Endocr Dev.* 2012;23:96-108. PMID: 23182824

Siklar Z, Tuna C, Dallar Y, Tanyer G. Zinc deficiency: a contributing factor of short stature in growth hormone deficient children. *J Trop Pediatr.* 2003;49(3):187-188. PMID: 12848213

73 ANSWER: A) *AIP*

This patient has both clinical evidence (growth acceleration, menstrual disruption, coarse facial features, hypertension) and biochemical evidence (elevated IGF-1, elevated random GH) of GH excess. When GH excess occurs in a patient with open epiphyses (gigantism), affected individuals, mostly children, experience brisk linear growth, often well above midparental potential and not aligned with typical timing, as in this case. When GH excess occurs in patients, mostly adults, with closed epiphyses (acromegaly), other clinical features predominate, including some of those this patient experienced, as well as others (eg, snoring and obstructive sleep apnea, arthralgias, and hyperglycemia).

Whereas acromegaly sometimes occurs as part of a genetic syndrome, many cases are sporadic. In contrast, nearly 50% of cases of gigantism have a genetic etiology. The rapidly evolving understanding of pituitary tumor genetics may demonstrate an even more substantial genetic contribution in the future.

This patient's gigantism occurred without any personal or family history suggestive of a particular genetic or familial tumor syndrome. In this setting, a pathogenic variant in the gene encoding aryl hydrocarbon receptor interacting protein (*AIP*) (Answer A) is the most likely identifiable variant (in one series, *AIP* pathogenic variants were the culprit in ~29% of patients).

Approximately 10% of gigantism cases are caused by pathogenic germline or somatic microduplications of Xq26.3 containing *GPR101* (Answer C), which are associated with X-linked acrogigantism (X-LAG). The median age of onset of GH excess in X-LAG is often before age 4 years, and this very young age is also associated with an aggressive presentation and limited treatment response. X-LAG can sometimes present with tumors that also contain some lactotrophs (vs stalk effect leading to modest prolactin elevation). However, this patient is much older than the typical age at which X-LAG is diagnosed.

While pathogenic variants in *GNAS* (Answer B) can lead to gigantism, they do so in the context of clinical McCune-Albright syndrome, and this patient has no evidence of this condition.

Multiple endocrine neoplasia type 1 (caused by *MEN1* pathogenic variants) (Answer D) and neurofibromatosis (caused by *NF1* pathogenic variants) (Answer E) can be associated with GH excess. There is no family or personal history to suggest these entities.

Unfortunately, pituitary gigantism usually presents with suprasellar extension and associated symptoms such as visual deficits. As is the case for acromegaly, surgical resection is the typical first management step. However, with these frequently aggressive tumors, multimodal therapy (surgery, medical management, radiation), informed by germline and tumor genetic studies, is often required. This patient underwent more than one surgical resection, and at various intervals she received a somatostatin analogue, GH-receptor antagonist, dopamine agonist, and proton-beam radiation therapy before she ultimately achieved remission.

**Image in the vignette reprinted from Galbiati F, Kaiser UB. Early onset GH excess: somatotroph adenoma in a young adult.* JCEM Case Rep. *2023;1(2):luad030.*

Educational Objective

Identify genetic causes of GH-secreting adenomas in childhood.

Reference(s)

Korbonits M, Blair JC, Boguslawska A, et al. Consensus guideline for the diagnosis and management of pituitary adenomas in childhood and adolescence: part 1, general recommendations. *Nat Rev Endocrinol.* 2024;20(5):278-289. PMID: 38336897

Galbiati F, Kaiser UB. Early onset GH excess: somatotroph adenoma in a young adult. *JCEM Case Rep.* 2023;1(2):luad030. PMID: 37908473

Rostomyan L, Daly AF, Petrossians P, et al. Clinical and genetic characterization of pituitary gigantism: an international collaborative study in 208 patients. *Endocr Relat Cancer.* 2015;22(5):745-757. PMID: 26187128

Stratakis CA. An update on, and genetics of refractory adenomas of childhood. *Pituitary.* 2023;26(3):281-287. PMID: 37318708

74 **ANSWER: C) Measure TSH in 4 to 6 months**

Hyperthyrotropinemia, also called subclinical hypothyroidism, is defined as a TSH elevation with normal free T_4 levels. TSH elevation is often considered the first sign of possible thyroid dysfunction. In adults, subclinical hypothyroidism is associated with adverse cardiovascular outcomes, including coronary heart disease, heart failure, and metabolic dysfunction-associated steatotic liver disease. There remains debate about the necessity or benefit of treatment for those with subclinical hypothyroidism with or without obesity. For both pediatric and adult patients, subclinical hypothyroidism has been frequently observed in those with elevated BMI and, in most cases, it is not autoimmune in nature. Multiple studies in both pediatric and adult patients have reported positive correlations between baseline TSH and BMI Z-score. The mechanisms by which obesity promotes subclinical hypothyroidism are imperfectly understood. However, TSH modulation by leptin or an adaptive response to increased energy expenditure has been considered.

There is often concern on the part of patients and families that subclinical hypothyroidism is driving weight gain, given the thyroid gland's role in regulating metabolism. However, a number of studies refute these concerns and support the claim that elevated TSH is a consequence, rather than the cause, of overweight/obesity. Studies have demonstrated that weight loss in most patients with isolated subclinical hypothyroidism leads to improvements in TSH without the need for medical therapy (Answer E). Given these data, the most appropriate next step in clinical management would be to monitor this patient's TSH trend over time (Answer C).

Ashwagandha (Withania somnifera) (Answer D) is an herb whose roots have been used in Ayurvedic medicine for centuries. Ashwagandha supplements, which contain the root powder, have become increasingly popular for their purported health benefits, including treatment of subclinical hypothyroidism. While one small study of adults with subclinical hypothyroidism reported improvements in TSH after 8 weeks of Ashwagandha treatment, the lack of regulatory oversight, as well as insufficient data on long-term safety and efficacy, means that supplementation should not be recommended to this patient and family.

In addition to TSH elevations that have been demonstrated in the setting of overweight/obesity, many studies have also reported elevations in free T_3 values. While an elevated free T_3 value could further support that the patient's subclinical hypothyroidism is related to weight status, it is not absolutely necessary for clinical care and its measurement (Answer A) contributes to health care expenses.

While autoimmune thyroiditis can present as subclinical hypothyroidism, this has not been commonly reported in patients with obesity and subclinical hypothyroidism. This patient does not have evidence of a goiter, which is common with autoimmune thyroiditis, and there is no relevant family history. While it would be reasonable to consider assessing thyroid antibodies in the future if an upward trend in TSH were noted, thyroglobulin antibodies alone (Answer B) are less reliable for diagnosis of autoimmune thyroiditis than measurement of TPO antibodies.

Educational Objective

Explain the association between pediatric obesity and abnormal thyroid function test results.

Reference(s)

Chen X, Deng S, Sena C, Zhou C, Thaker VV. Relationship of TSH Levels with Cardiometabolic risk factors in US youth and reference percentiles for thyroid function. *J Clin Endocrinol Metab.* 2021;106(3):e1221-e1230. PMID: 33274355

Grandone A, Santoro N, Coppola F, Calabrò P, Perrone L, Del Giudice EM. Thyroid function derangement and childhood obesity: an Italian experience. *BMC Endocr Disord.* 2010;10:8. PMID: 20441588

Krause AJ, Cines B, Pogrebniak E, et al. Associations between adiposity and indicators of thyroid status in children and adolescents. *Pediatr Obes.* 2016;11(6):551-558. PMID: 26910299

Matusik P, Gawlik A, Januszek-Trzciakowska A, Malecka-Tendera E. Isolated subclinical hyperthyrotropinemia in obese children: does levothyroxine (LT4) improve weight reduction during combined behavioral therapy? *Int J Endocrinol.* 2015;2015:792509. PMID: 26229533

75 ANSWER: A) Discontinue phosphate and calcitriol 1 week before starting burosumab

X-linked hypophosphatemia (XLH) is caused by pathogenic variants in the *PHEX* gene, which lead to elevated circulating FGF-23. This results in hypophosphatemia, a reduced active vitamin D concentration, and rickets in children. Conventional therapy for XLH includes oral phosphate and active vitamin D analogues, but these do not address the root cause of high FGF-23 levels. Additionally, conventional therapy has challenges such as frequent daily dosing and adverse effects such as gastrointestinal symptoms, secondary hyperparathyroidism, and nephrocalcinosis. Burosumab, a recombinant human IgG1 monoclonal antibody that binds to and inhibits FGF-23 activity, was approved in 2018 for the treatment of X-linked hypophosphatemic rickets. Burosumab is administered subcutaneously every 2 weeks in children and every 4 weeks in adults. In clinical trials, burosumab demonstrated consistent benefits over conventional therapy in improving rickets, skeletal deformities, growth, and biochemical markers in children with XLH. Burosumab should not be given alongside conventional treatment, as combined therapies (Answers C and E) can lead to high phosphorus levels. Calcitriol and phosphate treatment should be discontinued 1 week before starting burosumab to allow for a wash-out period (thus, Answer A is correct and Answers B and D are incorrect).

Educational Objective

Formulate optimal management strategies for X-linked hypophosphatemic rickets based on current clinical guidelines and evidence.

Reference(s)

Ackah SA, Imel EA. Approach to hypophosphatemic rickets. *J Clin Endocrinol Metab.* 2022;108(1):209-220. PMID: 35981346

Padidela R, Cheung MS, Saraff V, Dharmaraj P. Clinical guidelines for burosumab in the treatment of XLH in children and adolescents: British paediatric and adolescent bone group recommendations. *Endocr Connect.* 2020;9(10):1051-1056. PMID: 33112809

76 ANSWER: D) Recessive pathogenic variants in the IGF acid-labile subunit gene (*IGFALS*)

The patient described in this vignette has classic acid-labile subunit deficiency. In circulation, IGF-1 is bound in a ternary complex to an IGF-binding protein (most commonly IGFBP-3 or IGFBP-5) in conjunction with the acid-labile subunit. This ternary complex serves to increase the half-life of circulating IGF-1 from approximately 12 minutes in its free form to more than 12 hours in the ternary complex. Patients with recessive pathogenic variants in the IGF acid-labile subunit gene (*IGFALS*) (Answer D) present with relatively mild short stature that is out of proportion to the very low IGF-1 and IGFBP-3 levels. IGFBP-3 is characteristically much lower than IGF-1. The relatively mild short stature in the face of very low circulating IGF-1 levels speaks to the relative importance of local IGF-1 production at the growth plate compared with circulating IGF-1 levels. Patients with acid-labile subunit deficiency may also have insulin resistance with elevated fasting insulin levels. Delayed puberty is commonly seen in these patients, especially in males.

Interestingly, heterozygous carriers of pathogenic *IGFALS* variants are on average approximately 1 SD shorter than relatives who do not carry the variant. The patient's parents must be heterozygous carriers, as the patient is affected with a recessive disorder. Their children each have a 25% chance of being affected with acid-labile subunit deficiency, a 50% chance of being a heterozygous carrier, and a 25% chance of not inheriting either copy of the variant. This distribution is seen in the patient's siblings in the pedigree.

The other answer options are all genetic causes of GH insensitivity syndrome, which is characterized by short stature, low IGF-1 concentrations, and elevated GH secretion. STAT5b deficiency (Answer E), Laron syndrome (Answer C), and Kowarski syndrome (Answer A) are characterized by severe short stature, often with heights below −5 SD along with a subnormal growth velocity. A heterozygous pathogenic variant in the *IGF1* gene (Answer B) can lead to a wide clinical spectrum, but the pedigree is more suggestive of a recessive disorder. Also, IGFBP-3 would not be more severely affected in any of the other conditions.

Educational Objective

Diagnose acid-labile subunit deficiency based on clinical and biochemical findings and pedigree analysis.

Reference(s)

Domené HM, Bengolea SV, Martínez AS, et al. Deficiency of the circulating insulin-like growth factor system associated with inactivation of the acid-labile subunit gene. *N Engl J Med.* 2004;350(6):570-577. PMID: 14762184

Domené HM, Hwa V, Jasper HG, Rosenfeld RG. Acid-labile subunit (ALS) deficiency. *Best Pract Res Clin Endocrinol Metab.* 2011;25(1):101-113. PMID: 21396577

Fofanova-Gambetti OV, Hwa V, Wit JM, et al. Impact of heterozygosity for acid-labile subunit (IGFALS) gene mutations on stature: results from the international acid-labile subunit consortium. *J Clin Endocrinol Metab.* 2010;95(9):4184-4191. PMID: 20591980

Storr HL, Chatterjee S, Metherell LA, et al. Nonclassical GH insensitivity: characterization of mild abnormalities of GH action. *Endocr Rev.* 2019;40(2):476-505. PMID: 30265312

77 **ANSWER: E) Phosphate and calcitriol**

This patient has hypophosphatemic rickets, as evidenced by significant hypophosphatemia, elevated alkaline phosphatase and PTH, and signs of rickets on radiographs. Hypophosphatemic rickets are due to renal phosphate wasting and can be divided into 2 groups: FGF-23–mediated and non–FGF-23–mediated forms. FGF-23 is a phosphaturic hormone that is produced by osteocytes, and it reduces expression of the renal sodium-phosphate cotransporters, thereby reducing renal phosphate reabsorption in the proximal tubule. FGF-23 inhibits 1α-hydroxylase activity, and thus the synthesis of 1,25-dihydroxyvitamin D in the kidney. The most common form of FGF-23–mediated hypophosphatemic rickets is X-linked hypophosphatemic rickets (XLH) caused by loss-of-function pathogenic variants in *PHEX.* Other forms of FGF-23–mediated hypophosphatemic rickets are autosomal dominant caused by pathogenic variants in the *FGF23* gene and 3 autosomal recessive forms caused by pathogenic variants in *DMP1* (encodes dentin matrix acidic phosphoprotein 1), *ENPP1* (encodes the enzyme ectonucleotide pyrophosphatase/phosphodiesterase 1), and *FAM20C* (encodes a Golgi-localized protein kinase that phosphorylates protein and proteoglycans). It is important to perform genetic testing in patients with hypophosphatemic rickets to delineate the underlying genetic etiology.

Biallelic loss-of-function variants in the *ENPP1* gene are associated with 2 clinical phenotypes: generalized arterial calcification of infancy (GACI) and autosomal recessive hypophosphatemic rickets type 2 (ARHR2), both representing a spectrum of ENPP1 deficiency. GACI is a potentially life-threatening condition characterized by infantile-onset diffuse calcification of the arterial media and/or stenosis of large- and medium- sized arteries. This condition is primarily caused by pathogenic variants in *ENPP1* (type 1) in approximately 70% to 75% of cases, or less commonly, by pathogenic variants in *ABCC6* (type 2). These variants disrupt the normal function of inorganic pyrophosphate, a critical inhibitor of pathological calcification. Infants with GACI may present with respiratory distress due to pulmonary hypertension, arterial hypertension, or heart failure. The overall mortality is approximately 55% within the first 6 months of life. Most infants with GACI who survive develop ARHR2 later in life. Spontaneous resolution of arterial calcifications can be observed. Other individuals with ENPP1 deficiency are diagnosed with hypophosphatemic rickets type 2 without a previous GACI diagnosis (like this patient). ENPP1 deficiency is associated with elevated FGF-23, which leads to ARHR2. The mechanism underlying elevated FGF-23 in ENPP1 deficiency has not been elucidated, but it is speculated that it might be a protective response to counter extraskeletal calcification by inducing hypophosphatemia in individuals with *ENPP1* pathogenic variants.

Treatment of ARHR2 includes phosphate and calcitriol (Answer E), which have been shown to improve rickets and bone pain. This treatment requires close monitoring of biochemical parameters and signs of calcification.

Treatment with burosumab (Answer B), an anti–FGF-23 antibody, is not recommended in the setting of ARHR2, as reducing FGF-23 may negate its protective benefit in preventing calcification. Worsening of arterial or cardiac calcifications has been reported in patients treated with burosumab.

Bisphosphonates (Answer A) have been used in infants with GACI to reduce arterial calcifications. However, the benefits are not clear and remain controversial. A recent study indicated that bisphosphonate treatment to reduce calcifications may not be effective if started later than 7 days after birth. Bisphosphonate treatment is generally not recommended for hypophosphatemic rickets of any form, including ARHR2.

Cinacalcet (Answer C) is a calcimimetic agent that decreases PTH and calcium by enhancing the sensitivity of calcium-sensing receptors to extracellular calcium. It is used in secondary hyperparathyroidism in patients with chronic kidney disease on dialysis, as well as in hypercalcemia in patients with parathyroid carcinoma and primary hyperparathyroidism who are unable to undergo parathyroidectomy. Although PTH levels are often elevated in hypophosphatemic rickets, cinacalcet is not indicated because it does not address phosphate wasting.

Treatment with high-dosage cholecalciferol (Answer D) is not effective in hypophosphatemic rickets.

* *Image in vignette reprinted from Choe Y, Shin CH, Lee YA, Kim MJ, Lee YJ. Case report and review of literature: autosomal recessive hypophosphatemic rickets type 2 caused by a pathogenic variant in ENPP1 gene.* Front Endocrinol (Lausanne). *2022;13:911672.*

Educational Objective

Explain the risk of developing autosomal recessive hypophosphatemic rickets type 2 in survivors of generalized arterial calcification of infancy or in persons with *ENPP1* pathogenic variants and discuss the contraindication of burosumab in this setting.

Reference(s)

Ferreira CR, Kintzinger K, Hackbarth ME, et al. Ectopic calcification and hypophosphatemic rickets: natural history of ENPP1 and ABCC6 deficiencies. *J Bone Mine Res.* 2021;36(11):2193-2202. PMID: 34355424

Höppner J, Kornak U, Sinningen K, Rutsch F, Oheim R, Grasemann C. Autosomal recessive hypophosphatemic rickets type 2 (ARHR2) due to ENPP1-deficiency. *Bone.* 2021;153:116111. PMID: 34252603

Rutsch F, Böyer P, Nitschke Y, et al. Hypophosphatemia, hyperphosphaturia, and bisphosphonate treatment are associated with survival beyond infancy in generalized arterial calcification of infancy. Circ Cardiovasc Genet. 2008;1(2):133-140. PMID: 20016754

78 ANSWER: C) Bethesda III (>50% risk of malignancy)

This patient has a thyroid nodule with several suspicious characteristics on ultrasonography (solid and hypoechoic) and appropriately underwent FNA. The FNA results are consistent with Bethesda III with nuclear atypia. The most recent update to the Bethesda system for reporting thyroid cytopathology was published in 2023. One of the most significant differences is the recommendation that Bethesda III (atypia of undetermined significance [AUS]) be subdivided on the basis of where atypia is located: nuclear or "other." The presence of nuclear atypia is associated with a significantly higher risk of malignancy than other atypia. Several pediatric studies have shown the risk of malignancy for Bethesda III nodules with nuclear atypia is greater than 50% compared with 6% to 15% for AUS without nuclear atypia (thus, Answer B is correct).

The 2023 Bethesda system for reporting thyroid cytopathology has some simplifications and recommends that all cytology results be reported in 1 of the following 6 categories:

Bethesda category	Features	Risk of malignancy (pooled studies)
I	Nondiagnostic (eg, cyst fluid only, virtually acellular, artifacts from clotting or drying, obscured by blood)	0%-33%
II	Benign (eg, consistent with follicular nodular disease, chronic lymphocytic thyroiditis, or granulomatous thyroiditis)	0%-27%
III	Atypia of undetermined significance (should be specified whether the atypia is nuclear or nonnuclear "other" [architectural/oncocytic/lymphocytic])	11%-54% Nuclear atypia: >50% Nonnuclear atypia: 6%-15%
IV	Follicular neoplasm (should be specified if oncocytic type [formerly Hurthle cell])	28%-100%
V	Suspicious for malignancy (eg, papillary thyroid carcinoma/medullary thyroid carcinoma/metastatic carcinoma/lymphoma/other)	40%-100%
VI	Malignant (eg, papillary thyroid carcinoma/high-grade follicular-derived carcinoma/medullary thyroid carcinoma/squamous-cell carcinoma/carcinoma with mixed features/metastatic malignancy/lymphoma)	86%-100%

Based on Ali SZ et al. *Thyroid*, 2023; 33(9): 1039-1044. © Mary Ann Liebert, Inc.

The 2015 American Thyroid Association guidelines for management of pediatric thyroid nodules recommends surgery for all nodules with Bethesda III, IV, V, or VI cytopathology. Clearly, the risk of malignancy varies enormously between these groups, and many recommend that monitoring with repeat ultrasonography and FNA is a reasonable approach for some nodules with Bethesda III cytology deemed to have a lower risk of malignancy. This particular patient has a 3.2-cm nodule, which may or may not be bothering her cosmetically. The presence of nuclear atypia substantially increases her risk of malignancy. In this situation, surgery will be recommended, but shared decision-making with the patient and her family should be undertaken to determine next steps.

Answer A (Bethesda II [5%-15% risk of malignancy]]) is incorrect, as Bethesda II is benign cytology, which was not seen in this case. For Bethesda II cytology, pooled data from pediatric studies show 0% to 27% risk of malignancy.

Answer B (Bethesda III [10%-20% risk of malignancy]) is incorrect because the malignancy risk is greater than 50% in this case due to the presence of nuclear atypia. For all Bethesda III nodules (before the distinction of location of atypia), the malignancy risk is 11% to 54%.

Answers D and E are incorrect because the histology in this vignette is Bethesda III, not IV. The malignancy risk in nodules with Bethesda IV cytology in pooled pediatric studies is 28% to 100%.

Educational Objective

Describe the 2023 updates to the Bethesda system for reporting thyroid cytopathology.

Reference(s)

Ali SZ, Baloch ZW, Cochand-Priollet B, Schmitt FC, Vielh P, VanderLaan PA. The 2024 Bethesda System for Reporting Thyroid Cytopathology. *Thyroid.* 2023;33(9):1039-1044. PMID: 37427847

Ali SZ, VanderLaan PA, eds. *The Bethesda System for Reporting Thyroid Cytopathology: Definitions, Criteria, and Explanatory Notes.* 3rd ed. Springer; 2023.

Cherella CE, Hollowell ML, Smith JR, et al. Subtype of atypia on cytology and risk of malignancy in pediatric thyroid nodules. *Cancer Cytopathol.* 2022;130(5):330-335. PMID: 35119774

Jin X, Jing X, Smola B, Heider A. Malignant risk of pediatric Bethesda category III thyroid nodules subcategorized by nuclear atypia and other: a single institution experience. *Cancer Cytopathol.* 2024;132(9):564-568. PMID: 38771850

79 **ANSWER: D) Start intramuscular testosterone enanthate injections, 100 mg once monthly**

Klinefelter syndrome is a sex chromosome aneuploidy caused by an extra X chromosome (47,XXY) that occurs in approximately 1 in 600 males. In addition to physical features such as hypogonadism, gynecomastia, and tall stature, Klinefelter syndrome may be associated with a variety of behavioral findings, including language and learning problems, increased anxiety, and depressed mood. Hypogonadism may lead to changes in body composition and risk of developing metabolic syndrome and type 2 diabetes. Some evidence suggests that cognitive impairment may be affected by hypogonadism.

Medical treatment is mainly testosterone replacement therapy to alleviate acute and long-term consequences of hypogonadism, as well as to treat or prevent frequent comorbidities. This child has reached near-final adult height, and he is bothered by his appearance. The workup indicates that he has testicular failure. Low-dosage testosterone therapy will enhance his secondary sexual characteristics without adversely affecting his final height at this point. The typical treatment regimen for testicular failure in teens with Klinefelter syndrome who are 13 to 18 years old is intramuscular testosterone enanthate or cypionate (50 to 100 mg monthly) (Answer D) until growth ceases or until age 18 to 19 years.

Intramuscular testosterone, 25 mg once monthly (Answer E), would be a relatively low dosage, given that this child already has some pubertal development, his testicular volume is 8 cc, and his testosterone concentration is not extremely low.

Transdermal testosterone products and testosterone enanthate administered subcutaneously have not been approved for use in boys due to lack of efficacy and safety data. However, transdermal and subcutaneous formulations can be used off-label at low dosages (eg, one-half the usual adult dose) for adolescent males.

Although transdermal testosterone application obviates the need for injections, adherence to monthly injections might be easier for some patients. Very long-acting testosterone formulations (such as intramuscular testosterone undecanoate given every 12 weeks or testosterone pellets) are not recommended in teenage boys because low doses of these preparations cannot be delivered reliably.

Testosterone therapy can improve secondary sexual characteristics, such as facial hair growth and a deeper voice, can reduce gynecomastia and behavioral problems, and may improve psychosocial outcomes. Testosterone therapy can also improve bone mineral density. Erythrocytosis is a common adverse effect of testosterone therapy. Because the risk of venous thromboembolic disease is directly related to hematocrit, periodic complete blood cell count is recommended in patients on testosterone replacement. Prostate volumes and serum PSA increase in response to testosterone treatment is less of a concern in teenagers than in adults.

His condition is unlikely to reverse itself, so delaying treatment for another year (Answer B) is incorrect. This patient also has high LH levels and low-normal testosterone levels, indicating the need for exogenous replacement therapy.

There is no information in the stem indicating that testicular ultrasonography (Answer A) would offer useful information at this point. Individuals with Klinefelter syndrome are at high risk for germinomas, which may present as testicular tumors. However, this patient's testosterone concentration is not high, and testicular examination did not reveal any firm masses. Gonadal germ-cell tumors are rare in pediatric patients with Klinefelter syndrome. Individuals with Klinefelter syndrome have an increased risk of several malignancies, especially breast cancer and extragonadal germ-cell tumors, primarily localized in the mediastinum.

Individuals with Klinefelter syndrome can have mild learning disabilities. This particular patient does not appear to be extremely affected. Thus, cognitive evaluation (Answer C), while it could be helpful, would not be the most important next step in his management, as it would not address his concerns related to hypogonadism.

Educational Objective

Recommend the best treatment to address hypogonadism in a teenage boy with Klinefelter syndrome.

Reference(s)

Aksglaede L, Link K, Giwercman A, Jorgensen N, Skakkebaek NE, Juul A. 47,XXY Klinefelter syndrome: clinical characteristics and age-specific recommendations for medical management. *Am J Med Genet C Semin Med Genet.* 2013;163C(1):55-63. PMID: 23345262

Groth KA, Skakkebæk A, Høst C, Gravholt CH, Bojesen A. Clinical review: Klinefelter syndrome—a clinical update. *J Clin Endocrinol Metab.* 2013;98(1):20-30. PMID: 23118429

80 ANSWER: B) Current treatment with megestrol

Many survivors of childhood cancer develop endocrine comorbidities from either the cancer itself and/or from the myriad anticancer treatments they receive. As more and more children are successfully treated for cancer, a growing number will need lifelong multidisciplinary care to manage the lasting effects on diverse health outcomes. From an endocrine perspective, risks include pituitary hormone deficiencies, infertility, impaired bone health, increased cardiometabolic risk, and secondary malignancies (eg, thyroid). In some individuals, the effects of these treatments are apparent immediately, whereas in others, it may take time, even years, for health problems to emerge. Thus, careful evaluation of risk and ongoing evidence-supported surveillance are essential.

This patient has hyponatremia related to adrenal insufficiency, as supported by a cortisol concentration that was below the assay's lower limit. Megestrol treatment (Answer B) is the most likely culprit. Megestrol is a progestin analogue that is used for palliation in some gynecological malignancies, and it is often prescribed to patients with cancer who have cachexia because it also increases appetite. Megestrol also has activity at the glucocorticoid receptor and is thus a known precipitant of symptomatic iatrogenic adrenal insufficiency, in particular during illness with impaired enteral intake, as in this vignette. In previous studies, results of provocative testing (eg, low-dose cosyntropin-stimulation testing) in individuals taking megestrol have been consistent with secondary adrenal insufficiency. With time off megestrol, function of the hypothalamic-pituitary-adrenal axis is expected to be restored. In the interim, treatment with stress-dose glucocorticoid replacement is indicated, in particular if enteral intake is compromised. Also, similar to glucocorticoid treatment, abrupt withdrawal of megestrol can precipitate pseudotumor cerebri syndrome. Unfortunately, systematic investigations have found that adrenal insufficiency is a common complication of megestrol, which may limit enthusiasm for its use, despite its benefits with respect to weight gain. At minimum, practitioners should be aware of and vigilant for this potential complication, since scenarios like the one in this vignette have been reported by multiple groups.

All of the listed treatment modalities could affect this patient's endocrine health. The effects of total-body irradiation (Answer E) are being appreciated. However, at the dose received by this patient, there would not be an expected effect on either the pituitary (to produce secondary adrenal insufficiency) or the adrenal glands (to cause primary adrenal insufficiency). Higher doses (≥30 Gy) to the hypothalamus/pituitary can cause secondary adrenal insufficiency.

Previous treatment with cyclophosphamide (Answer C) is a risk for primary gonadal, not adrenal, insufficiency.

While previous glucocorticoid therapy (Answer D) often produces iatrogenic adrenal insufficiency, the duration (1.5 years) since the last prednisone dose makes this a less likely etiology.

Similarly, while inhaled glucocorticoids (Answer A) can impact the hypothalamic-pituitary-adrenal axis, the effect is not typically to this extent, and megestrol is much more likely to be the cause.

Educational Objective

Recognize the potential for megestrol to cause secondary adrenal insufficiency.

Reference(s)

Chidakel AR, Zweig SB, Schlosser JR, Homel P, Schappert JW, Fleckman AM. High prevalence of adrenal suppression during acute illness in hospitalized patients receiving megestrol acetate. *J Endocrinol Invest.* 2006;29(2):136-140. PMID: 16610239

Children's Oncology Group. Long-Term Follow-Up Guidelines for Survivors of Childhood, Adolescent, and Young Adult Cancer. Available at: http://www.survivorshipguidelines.org/pdf/2023/COG_LTFU_Guidelines_Comprehensive_v6.pdf.

Meacham LR, Mazewski C, Krawiecki N. Mechanism of transient adrenal insufficiency with megestrol acetate treatment of cachexia in children with cancer. *J Pediatr Hematol Oncol.* 2003;25(5):414-417. PMID: 12759631

Orme LM, Bond JD, Humphrey MS, et al. Megestrol acetate in pediatric oncology patients may lead to severe, symptomatic adrenal suppression. *Cancer.* 2003;98(2):397-405. PMID: 12872362

Ron IG, Soyfer V, Goldray D, Inbar MJ, Weisman Y. A low-dose adrenocorticotropin test reveals impaired adrenal function in cancer patients receiving megestrol acetate therapy. *Eur J Cancer.* 2002;38(11):1490-1494. PMID: 12110495

81 ANSWER: C) 17α-Hydroxylase/17,20-lyase deficiency (P450c17)

Phenotypic females with a 46,XY karyotype due to complete 17α-hydroxylase/17,20-lyase deficiency (Answer C), caused by *CYP17A1* gene pathogenic variants, have absent adrenal and testicular steroidogenesis. Affected individuals have no wolffian ducts because of absent testosterone synthesis in utero and no müllerian structures due to antimüllerian hormone secreted by the Sertoli cells. Presenting symptoms can include a hernia or inguinal mass, primary amenorrhea, lack of secondary sex development (including pubic and axillary hair) due to hypergonadotropic hypogonadism, and low renin hypertension due to elevated 11-deoxycorticosterone levels. Affected individuals do not typically develop salt-wasting or adrenal crisis because elevated precursors 11-deoxycorticosterone and corticosterone have mineralocorticoid and glucocorticoid activity, respectively (*figure 1*). Progesterone levels are characteristically elevated. In addition, increased ACTH stimulation of the zona fasciculata leads to increased production of 11-deoxycorticosterone, a steroid with mineralocorticoid activity, and corticosterone, a steroid with glucocorticoid activity, through the 17-deoxylation pathway that does not require 17α-hydroxylation. The sodium retention and subsequent plasma volume expansion suppress plasma renin activity and inhibit aldosterone synthesis at the zona glomerulosa through the renin-angiotensin-aldosterone axis. Of note, although affected individuals are cortisol-deficient; they do not develop symptoms of adrenal insufficiency because corticosterone has some glucocorticoid activity, which, at elevated levels (50-100 times normal) prevents adrenal insufficiency.

Figure 1. Steroidogenesis in 17α-hydroxylase/17,20-lyase deficiency (P450c17)

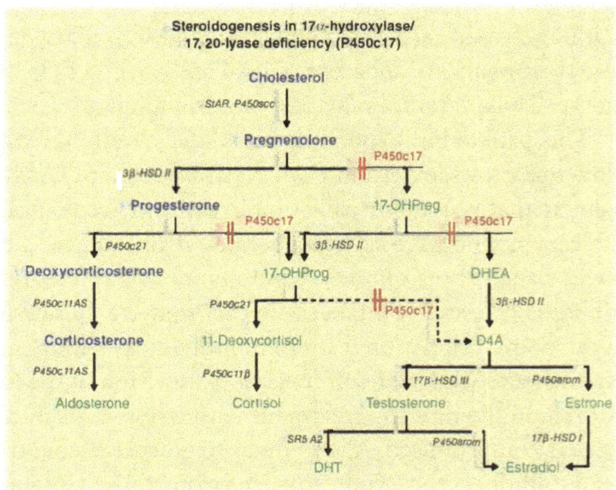

Red bars represent the enzyme block. Increased metabolites are blue. Metabolites that may be deficient are green. Reprinted with permission from Sarafoglou K, Hoffmann GF & Roth KS, eds. *Pediatric Endocrinology and Inborn Errors of Metabolism*. 2nd edition. New York, NY: McGraw-Hill Education; 2017. © The McGraw-Hill Companies, Inc.

Individuals with a 46,XY karyotype due to classic 3β-hydroxysteroid dehydrogenase deficiency type II (Answer E), caused by pathogenic variants in the *HSD3B2* gene, have elevated DHEA-S, decreased synthesis of adrenal androgens, and undervirilized male genitalia ranging from hypospadias and micropenis to penoscrotal hypospadias and bifid scrotum. They typically present with adrenal/salt-wasting crisis during infancy and do not have elevated progesterone levels. They have testes and no uterus. Because of decreased sex steroid synthesis, gonadotropin concentrations are elevated (*figure 2*).

Individuals with a 46,XY karyotype due to lipoid adrenal hyperplasia (Answer B) present during the first months of life with salt-wasting and adrenal crisis. Most cases of lipoid CAH are caused by recessive pathogenic variants in the gene encoding steroidogenic acute regulatory protein (*STAR*). A few patients with lipoid CAH have been reported to have pathogenic variants in the *CYP11A1* gene (aka P450scc). They have hypergonadotropic hypogonadism because both the adrenal glands and the testes have impaired sex hormone steroidogenesis (*figure 3*). Genital atypia in males can range from phenotypic female external genitalia to hypospadias and micropenis to penoscrotal hypospadias and bifid scrotum. They have testes and no uterus.

Individuals with 17β-hydroxysteroid dehydrogenase type III deficiency, caused by pathogenic variants in the *HSD17B3* gene (Answer D) have undervirilized external genitalia, elevated androstenedione, and low testosterone. The diagnosis may require measurement of testosterone and androstenedione after a β-hCG-stimulation test (abnormal if ratio >15:1). Affected individuals have testes and no uterus. LH and FSH are typically elevated.

Patients with a 46,XY difference of sex development due to heterozygous pathogenic variants in the *NR5A1* (*SF-1*) gene (Answer A) have varying degrees of gonadal dysgenesis, normal adrenal function, and no hypertension or elevated progesterone levels.

Educational Objective

Identify adrenal disorders that result in a female phenotype in individuals with a 46,XY karyotype.

Figure 2. Steroidogenesis in 3β-hydroxysteroid dehydrogenase deficiency type II

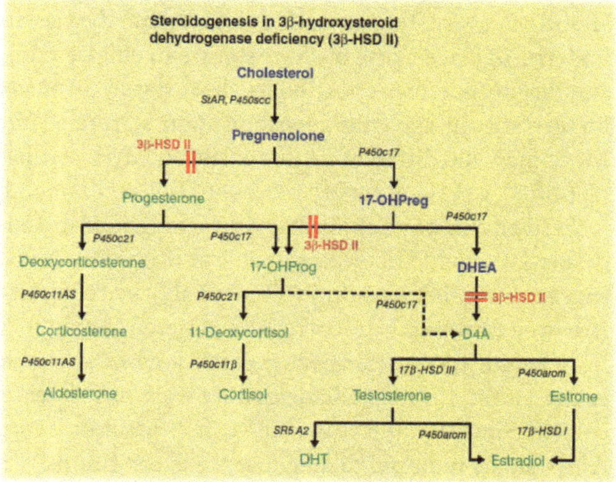

Red bars represent the enzyme block. Increased metabolites are blue. Metabolites that may be deficient are green. Reprinted with permission from Sarafoglou K, Hoffmann GF & Roth KS, eds. *Pediatric Endocrinology and Inborn Errors of Metabolism*. 2nd edition. New York, NY: McGraw-Hill Education; 2017. © The McGraw-Hill Companies, Inc.

Figure 3. Steroidogenesis in congenital lipoid adrenal hyperplasia

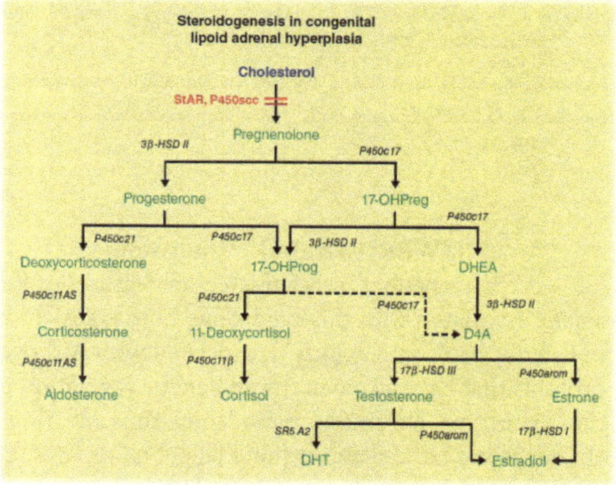

Red bars represent the enzyme block. Increased metabolites are blue. Metabolites that may be deficient are green. Reprinted with permission from Sarafoglou K, Hoffmann GF & Roth KS, eds. *Pediatric Endocrinology and Inborn Errors of Metabolism*. 2nd edition. New York, NY: McGraw-Hill Education; 2017. © The McGraw-Hill Companies, Inc.

Reference(s)

Claahsen-van der Grinten HL, Speiser PW, Ahmed SF, et al. Congenital adrenal hyperplasia-current insights in pathophysiology, diagnostics, and management. *Endocr Rev*. 2022;43(1):91-159. PMID: 33961029

Monig I, Schneidewind J, Johannsen TH, et al. Pubertal development in 46,XY patients with NR5A1 mutations. *Endocrine*. 2022;75(2):601-613. PMID: 34613524

Sarafoglou K, Reiner W, Hindmarsh PC. Congenital adrenal hyperplasia. In: Sarafoglou K, Hoffmann GF, Roth KS, eds. *Pediatric Endocrinology and Inborn Errors of Metabolism*. 2nd edition. New York, NY: McGraw-Hill Education; 2017:533-559.

82 ANSWER: D) Skeletal survey

This patient has extreme short stature and is late in puberty without a delayed bone age. His adult height will be significantly below his midparental height percentile. His sitting height-to-standing height ratio is abnormal, suggesting an underlying skeletal dysplasia as the etiology of his short stature. Skeletal dysplasia is an underrecognized cause of short stature in children, highlighting the need for a structured approach to identifying and diagnosing disproportionate short stature. Approximately 15% to 20% of children characterized as being small-for-gestational-age with persistent short stature or idiopathic short stature have an underlying genetic diagnosis. More than 460 different causes of skeletal dysplasia have been identified. When disproportionate short stature is identified, a skeletal survey (Answer D) is recommended as the next step.

Given this boy's abnormal sitting height ratio and clinical phenotype, requesting a genetic panel for skeletal dysplasias would also be reasonable at this point. Not all cases of skeletal dysplasia are identified on skeletal survey, and genetic testing will inevitably be required to make the diagnosis. However, whole-exome sequencing (Answer E) would be incorrect, as targeted testing focused on the clinical phenotype would be preferred.

Genetic testing for specific conditions would be indicated if a diagnosis is suggested by imaging or clinical examination. If Madelung deformity were noted, testing for *SHOX* gene haploinsufficiency (Answer C) would be correct. Similarly, if features of Russell-Silver or Temple syndromes were noted, DNA methylation studies (Answer A) would be required to diagnose these conditions.

In persons with GH deficiency, short stature is not disproportionate. Thus, GH-stimulation testing or IGF-1 measurement (Answer B) is not the appropriate next assessment in this case.

Educational Objective

Guide the workup for disproportionate short stature in a child.

Reference(s)

Freire BL, Homma TK, Funari MFA, et al. Multigene sequencing analysis of children born small for gestational age with isolated short Stature. *J Clin Endocrinol Metab.* 2019;104(6):2023-2030. PMID: 30602027

Hauer NN, Popp B, Schoeller E, et al. Clinical relevance of systematic phenotyping and exome sequencing in patients with short stature. *Genet Med.* 2018;20(6):630-638. PMID: 29758562

Hawkes CP, Mostoufi-Moab S, McCormack SE, Grimberg A, Zemel BS. Sitting Height to standing height ratio reference charts for children in the United States. *J Pediatr.* 2020;226:221-227.e15. PMID: 32579888

Mintz CS, Seaver LH, Irons M, et al. Focused revision: ACMG practice resource: Genetic evaluation of short stature. *Genet Med.* 2021;23(5):813-815. PMID: 33514815

Mortier GR, Cohn DH, Cormier-Daire V, et al. Nosology and classification of genetic skeletal disorders: 2019 revision. *Am J Med Genet A.* 2019;179(12):2393-2419. PMID: 31633310

83 ANSWER: C) Kabuki syndrome

This patient has characteristic features of Kabuki syndrome (Answer C) and has a pathogenic variant in a gene associated with this syndrome. Both transient neonatal and persistent hyperinsulinism have been described in Kabuki syndrome, which is associated with pathogenic variants in *KMT2D* and *KDM6A*. These 2 genes encode proteins that have a role in the epigenetic regulation of transcriptionally active chromatin; pathogenic variants cause abnormal chromatin remodeling, thus affecting multiple organ systems. Hallmark manifestations include characteristic facial features (long palpebral fissures, eversion of the lower lateral lid, long eyelashes, arched and broad eyebrows, depressed nasal tip, prominent ears), craniofacial/skeletal abnormalities, dermatoglyphic abnormalities, mild to moderate intellectual disability, and postnatal growth deficiency. Up to 70% of children with Kabuki syndrome have hyperinsulinism. Other features include congenital heart defects, congenital hypothyroidism, seizures, hypotonia, feeding difficulties, and increased susceptibility to infections.

Most individuals with molecularly confirmed Kabuki syndrome have pathogenic variants in *KMT2D*. While the overall frequency of pathogenic variants in *KDM6A* is about 2% to 8% in individuals with Kabuki syndrome, *KDM6A* variants were found in 5 of 11 children with hyperinsulinism due to Kabuki syndrome in a series reported by Yap et al. The authors also described a good response to medical treatment; 9 of 10 affected patients achieved normal glycemic control with diazoxide, while 1 patient required 98% pancreatectomy at 3 years of age. Kabuki syndrome may be underdiagnosed in infants with hyperinsulinism because this condition has not been included in hyperinsulinism gene panels and typical facial features of this syndrome may not be evident in infants. Although

1 patient in the Yap et al series received an early genetic diagnosis, others were diagnosed with Kabuki syndrome between 6 and 18 months of age.

Typical features of Beckwith-Wiedemann syndrome (Answer A) include neonatal macrosomia, hemihypertrophy, macroglossia, omphalocele, and enlarged organs. Beckwith-Wiedemann syndrome is caused by epigenetic or genetic variants resulting in abnormal methylation in the chromosome 11p15.5 region. Neonatal hypoglycemia is common (~50%), but most patients with persistent hyperinsulinism are unresponsive to diazoxide.

Sotos syndrome (Answer D) is caused by pathogenic variants in *NSD1* or deletions containing *NSD1* and is characterized by macrosomia, developmental delay, and distinctive facial characteristics (eg, prominent forehead, dolichocephaly, and downslanting palpebral fissures). Neonatal hypoglycemia is seen in less than 15% of affected individuals and is most often transient. In persistent cases, the hypoglycemia is responsive to diazoxide.

Costello syndrome (Answer B) is caused by pathogenic variants in components or modulators of the RAS-MAPK pathway and is characterized by heart problems (arrhythmias, structural heart defects, hypertrophic cardiomyopathy), developmental delay, postnatal growth failure, and predisposition to tumors (most commonly papillomas and rhabdomyosarcoma). Distinctive facial features include prominent forehead, full cheeks, and full lips. Neonatal hypoglycemia occurs in nearly half of infants with Costello syndrome. The hypoglycemia is usually diazoxide-responsive and typically resolves by 6 months of age.

Usher-congenital hyperinsulinism syndrome (Answer E) is caused by a homozygous contiguous gene deletion encompassing parts of the *ABCC8* and *USH1C* genes. Features include congenital sensorineural deafness, developmental delay, enteropathy, and renal tubular dysfunction. Hyperinsulinism due to *ABCC8* deletion in these patients is diffuse and most often diazoxide-resistant.

Educational Objective

Identify Kabuki syndrome as a potential cause of syndromic hyperinsulinism.

Reference(s)

Yap KL, Johnson AEK, Fischer D, et al. Congenital hyperinsulinism as the presenting feature of Kabuki syndrome: clinical and molecular characterization of 9 affected individuals. *Genet Med.* 2019;21(1):233-242. PMID: 29907798

Zenker M, Mohnike K, Palm K. Syndromic forms of congenital hyperinsulinism. *Front Endocrinol.* 2023;14:1013874. PMID: 37065762

84 ANSWER: D) Perform thyroid scintigraphy

This adolescent has a thyroid nodule and subclinical hyperthyroidism. The differential diagnosis includes an autonomous (toxic) thyroid nodule or a nonautonomous nodule in the setting of another cause of hyperthyroidism such as Graves disease or transient thyroiditis. In this case, the absence of TSH receptor antibodies or diffuse goiter indicates that Graves disease is unlikely. Although positive TPO antibodies indicate the presence of autoimmune thyroiditis, this does not explain the thyroid asymmetry. Rather, the thyroid asymmetry suggests a possible autonomous nodule causing low TSH, leading to atrophy of the contralateral lobe.

For evaluation of a thyroid nodule, thyroid ultrasonography is recommended to confirm the nodule's presence and sonographic characteristics. In addition, if the TSH concentration is below the reference range, thyroid scintigraphy (uptake and scan) (Answer D) should be performed to determine whether the nodule is autonomous. Criteria for diagnosing an autonomous nodule are focal uptake in the nodule with suppression of uptake in the surrounding thyroid in the setting of low TSH. Autonomous nodules have a very low risk of malignancy (around 2%-3%), and therefore further diagnostic evaluation with FNA (Answer C) generally is not required.

Methimazole (Answer B) may be used to treat hyperthyroidism caused by an autonomous nodule, particularly if the patient is symptomatic, or as a bridge to definitive therapy with surgical resection or radioactive iodine ablation. Atenolol (Answer A) can be used to treat symptoms of hyperthyroidism of any etiology. However, in this asymptomatic patient with subclinical hyperthyroidism, treatment with atenolol or methimazole is not needed immediately, and initial management should focus on evaluation and correct diagnosis of the thyroid nodule.

Referral for surgical consultation (Answer E) may be considered for definitive therapy of an autonomous nodule, but it would be premature at this point in the evaluation.

Educational Objective

Evaluate a thyroid nodule in the setting of hyperthyroidism.

Reference(s)

Francis GL, Waguespack SG, Bauer AJ, et al; American Thyroid Association Guidelines Task Force. Management guidelines for children with thyroid nodules and differentiated thyroid cancer. *Thyroid.* 2015;25(7):716-759. PMID: 25900731

Ly S, Frates MC, Benson CB, et al. Features and outcome of autonomous thyroid nodules in children: 31 consecutive patients seen at a single center. *J Clin Endocrinol Metab.* 2016;101(10):3856-3862. PMID: 27501280

85 **ANSWER: A) Determine the average of 2 auscultatory measurements**

The prevalence of hypertension in children and adolescents ranges from 5% to 30%, with greater prevalence seen in those with higher BMI values. In fact, obesity is considered the strongest risk factor for elevated blood pressure in childhood. Hypertension in childhood and adolescence increases risk for adult hypertension and cardiovascular disease. Therefore, it is recommended that blood pressure be checked in all children and adolescents 3 years of age and older at every health care encounter if they have obesity.

Given lack of outcome data, the current definition of hypertension in children and adolescents is based on the normative distribution of blood pressure in healthy children. The 2017 American Academy of Pediatrics (AAP) clinical practice guideline introduced new age-, sex-, and height-specific normative percentile tables based on the distribution of blood pressure among normal-weight children and adolescents, using the auscultatory technique (*table 1*).

Table 1. Updated Definitions of Blood Pressure Categories and Stages

Children aged 1 to <13 years	Children aged ≥13 years
Normal blood pressure: <90th percentile	Normal blood pressure: <120/<80 mm Hg
Elevated blood pressure: ≥90th percentile to <95th percentile or 120/80 mm Hg to <95th percentile (whichever is lower)	Elevated blood pressure: 120/<80 to 129/<80 mm Hg
Stage 1 hypertension: ≥95th percentile to <95th percentile + 12 mm Hg, or 130/80 to 139/89 mm Hg (whichever is lower)	Stage 1 hypertension: 130/80 to 139/89 mm Hg
Stage 2 hypertension: ≥95th percentile + 12 mm Hg, or ≥140/90 mm Hg (whichever is lower)	Stage 2 hypertension: ≥140/90 mm Hg

Reprinted from Flynn JT et al. Pediatrics, 2017; 140(3): e20171904. © The American Academy of Pediatrics.

Although oscillometric device–determined blood pressure may be suitable for screening, the 2017 AAP clinical practice guideline recommends confirmation of an elevated blood pressure measurement by averaging 2 additional measurements using the auscultatory technique and repeating blood pressure measurements at an interval determined by the severity of the elevation. Even though this patient had blood pressure values at or greater than the 90th percentile for age, sex, and height, the best initial step in management is to obtain at least 2 auscultatory measurements and average these values (Answer A) to define his blood pressure category (*table 1*). Subsequent evaluation and management are outlined according to the AAP clinical practice guideline (*table 2*).

It is critical to obtain multiple blood pressure measurements over time to avoid overdiagnosis and unnecessary treatment. Blood pressure can vary significantly between visits and even during the same visit. Isolated elevated blood pressure can be due to factors such as recent caffeine intake, anxiety, stress, and improper measurement technique. The phenomena of white-coat and masked hypertension are also common in children and adolescents. Therefore, a child or adolescent should only be diagnosed with hypertension when their average blood pressure is at or above the 95th percentile for their age, sex, and height when measured multiple times over the span of several visits, the frequency of which depends on their initial blood pressure category (*table 2*).

Table 2. Patient Evaluation and Management According to Blood Pressure

BP Category (See Table 3)	BP Screening Schedule	Lifestyle Counseling (Weight and Nutrition)	Check Upper and Lower Extremity BP	ABPM[a]	Diagnostic Evaluation[b]	Initiate Treatment[c]	Consider Subspecialty Referral
Normal	Annual	X	—	—	—	—	—
Elevated BP	Initial measurement	X	—	—	—	—	—
	Second measurement: repeat in 6 mo	X	X	—	—	—	—
	Third measurement: repeat in 6 mo	X	—	X	X	—	X
Stage 1 HTN	Initial measurement	X	—	—	—	—	—
	Second measurement: repeat in 1-2 wk	X	X	—	—	—	—
	Third measurement: repeat in 3 mo	X	—	X	X	X	X
Stage 2 HTN[d]	Initial measurement	X	X	—	—	—	—
	Second measurement: repeat, refer to specialty care within 1 wk	X	—	X	X	X	X

Reprinted from Flynn JT et al. *Pediatrics*, 2017; 140(3): e20171904. © The American Academy of Pediatrics.

While lifestyle modifications, including reduction of dietary salt intake (Answer E), are associated with lower blood pressure and would most likely benefit this patient, repeating blood pressure via auscultatory techniques is still the recommended first step.

Electrocardiography (Answer C) takes minimal time and is a relatively low-cost test. While electrocardiography has high specificity, it has poor sensitivity for identifying children and adolescents with left ventricular hypertrophy, which can be caused by chronic hypertension. Therefore, the 2017 clinical practice guideline does not recommend performing electrocardiography in hypertensive children and adolescents, even in those being evaluated for left ventricular hypertrophy.

While an ACE inhibitor (Answer D) or other hypertensive agent may be appropriate to prescribe in certain situations, pharmacotherapy is typically reserved for children and adolescents who remain hypertensive despite lifestyle modifications, those with symptomatic hypertension, those with stage 2 hypertension without a clearly modifiable risk factor such as obesity, or any stage of hypertension that is associated with chronic kidney disease or diabetes.

Ambulatory blood pressure monitoring (ABPM) (Answer B) records blood pressure periodically (usually every 20 to 30 minutes) throughout the day and night with the data downloaded for later analysis. While ABPM has been recommended for the confirmation of hypertension in adults before starting treatment, there are still gaps in access and knowledge on how best to incorporate ABPM into the evaluation of elevated blood pressure in children and adolescents. However, ABPM has been shown to be more accurate than in-office measurements and is more predictive of future blood pressure. Therefore, the 2017 clinical practice guideline does recommend ABPM, when possible, for confirmation of hypertension in children and adolescents who have office blood pressure measurements in the elevated category for 1 or more years or those who have stage 1 hypertension over 3 clinic visits. The guideline also recommends that ABPM be strongly considered in those with high-risk conditions. ABPM would not be the appropriate next step for the boy in this vignette for whom the diagnosis of hypertension is not yet established.

Educational Objective

Diagnose obesity-related hypertension in pediatric patients and anticipate challenges associated with the diagnosis.

Reference(s)

Flynn JT, Kaelber DC, Baker-Smith CM, et al; Subcommittee on Screening and Management of High Blood Pressure in Children. Clinical practice guideline for screening and management of high blood pressure in children and adolescents. *Pediatrics.* 2017;140(3):e20171904. PMID: 28827377

Hampl SE, Hassink SG, Skinner AC, et al. Clinical practice guideline for the evaluation and treatment of children and adolescents with obesity. *Pediatrics.* 2023;151(2):e2022060640. PMID: 36622115

Hardy ST, Urbina EM. Blood pressure in childhood and adolescence. *Am J Hypertens.* 2021;34(3):242-249. PMID: 33821942

86 ANSWER: E) Suggest a therapeutic trial of combination therapy with levothyroxine, 112 mcg daily, and liothyronine, 2.5 mcg twice daily

This patient has postsurgical hypothyroidism, and despite TSH normalization she continues to struggle with symptoms. This is a very common issue in adults, and it is gaining more attention in pediatrics. No pediatric studies have been conducted that describe outcomes of combination levothyroxine and liothyronine or desiccated thyroid extract compared with outcomes of levothyroxine monotherapy. However, families often ask about alternative therapies, and physicians should engage in shared decision-making and offer families safe options coupled with appropriate monitoring.

Animal and human studies show that compared with euthyroid individuals, hypothyroid patients treated with levothyroxine monotherapy have higher free T_4 levels and free T_4-to-T_3 ratios, which are associated with lower T_3 levels. Multiple studies show that even when TSH normalizes, the T_3 concentration is frequently in the lower end of the reference range or even below the reference range. Therefore, normalization of TSH and free T_4 does not necessarily normalize all thyroid hormone concentrations in the blood or in all tissues. T_4-to-T_3 conversion occurs predominantly through the action of deiodinase 2 (D2) and is inhibited by the presence of T_4. This negative regulation occurs more slowly in the hypothalamus and pituitary than in peripheral tissues. There is more efficient conversion of T_4 to T_3 centrally and resultant TSH normalization before peripheral T_3 levels normalize.

Many groups have advocated for use of combination levothyroxine/liothyronine therapy with a goal of normalizing TSH, free T_4, and T_3 levels. Multiple randomized clinical trials have been performed in adults, which show no overall benefit of combination therapy over levothyroxine monotherapy. These studies have included numerous populations and widely variable dosing regimens, monitoring, and outcome measures. Despite these flaws and lack of evidence of superiority, several blinded randomized trials have shown a patient preference for combination therapy (levothyroxine/liothyronine) over levothyroxine monotherapy.

When a patient requests combination dosing, several things should be considered:

- In vivo, the thyroid gland produces T_4 and T_3 in a 14:1 ratio. Previous clinical trials have used ratios of levothyroxine-to-liothyronine ranging from 4:1 to 19:1.
- The pharmacologic equivalence of liothyronine to levothyroxine is approximately 1:3.
- T_3 in vivo remains at a steady level, and liothyronine has a short half-life; therefore, to mimic physiologic levels, it should be given as a slow-release pill (not available) or multiple times daily. In practical terms, studies have used twice-daily dosing, although this still results in marked variability in levels throughout the day.
- Combination therapy can be considered for patients who remain symptomatic and who have low T_3 levels.

This pediatric patient has stable TSH levels on levothyroxine, 125 mcg daily. The levothyroxine dosage must be reduced if liothyronine is added. One potential option is levothyroxine, 112 mcg daily, and liothyronine, 2.5 mcg twice daily (Answer E). The 5 mcg per day of liothyronine is pharmacologically equivalent to 15 mcg of levothyroxine. This, plus 112 mcg levothyroxine, is similar to the current levothyroxine dosage of 125 mcg daily. The ratio of levothyroxine-to-liothyronine is 22:1. The dosage can certainly be adjusted based on therapeutic response.

A regimen of levothyroxine, 100 mcg daily, and liothyronine, 25 mcg daily (Answer C), is incorrect for 2 reasons: the overall combined dose equivalent of thyroid hormone replacement far exceeds the previous levothyroxine dosage, and liothyronine should be administered at least twice daily.

Recommending that she continue current therapy (Answer D) is incorrect in this particular case. The patient's family is informed and highly motivated to switch therapy. The risk of refusing to engage with the family is that they may choose to seek care from someone willing to prescribe the alternative treatment, perhaps without appropriate dosing and/or follow-up monitoring.

Treatment with a desiccated thyroid preparation is typically not preferred by thyroid and endocrine societies for a variety of reasons:

- Variability in medication content
- Higher content of T_3 relative to T_4
- Once-daily preparation

However, desiccated thyroid preparations have not been proven harmful (Answer A). Some argue that future well-designed trials of combination thyroid hormone treatment should also include an arm randomly assigned to receive a desiccated thyroid preparation.

Measuring reverse T_3 (Answer B) would not help determine whether a trial of combination therapy may be helpful. Total (and free) T_3 (not reverse T_3) is low in many patients on levothyroxine monotherapy. The goal of combination levothyroxine/liothyronine therapy is to normalize T_4, T_3, and TSH levels. If all levels are well within normal limits on monotherapy, there may not be justification for combination therapy.

Educational Objective

Explain the potential rationale for combination levothyroxine/liothyronine therapy in the setting of hypothyroidism and guide appropriate management.

Reference(s)

Jonklaas J, Bianco AC, Coppola AR, et al. Evidence-based use of levothyroxine/liothyronine combinations in treating hypothyroidism: a consensus document. *Thyroid.* 2021;31(2):156-182. PMID: 33276704

Millan-Alanis JM, Gonzalez-Gonzalez JG, Flores-Rodríguez A, et al. Benefits and harms of levothyroxine/L-triiodothyronine versus levothyroxine monotherapy for adult patients with hypothyroidism: systematic review and meta-analysis. *Thyroid.* 2021;31(11):1613-1625. PMID: 34340589

Rii KR, Larsen CB, Bonnema SJ. Potential risks and benefits of desiccated thyroid extract for the treatment of hypothyroidism: a systematic review. *Thyroid.* 2024;34(6):687-701. PMID: 38526391

Shakir MKM, Brooks DI, McAninch EA, et al. Comparative effectiveness of levothyroxine, desiccated thyroid extract, and levothyroxine+liothyronine in hypothyroidism. *J Clin Endocrinol Metab.* 2021;106(11):e4400-e4413. PMID: 34185829

87 ANSWER: A) Gain-of-function pathogenic variant in the *FGFR3* gene (fibroblast growth factor receptor 3)

The physical and radiographic descriptions in this case are consistent with achondroplasia, the most common type of skeletal dysplasia resulting in marked short stature. Most individuals with achondroplasia are diagnosed in early infancy, although prenatal recognition has become more frequent and more accurate. It is critical that the diagnosis be made as early as possible because certain complications can only be prevented through evaluation in early infancy. Well-defined clinical and radiologic characteristics of achondroplasia usually allow for a clinical diagnosis with virtual certainty.

While small size is not a constant feature in newborns, who may have lengths within the normal range, rhizomelic (proximal) shortening is uniformly present, at least in the arms. Macrocephaly is usually present at birth and remains so throughout life. Underdevelopment of cartilaginous bones of the face results in flattening of the entire midface and a flat nasal bridge, a short nasal spine, and anteversion of the nose. Short fingers and a trident configuration (excess separation between the third and fourth fingers; *see image*) of the hands are distinct features. Other physical features include a small chest, hypermobility of the hips and knees, and hypotonia. Diagnostic confirmation requires radiographic assessment. Helpful diagnostic features include short tubular long bones, squared-off iliac wings, flat and horizontal acetabula, marked narrowing of the sacrosciatic notch, characteristic proximal femoral radiolucency, narrowing of the interpediculate distance of the caudal spine (which may not be present in the neonate), and short proximal and middle phalanges.

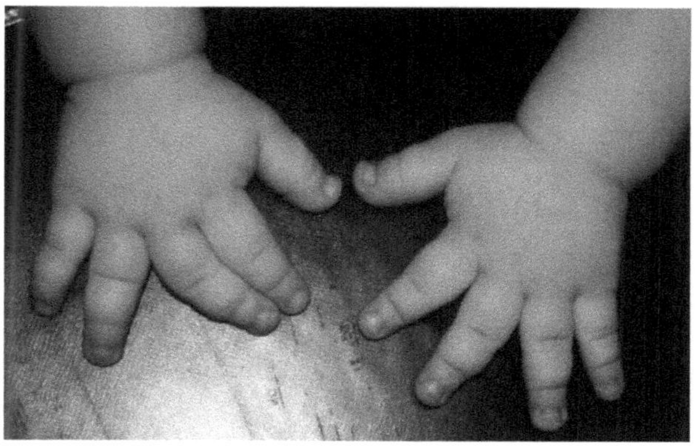

Reprinted from Pauli RM. *Orphanet J Rare Dis*, 2019; 14(1): 1. © The Authors. Published by BioMed Central Ltd., a part of Springer Nature.

Achondroplasia is caused by gain-of-function pathogenic variants in the FGF receptor 3 gene (*FGFR3*) (Answer A). FGFR3 is a tyrosine kinase receptor that normally acts as a negative regulator of bone growth by inhibiting the proliferation and differentiation of chondrocytes. The most common (98%) variant in *FGFR3* is a point variant where glycine is replaced by arginine at position 380 (G380R) in the transmembrane domain of the FGFR3 protein. This variant leads to constitutive activation of FGFR3, meaning the receptor is always "on," even in the absence of its ligand (FGF). This constant activation results in excessive inhibition of chondrocyte proliferation and differentiation, disrupting the normal process of endochondral ossification and leading to the characteristic skeletal features of achondroplasia.

Approximately 80% of achondroplasia cases result from spontaneous (de novo) pathogenic variants in the *FGFR3* gene, rather than being inherited from a parent. This means that in about 4 out of 5 cases, neither parent has achondroplasia nor carries the pathogenic variant. Advanced paternal age is considered a contributing factor in cases of spontaneous achondroplasia. This high rate of spontaneous mutation makes achondroplasia unique among many genetic disorders and contributes to its relatively stable prevalence in the population despite potential reproductive challenges for affected individuals.

C-type natriuretic peptide (CNP) has a crucial role in stimulating endochondral ossification and bone growth. CNP binds to its receptor, natriuretic peptide receptor-B (NPR-B), which is encoded by the *NPR2* gene. This receptor is expressed on growth plate chondrocytes. The binding of CNP to NPR-B stimulates the production of cyclic guanosine monophosphate (cGMP), initiating a signaling cascade that promotes bone growth. CNP signaling through NPR-B can antagonize the growth-inhibitory effects of FGFR3 activation. This is particularly relevant in achondroplasia, where FGFR3 is constitutively activated. CNP is elevated in achondroplasia, which is thought to be a compensatory mechanism counteracting the growth inhibiting effects of FGFR3, as CNP is a positive regulator of bone growth. Treatment with CNP analogues aims to enhance this effect.

Pathogenic variants in the CNP/NPR2 system can lead to various growth disorders. Loss-of-function variants (Answer E) cause short stature, while gain-of-function variants (Answer C) result in tall stature. Autosomal dominant heterozygous loss-of-function variants in the *NPR2* gene are associated with short stature without overt skeletal dysplasia and have been identified in 2% to 6% of individuals with idiopathic short stature. Homozygous loss-of-function variants in the *NPR2* gene cause acromesomelic dysplasia, Maroteaux type (AMDM), a skeletal dysplasia characterized by extreme short stature and disproportionate shortening of the middle and distal segments of the limbs (mesomelia) (unlike achondroplasia which affects the proximal segments of the limbs [rhizomelia]). Individuals with AMDM generally have normal facial features, whereas achondroplasia is characterized by distinct facial features, including a large head, prominent forehead, and midface hypoplasia.

Gain-of-function pathogenic variants in the *FGF23* gene (Answer B) cause autosomal dominant hypophosphatemic rickets, a disorder characterized by low serum phosphorus levels, rickets, and genu varum or valgum—features that are not consistent with the patient in this vignette.

Loss-of-function pathogenic variants in the *FGFR3* gene (Answer D) cause camptodactyly, tall stature, and hearing loss (CATSHL) syndrome. The *FGFR3* gene normally acts as a negative regulator of bone growth. Therefore, loss-of-function pathogenic variants in *FGFR3* lead to reduced function of the FGFR3 protein, resulting in enhanced proliferation of growth plate chondrocytes, which explains the tall stature in affected individuals.

* *Images in the vignette reprinted from Llerena Jr J, Kim CA, Fano V, et al. Achondroplasia in Latin America: practical recommendations for the multidisciplinary care of pediatric patients.* BMC Pediatr. *2022;22(1):492.*

Educational Objective

Describe the clinical manifestations and characteristic features of achondroplasia and explain the molecular basis of this condition.

Reference(s)

Llerena Jr J, Kim CA, Fano V, et al. Achondroplasia in Latin America: practical recommendations for the multidisciplinary care of pediatric patients. *BMC Pediatr.* 2022;22(1):492. PMID: 35986266

Lui JC, Baron J. CNP-related short and tall stature: a close-knit family of growth disorders. *J Endocr Soc.* 2022;6(6):bvac064. PMID: 35528827

Pauli RM. Achondroplasia: a comprehensive clinical review. *Orphanet J Rare Dis.* 2019;14(1):1. PMID: 30606190

Vasques GA, Arnhold IJP, Jorge AAL. Role of the natriuretic peptide system in normal growth and growth disorders. *Horm Res Paediatr.* 2014;82(4):222-229. PMID: 25196103

88 **ANSWER: E) Start GH treatment**

The child in this vignette meets criteria to be classified as being small-for-gestational-age based on both weight and length at birth. The etiology can be due to maternal factors (eg, inadequate nutrition, chronic disease in the mother, multiple births, parental genetic factors), placental insufficiency, fetal syndromes, and/or environmental factors (eg, adolescent pregnancy, maternal cigarette smoking or substance abuse, high altitude). Most children born small-for-gestational-age (~90%) undergo linear growth acceleration in the first year of life, so-called catch-up growth that is mostly completed by 2 years of age. However, approximately 10% of children born small-for-gestational-age do not display such acceleration and fail to catch up. GH treatment (Answer E) is approved by the US FDA for the management of short stature in children born small-for-gestational-age when catch-up growth has not occurred by 2 years of age and is approved by the European Medicines Agency if catch-up growth has not occurred by 4 years of age. As such, the best course of action is to start GH treatment for this patient.

He has a family history of constitutional delay, which is a common explanation for short stature in childhood. However, his bone age is equivalent to chronological age, which is not consistent with constitutional delay and indicates a low likelihood of catch-up growth without intervention. Midparental height, GH dosage, age, and height SDS at the start of therapy are associated with response to GH treatment. Late initiation of GH therapy in children who are small-for-gestational-age without catch-up growth would be suboptimal, as earlier treatment initiation is associated with better outcomes. Thus, simply following this patient's height velocity (Answer A) is incorrect.

While mean circulating IGF-1 and IGFBP-3 levels are somewhat lower in children who are small-for-gestational-age, classic GH deficiency is rare in this population. This patient's IGF-1 and IGFBP-3 values are not suggestive of GH deficiency and his height velocity is normal; thus, performing a GH-stimulation test (Answer B) is not indicated. Also, GH-stimulation testing is not required before initiating treatment in children who are small-for-gestational-age.

Although this patient did not demonstrate linear growth acceleration seen in approximately 90% of children born small-for-gestational-age, his weight progressed to the third percentile, resulting in normal BMI. His linear growth failure is not related to poor weight gain, so referral to gastroenterology (Answer D) is not the best answer.

Birth length in SHOX deficiency (Answer C) is only mildly reduced. Children younger than 6 years who have SHOX insufficiency may not yet have developed characteristic features such as Madelung deformity and mesomelic limb shortening, but short stature is typically already evident by preschool age, indicating an abnormal growth rate in early childhood. The presentation in this vignette is not consistent with SHOX deficiency.

Educational Objective

Identify indications for GH treatment in children born small-for-gestational-age who do not display catch-up growth in the first 3 years of life.

Reference(s)

Clayton PE, Cianfarani S, Czernichow P, Johannsson G, Rapaport R, Rogol A. Management of the child born small for gestational age through adulthood: a consensus statement of the International Societies of Pediatric Endocrinology and the Growth Hormone Research Society. *J Clin Endocrinol Metab.* 2007;92(3):804-810. PMID: 17200164

Houk CP, Lee PA. Early diagnosis and treatment referral of children born small for gestational age without catch-up growth are critical for optimal outcomes. *Int J Pediatr Endocrinol.* 2012(1):11. PMID: 22559301

89 **ANSWER: B) Continue activity/exercise mode until bedtime on gymnastics days**

Individuals with type 1 diabetes are often less active than their peers without diabetes due to challenges of glycemic management with exercise. Automated insulin delivery (AID) systems (ie, hybrid closed-loop pumps) have made exercise safer but require different strategies to prevent excessive glucose variability. AID systems allow for more flexibility than multiple daily injections or traditional pumps, but during exercise, reductions in insulin delivery via AID systems still cannot match the rapid changes in blood glucose levels. Strategies for using AID systems with exercise include minimizing insulin on board during exercise, adding extra carbohydrates to balance the increase in glucose use, and setting a higher blood glucose target to reduce risk of hypoglycemia.

In general, insulin sensitivity is increased for up to 11 hours after exercise. Prolonged or intensive exercise such as gymnastics may cause delayed hypoglycemia many hours later. Research shows that setting a higher glucose target starting 1 to 2 hours before exercise and extending the higher target into postexercise recovery (Answer B) can reduce the risk of delayed hypoglycemia.

Additional strategies may be used, including consuming additional carbohydrates. While consuming a 15 g snack before exercise along with use of activity mode during exercise (Answer A) would increase the likelihood that glucose is in range during exercise, this approach does not address the issue of delayed hypoglycemia.

Reducing basal insulin rates (Answer E) is an effective strategy for open-loop pumps, but for those using AID systems this requires the user to exit automated mode. This creates the risk of forgetting to resume automated mode after exercise. Likewise, prolonged pump suspension may not be as effective as setting a higher exercise target 1 to 2 hours before the start of activity, and it also increases the risk of forgetting to resume insulin delivery after exercise.

Reducing mealtime bolus insulin, along with use of a higher blood glucose target, can reduce time in hypoglycemia vs just changing the blood glucose target. However, optimal timing for this strategy requires exercise about 90 minutes after the meal. If exercise occurs later, there may be more insulin on board at the time of exercise, as the reduced mealtime bolus is likely to elicit an increase in insulin delivery by the AID system. In this vignette, gymnastics after school is taking place several hours after lunch. Thus, entering half the carbohydrates at lunch (Answer C) is likely to be counterproductive, as the resulting hyperglycemia would trigger additional automated insulin delivery.

Several AID systems use learning algorithms that can respond to the user's insulin requirements to adapt automated insulin delivery. However, these systems still require adjustments for exercise (thus, Answer D is incorrect). For AID systems that do not rely on user-programmed settings, the user can raise the blood glucose target while exercising or disconnect from the pump during exercise and reconnect after. Users can also consume carbohydrates after disconnecting, so the pump does not deliver insulin.

Educational Objective

Prevent exercise-related hypoglycemia with hybrid closed-loop automated insulin delivery systems.

Reference(s)

Paldus B, Morrison D, Lee M, et al. Strengths and challenges of closed-loop insulin delivery during exercise in people with type 1 diabetes: potential future directions. *J Diabetes Sci Technol.* 2023;17(4):1077-1084. PMID: 35466723

Zaharieva DP, Morrison D, Paldus B, et al. Practical aspects and exercise safety benefits of automated insulin delivery systems in type 1 diabetes. *Diabetes Spectr.* 2023;36(2):127-136. PMID: 37193203

90 ANSWER: E) Repeat newborn screening at 2 weeks of age

Newborn screening for congenital hypothyroidism is recommended for all newborns between 24 hours of life and hospital discharge or 1 week of age, whichever is sooner. Repeating newborn screening at 2 to 4 weeks of age (Answer E) is recommended for specific categories of babies who are at risk of hypothyroidism that may not be detected on initial screening, including same-sex twins (or higher-order multiple births). In most sets of twins in which one baby has congenital hypothyroidism, the other twin is unaffected. Repeating newborn screening is recommended for same-sex twins because possible fetal blood mixing (particularly in monochorionic twins) may allow normal thyroid function in an unaffected twin to compensate for congenital hypothyroidism in the other, causing newborn screening to be normal in both twins immediately after birth, before hypothyroidism develops in the affected twin. Repeating newborn screening is also recommended in neonates who are preterm (<32 weeks), have very low birth weight (<1500 g), are acutely ill, or have trisomy 21.

Hypothyroidism is common in individuals of reproductive age. In most cases, the presence of treated maternal hypothyroidism does not significantly increase the risk of hypothyroidism in a newborn. The most common cause of maternal hypothyroidism is autoimmune thyroiditis, which in many cases is associated with the presence of TPO antibodies. TPO antibodies are a marker of autoimmune thyroid inflammation, but they do not have a significant direct pathogenic role. Although TPO antibodies are of the IgG class and can cross the placenta, they do not cause fetal or neonatal hypothyroidism. Therefore, measurement of TPO antibodies in these newborn twins (Answer A) would not be clinically useful.

A small percentage of individuals with autoimmune thyroiditis may have TRAb that can cross the placenta and cause fetal or neonatal hypothyroidism that resolves over the first months of life as the maternal antibodies are cleared. Measurement of TRAb may be indicated in babies with congenital hypothyroidism or in their mother when this etiology is suspected, but it is not necessary in babies with normal thyroid function on newborn screening (Answers B and C).

Educational Objective

Recommend repeating newborn screening for hypothyroidism in same-sex twins.

Reference(s)

Rose SR, Wassner AJ, Wintergerst KA, et al; Section on Endocrinology Executive Committee; Council on Genetics Executive Committee. Congenital hypothyroidism: screening and management. *Pediatrics.* 2023;151(1):e2022060419. PMID: 36827523

van Trotsenburg P, Stoupa A, Léger J, et al. Congenital hypothyroidism: a 2020-2021 consensus guidelines update-an ENDO-European Reference Network Initiative endorsed by the European Society for Pediatric Endocrinology and the European Society for Endocrinology. *Thyroid.* 2021;31(3):387-419. PMID: 33272083

91 **ANSWER: B) Enhanced glucagon secretion**

Glucose-dependent insulinotropic polypeptide (GIP) and GLP-1 are peptides known as incretins. They are secreted from the gastrointestinal tract into the circulation when nutrients are ingested, leading to increased insulin secretion in a glucose-dependent manner. Native GIP is released from K cells in the duodenum and upper jejunum, but it is also found throughout the small intestine. Fat is the most potent stimulator of GIP secretion in humans. GLP-1 is a posttranslational product of proglucagon released from intestinal L cells, located primarily in the distal ileum and colon, in response to nutrient ingestion that enhances glucose-stimulated insulin secretion. Ingestion of meals, particularly those rich in fats and carbohydrates, is the primary stimulus for GLP-1 secretion. The 2 incretins synergistically lower blood glucose levels by stimulating insulin secretion from β cells and jointly account for the incretin effect in humans, which is the phenomenon where oral glucose consumption leads to higher insulin production compared with that induced by intravenous glucose. The half-life of native GLP-1 in the circulation is less than 2 minutes due to rapid inactivation by the enzyme DPP-4. The half-life of native GIP is only slightly longer than that of GLP-1: 7 minutes in healthy individuals and 5 minutes in those with type 2 diabetes.

Tirzepatide is distinct from other GLP-1 therapies in that it targets not only the GLP-1 receptor, but also the GIP receptor. Its half-life is 5 days, which allows for once-weekly dosing. Semaglutide is a GLP-1 receptor analogue with 94% homology to human GLP-1. Importantly, due to structural modifications, it has a much longer half-life than native GLP-1 (165 to 184 hours), which also allows for once-weekly dosing. In addition to blood glucose lowering, both agents also promote weight loss through beneficial effects on metabolic rate, appetite reduction, and reduction in energy intake. This has contributed to their use as antiobesity medications.

In contrast to GLP-1 action, GIP receptor agonism stimulates α cells in the pancreas to promote glucagon secretion (Answer B). GLP-1, however, is inhibitory.

While native GIP is secreted from K cells in the duodenum and upper jejunum, there is no evidence that tirzepatide enhances native GIP secretion (thus, Answer D is incorrect). Rather, it is a dual GIP/GLP-1 receptor co-agonist with a similar affinity for GIP receptors as native GIP.

Although treatment with either tirzepatide or semaglutide leads to weight reduction in randomized controlled trials, studies have consistently reported that tirzepatide treatment results in a greater percentage weight loss, likely because of its dual agonist effects (thus, Answer E is incorrect).

GIP also exhibits unique actions in extrapancreatic tissues, including bone. There is significant expression of the GIP receptor in mature human osteoclasts. Through multiple signaling pathways, GIP works to reduce osteoclast differentiation and impair bone resorption (thus, Answer A is incorrect).

Both GLP-1 and GIP affect insulin secretion in a glucose-dependent fashion (thus, Answer C is incorrect).

Educational Objective

Explain differences in mechanism of action between tirzepatide and semaglutide.

Reference(s)

Baggio LL, Drucker DJ. Biology of incretins: GLP-1 and GIP. *Gastroenterology.* 2007;132(6):2131-2157. PMID: 17498508

Frías JP, Davies MJ, Rosenstock J, et al; SURPASS-2 Investigators. Tirzepatide versus semaglutide once weekly in patients with type 2 diabetes. *N Engl J Med.* 2021;385(6):503-515. PMID: 34170647

Heise T, DeVries JH, Urva S, et al. Tirzepatide reduces appetite, energy intake, and fat mass in people with type 2 diabetes. *Diabetes Care.* 2023;46(5):998-1004. PMID: 36857477

Lempesis IG, Liu J, Dalamaga M. The catcher in the gut: tirzepatide, a dual incretin analog for the treatment of type 2 diabetes mellitus and obesity. *Metabol Open.* 2022;16:100220. PMID: 36530219

92 **ANSWER: D) Somatostatin analogue therapy**

This patient has evidence of GH excess on a background of neurofibromatosis type 1 (NF 1) with optic pathway gliomas (OPGs). Specifically, she has clinical and biochemical evidence of GH excess (accelerating height Z-score far exceeding midparental height, increased growth velocity not explained by precocious puberty, new obesity, glucose intolerance, elevated IGF-1, and post–oral glucose tolerance test GH value not suppressed below 1 ng/mL [<1 μg/L]). This entity has been described in individuals with NF 1, mostly in those with OPGs. Multiple mechanism(s) have been proposed, but no unifying explanation has clear evidence. OPGs could plausibly interrupt hypothalamic somatostatinergic inhibition of GH secretion, but again, not all patients even have OPGs, and not all of those OPGs are hypothalamic. Alternatively, OPGs can produce GHRH. However, limited studies, including immunocytochemical staining, do not support this hypothesis. Intriguingly, tumor overexpression of GPR101, the G-protein–coupled receptor that is pathogenic in genetic X-linked acrogigantism (X-LAG) (at least in part by causing increased GHRH production), has been reported in at least 1 individual. A subset of OPGs may overexpress GPR101, leading to GH excess via the same mechanism(s) as in X-LAG. These mechanisms remain the focus of investigation and include activation of G_s, $G_{q/11}$, and $G_{12/13}$, causing GH secretion.

Most relevant to the management of affected individuals, natural history studies have shown that this phenomenon can be transient and resolve within several years of initial presentation even with no treatment. Thus, while surgical resection (Answer E) is the initial approach to manage pituitary somatotroph adenomas with clinical GH excess, operative resection is not the most appropriate first step. Instead, if there are observable clinical effects of GH excess, such as those in this patient (excess linear growth, obesity, glucose intolerance) or others (cardiomegaly, hypertension, concern for any associated tumor progression), then medical management with somatostatin analogue therapy (Answer D) is a reasonable first step. Other medical management options include GH receptor antagonist or dopamine agonist (usually in combination with a somatostatin analogue), which can be targeted to achieve IGF-1 and growth velocity Z-scores in the reference range. Given the often transient nature of this problem, dose titration downward and eventual discontinuation of medical therapy is often possible.

While precocious puberty can complicate NF 1, with or without OPGs, and lead to excess linear growth and a high IGF-1 concentration for chronologic age, this patient has neither clinical nor laboratory evidence of early puberty. Thus, gonadotropin-releasing hormone analogue therapy (Answer B) is incorrect.

Chemotherapy (Answer C) is typically reserved for OPGs that convey a visual threat, and it would not be required in this scenario. Even if the tumor is the culprit with respect to excess GH production, there are other management options.

Finally, while OPGs themselves may overproduce GPR101, germline genetic testing (Answer A) is unlikely to reveal an additional problem (X-LAG) in this child with established NF 1.

Educational Objective

Formulate an approach to manage GH excess in the setting of neurofibromatosis type 1.

Reference(s)

Cambiaso P, Galassi S, Palmiero M, et al. Growth hormone excess in children with neurofibromatosis type-1 and optic glioma. *Am J Med Genet A*. 2017;173(9):2353-2358. PMID: 28631895

Drimmie FM, MacLennan AC, Nicoll JA, Simpson E, McNeill E, Donaldson MD. Gigantism due to growth hormone excess in a boy with optic glioma. *Clin Endocrinol (Oxf)*. 2000;53(4):535-538. PMID: 11012581

Hannah-Shmouni F, Trivellin G, Beckers P, et al. Neurofibromatosis type 1 has a wide spectrum of growth hormone excess. *J Clin Med*. 2022;11(8):2168. PMID: 35456261

Josefson J, Listernick R, Fangusaro JR, Charrow J, Habiby R. Growth hormone excess in children with neurofibromatosis type 1-associated and sporadic optic pathway tumors. *J Pediatr*. 2011;158(3):433-436. PMID: 21030036

93 **ANSWER: D) Pseudohypoaldosteronism type 1, autosomal recessive**

Pseudohypoaldosteronism is a heterogeneous group of rare inherited disorders with end-organ resistance to aldosterone, resulting in hyponatremia, hyperkalemia, and metabolic acidosis. Autosomal recessive pseudohypoaldosteronism (PHA) type 1 (Answer D) presents during the neonatal period with feeding difficulties and salt-wasting, leading to severe hyponatremia and hyperkalemia that typically persist during adulthood. Both aldosterone and plasma renin are significantly elevated. Pathogenic variants in the *SCNN1A*, *SCNN1B*, and *SCNN1G* genes, encoding 3 subunits (α-, β-, and γ-subunits, respectively) of the endothelial sodium transport channels (ENaC) of the kidney, colon, and sweat and salivary glands lead to inappropriate sodium loss and potassium retention. Infants presenting with hyponatremia and hyperkalemia and salt-wasting should be screened for primary adrenal insufficiency due to either congenital adrenal hypoplasia or salt-wasting forms of congenital adrenal hyperplasia (CAH) such as 21- hydroxylase deficiency, 3β-hydroxysteroid dehydrogenase type II, and lipoid CAH, as it is associated with PHA-like electrolyte imbalance. In fact, they should be treated as such while waiting for results of plasma aldosterone and plasma renin measurements, which both would be significantly elevated. Before administration of hydrocortisone and fludrocortisone, diagnostic laboratory tests should include ACTH and cortisol measurement and a complete adrenal steroid profile including 17-hydroxyprogesterone, 17-hydroxypregenolone, and adrenal androgen measurements. PHA type 1 requires aggressive and intensive fluid and electrolyte management. Treatment includes sodium chloride supplementation and potassium-binding resins such as kayexalate to address severe hyperkalemia. For persistent hyperkalemia, a thiazide diuretic may be added.

Autosomal dominant (or renal) PHA type 1 (Answer C) is caused by pathogenic variants in the *NR3C2* gene, which encodes the mineralocorticoid receptor. Although both aldosterone and plasma renin are elevated in individuals with autosomal dominant PHA type 1, this condition has a milder clinical presentation than autosomal recessive PHA type 1, with less severe salt-wasting restricted to the kidneys, and it typically presents later in infancy. Due to variable penetrance, some family members are asymptomatic and may be identified only after family studies.

PHA type 2 (Answer E), also called Gordon syndrome, is frequently inherited in an autosomal dominant manner. PHA type 2, caused by pathogenic variants in the *KLHL3* gene, may also be inherited in an autosomal recessive manner. Clinical presentation is variable with hyperkalemia being the most consistent clinical feature in both children and young adults. As with essential hypertension, blood pressure is usually normal in young people and hypertension develops later in life. PHA type 2 is genetically heterogeneous and is associated with pathogenic variants in at least 4 genes (*WNK1, WNK4, CUL3,* and KLHL3), which lead to excessive sodium and chloride reabsorption in the distal convoluted tubule with intravascular volume expansion. Plasma renin is suppressed with highly variable plasma aldosterone concentrations, but aldosterone is relatively low given the degree of hyperkalemia (elevated serum potassium is a potent stimulus for aldosterone secretion). Mild hyperchloremia and metabolic acidosis are associated findings. Hypercalciuria has been described with normal calcium and PTH concentrations. Initial treatment includes thiazide diuretics.

Infants with lipoid congenital adrenal hyperplasia (CAH) (Answer B) present with hyponatremia, hyperkalemia, hypoglycemia, and adrenal crisis. Plasma renin is elevated, but aldosterone levels are low or normal. Most cases of lipoid CAH are caused by recessive pathogenic variants in the gene encoding steroidogenic acute regulatory protein (*STAR*). A few patients with lipoid CAH have been reported to have pathogenic variants in the *CYP11A1* gene. Genetic males (46,XY) are undervirilized or are phenotypic females due to impaired production of sex steroids in the adrenal glands and gonads.

Infants with aldosterone synthase deficiency type 1 due to *CYP11B2* gene pathogenic variants (Answer A) present during infancy with frequent vomiting, a variable degree of hyponatremia, hyperkalemia, and metabolic acidosis, and poor growth. Aldosterone is undetectable and plasma renin is elevated.

Educational Objective

Suspect autosomal recessive pseudohypoaldosteronism type 1 based on presentation in the first week of life with severe salt-wasting and markedly elevated plasma renin and aldosterone levels.

Reference(s)

Altinkilic EM, Augsburger P, Pandey AV, Flück CE. Clinical spectrum of human STAR variants and their genotype-phenotype correlation. *J Endocrinol.* 2024;262(3):e240078. PMID: 38913505

Sarafoglou K, Reiner W, Hindmarsh PC. Congenital adrenal hyperplasia. In: Sarafoglou K, Hoffmann GF, Roth KS, eds. *Pediatric Endocrinology and Inborn Errors of Metabolism.* 2nd edition. New York, NY: McGraw-Hill Education; 2017:533-559.

Tajima t, Morikawa S, Nakamura A. Clinical features and molecular basis of pseudohypoaldosteronism type 1. *Clin Pediatr Endocrinol.* 2017;26(3):109-117.

94 ANSWER: C) Later peak height velocity

Attention-deficit/hyperactivity disorder (ADHD) affects approximately 10% of children in the United States, and two-thirds of those with this diagnosis are treated with stimulant medications. The most commonly reported adverse effects of stimulant treatment are reduced appetite and weight loss, affecting approximately 70% of children within 2 months of starting treatment. Weight loss is more common in prepubertal children than in pubertal adolescents.

The relationship between stimulant treatment and linear growth has been evaluated in multiple longitudinal observational studies. Studies on the effect of stimulant treatment on growth trajectories, however, have demonstrated conflicting results. A reduction in height velocity during the first year of treatment is commonly seen, but timing of pubertal development (Answer B) and magnitude of peak height velocity (Answer E) do not appear to be affected. However, one large longitudinal study (Harstad et al) demonstrated that prepubertal boys treated with stimulants have a later peak height velocity (13.5 years vs 12.9 years) (Answer C). Despite the possible slowing of height velocity in the first year of treatment, the impact on adult height is unclear. One large meta-analysis (Carucci et al) that included 18 studies and followed children 21 to 72 months from the start of treatment demonstrated a small but significant standard mean difference in height Z-scores of –0.27 (95% CI, 0.16-0.38) between the start and end of observation.

Many children take medication "holidays" over the summer months, and increased height velocity with weight gain have been demonstrated during these breaks from medication (thus, Answer D is incorrect).

Educational Objective

Review the effects of stimulants on growth in children.

Reference(s)

Biederman J, Spencer TJ, Monuteaux MC, Faraone SV. A naturalistic 10-year prospective study of height and weight in children with attention-deficit hyperactivity disorder grown up: sex and treatment effects. *J Pediatr.* 2010;157(4):635-640, 640.e1. PMID: 20605163

Carucci S, Balia C, Gagliano A, et al. Long term methylphenidate exposure and growth in children and adolescents with ADHD. A systematic review and meta-analysis. *Neurosci Biobehav Rev.* 2021;120:509-525. PMID: 33080250

Harstad EB, Weaver AL, Katusic SK, et al. ADHD, stimulant treatment, and growth: a longitudinal study. *Pediatrics.* 2014;134(4):e935-e944. PMID: 25180281

Ibrahim K, Donyai P. Drug holidays from ADHD medication: international experience over the past four decades. *J Atten Disord.* 2015;19(7):551-568. PMID: 25253684

Poulton AS, Bui Q, Melzer E, Evans R. Stimulant medication effects on growth and bone age in children with attention-deficit/hyperactivity disorder: a prospective cohort study. *Int Clin Psychopharmacol.* 2016;31(2):93-99. PMID: 26544899

Zachor DA, Roberts AW, Hodgens JB, Isaacs JS, Merrick J. Effects of long-term psychostimulant medication on growth of children with ADHD. *Res Dev Disabil.* 2006;27(2):162-174. PMID: 15955659

95 ANSWER: C) Genetic testing for pathogenic variants in the LH receptor gene (*LHCGR*)

This boy has GnRH-independent precocious puberty. GnRH-independent precocious puberty in males is suggested by the presence of virilization, usually in the absence of marked testicular enlargement. However, some mild enlargement is expected if there is significant testosterone production by the testes, as in this case. Despite having a testicular volume of 5 cc, this child has low gonadotropins and normal results on GnRH-stimulation testing, indicating this is GnRH-independent precocious puberty.

This boy's maternal grandfather is very short (60 in [152.4 cm]). The patient most likely inherited a pathogenic variant in the gene encoding the LH receptor (*LHCGR*) from his mother. Activating pathogenic variants in *LHCGR* can cause a form of GnRH-independent precocious puberty in boys (familial male-limited precocious puberty). This is inherited in an autosomal dominant manner, but it may occur sporadically. Female carriers of the pathogenic variant do not have a specific phenotype. Affected males usually have symptoms of early puberty by 1 to 3 years of age. In the absence of treatment, this is followed by rapid virilization and premature epiphyseal fusion, which leads to compromised final adult height. The best next step in this patient's management is genetic testing (Answer C).

Other forms of GnRH-independent precocious puberty include McCune-Albright syndrome and hCG-secreting tumors. McCune-Albright syndrome can usually be ruled out by the absence of fibrous bony dysplasia and cafe-au-lait spots, and hCG-secreting tumors can be ruled out by documenting a normal hCG concentration.

Karyotype analysis (Answer E) cannot detect pathogenic variants in the LH receptor gene.

The GnRH-stimulation testing is useful in cases of central precocious puberty, but this child already had one test with a negative result. Waiting 6 months to repeat GnRH-stimulation testing (Answer D) would not be beneficial.

Brain MRI (Answer B) is indicated in all boys with central precocious puberty, which this patient does not have.

Adrenal tumors can lead to peripheral precocious puberty; however, this patient's DHEA-S concentration is normal, so this is less likely to be the case. Also, this diagnosis would not explain why the maternal grandfather is very short. Adrenal CT (Answer A) is not indicated.

Educational Objective

Explain the pathogenesis of LH receptor defects and describe the associated clinical manifestations.

Reference(s)

Leschek, Ellen Werber MD. Familial male-limited precocious puberty. *Endocrinologist.* 2004;14(3):148-151.

96 ANSWER: C) Induction of skeletal muscle iodothyronine deodinase type 3

The patient in this vignette has severe critical illness, and his thyroid function test results are most consistent with nonthyroidal illness syndrome (sick euthyroid syndrome). His laboratory findings are typical of individuals with acute critical illness: a decrease in T_3 (total and free) and, with more severe illness, a decrease in T_4 and TSH. Reverse T_3 levels are elevated, although measurement of reverse T_3 is not necessary to make the diagnosis. Thyroid hormone metabolism is complex, and critical illness can affect laboratory results through multiple mechanisms. The extent of nonthyroidal illness (based on abnormalities in laboratory analytes, including how low T_3 is) often correlates with disease severity.

Thyroid hormone deodinases are enzymes that have a very important role in permitting tissue-specific thyroid hormone signaling and in the fine regulation of thyroid hormone homeostasis.

Thyroid hormone deodinases are preferentially expressed in different body tissues.

- Type 1 (D1) present in the liver, kidney, and thyroid catalyzes deiodination of T_4 at both inner ($T_4 \rightarrow$reverse T_3, $T_3 \rightarrow T_2$) and outer ($T_4 \rightarrow T_3$, reverse $T_3 \rightarrow T_2$) rings
- Type 2 (D2) present in brain, pituitary, thyroid, and skeletal muscle catalyzes deiodination of T_4 at the outer ring only ($T_4 \rightarrow T_3$, reverse $T_3 \rightarrow T_2$)
- Type 3 (D3) present in brain, skin, placenta, pregnant uterus, and fetal tissues catalyzes deiodination of T_4 at the inner ring only ($T_4 \rightarrow$reverse T_3, $T_3 \rightarrow T_2$)

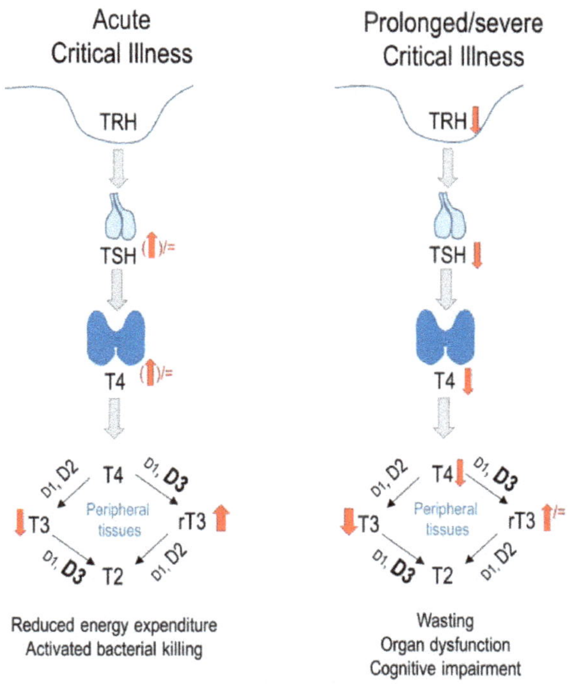

Figure 1. Schematic diagram of the biphasic changes observed in NTIS present in response to critical illness. Changes in the hypothalamus–pituitary–thyroid axis and in peripheral thyroid hormone metabolism. D1, D2, and D3 are iodothyronine deiodinase type 1, type 2, and type 3, respectively.

While all T_4 is produced in the thyroid gland, most circulating T_3 (approximately 80%) is produced by deiodination in the peripheral tissues (liver, kidney, skeletal muscle). Acute illness downregulates D1 expression in the liver and D2 in skeletal muscle, resulting in decreased T_3 production and decreased reverse T_3 clearance. In addition, D3 is induced in the liver and skeletal muscle, which causes more inactivation of T_4 (to reverse T_3) and T_3 (to T_2). D3 is not typically present in skeletal muscle; however, in states of severe illness, it is induced and contributes to the thyroid hormone laboratory changes seen in nonthyroidal illness (Answer C).

In the hypothalamus, the opposite occurs. Hypothalamic D2 is induced while D3 is inhibited (thus, Answers A and B are incorrect). These changes result in increased hypothalamic thyroid hormone availability and decreased TSH production through negative feedback.

Thyrotropin-releasing hormone expression is downregulated in critical illness, not upregulated (Answer E). The higher local hypothalamic availability of T_4 and T_3 results in decreased expression of thyrotropin-releasing hormone and pituitary TSH production. TSH is often low in the setting of nonthyroidal illness, but it is typically not as low as in patients with hyperthyroidism.

Many drugs can interfere with thyroid hormone metabolism. Induction of TSH secretion by dobutamine (Answer D) is incorrect because dobutamine suppresses the pituitary response to thyrotropin-releasing hormone. Other drugs commonly used in the intensive care unit setting can also affect thyroid hormone metabolism as follows:

- Iodine (eg, in topical antiseptic agents or intravenous contrast) can cause temporary hyperthyroidism or hypothyroidism
- Amiodarone can cause hypothyroidism, hyperthyroidism, and impaired conversion of T_4 to T_3
- β-Adrenergic blockers (eg, nadolol and propranolol) can cause impaired conversion of T_4 to T_3
- Glucocorticoids lower thyroid-binding globulin and can cause low total T_4 with normal free T_4 and also suppress TSH secretion by decreasing the pituitary response to thyrotropin-releasing hormone

Educational Objective

Describe the mechanism of laboratory changes seen in nonthyroidal illness.

Reference(s)

Fliers E, Boelen A. An update on non-thyroidal illness syndrome. *J Endocrinol Invest.* 2021;44(8):1597-1607. PMID: 33320308

Langouche L, Jacobs A, Van den Berge G. Nonthyroidal illness syndrome across the ages. *J Endocr Soc.* 2019;3(12):2313-2325. PMID: 31745528

Peeters RP, Wouters PJ, Kaptein E, van Toor H, Visser TJ, Van den Berghe G. Reduced activation and increased inactivation of thyroid hormone in tissues of critically ill patients. *J Clin Endocrinol Metab.* 2003;88(7):3202-3211. PMID: 12843166

Sahoo B, Dabas A, Goswami B, Agarwal A, Kurian S. Non-thyroidal illness in children with congestive heart failure. *J Clin Res Pediatr Endocrinol.* 2024;16(2):192-199. PMID: 38347684

97 **ANSWER: C) Glucocorticoid-remediable hyperaldosteronism**

Glucocorticoid-remediable hyperaldosteronism (GRA) (Answer C) is a rare autosomal dominant form of primary hyperaldosteronism. It is caused by a chimeric gene in which the 5′ regulatory sequences of the *CYP11B1* gene (encoding 11β-hydroxylase) are fused to the coding region of the *CYP11B2* gene (encoding aldosterone synthase), resulting in ectopic expression of aldosterone synthase in the zona fasciculata. As a result, the aldosterone synthase gene becomes abnormally regulated by ACTH because it is under the control of the *CYP11B1* gene promoter, which is under ACTH control for cortisol synthesis. Affected individuals can present with treatment-resistant hypertension, hypokalemia, and an aldosterone-to-plasma renin ratio greater than 30. Cerebral stroke or aneurysms are associated comorbidities during adulthood. GRA is typically treated with low doses of long-acting glucocorticoids at bedtime, such as dexamethasone or prednisone, to suppress ACTH secretion and ACTH-driven aldosterone production. As treatment with a glucocorticoid does not always normalize blood pressure, mineralocorticoid antagonists such as spironolactone and eplerenone can be used. Eplerenone may be preferred in affected children who are still growing.

Apparent mineralocorticoid excess (Answer A) is a rare autosomal recessive form of low-renin hypertension, marked hypokalemic alkalosis, low aldosterone levels, and high ratios of cortisol-to-cortisone metabolites. It is caused by pathogenic variants in the *HSD11B2* gene, encoding the enzyme 11β-hydroxysteroid dehydrogenase type 2 (11β-HSD2), which is primarily involved in the peripheral conversion of cortisol to cortisone. Affected children can present with poor growth, polydipsia, polyuria, and hypertension.

Congenital adrenal hyperplasia due to 17α-hydroxylase deficiency/17,20-lyase deficiency (Answer E) is caused by pathogenic variants in the *CYP17A1* gene and is characterized by low renin, low aldosterone, low 11-deoxycortisol, elevated 11-deoxycorticosterone, and low cortisol.

Congenital adrenal hyperplasia due to 11β-hydroxylase deficiency (Answer B) is caused by pathogenic variants in the *CYP11B1* gene and is characterized by low renin, low aldosterone, elevated 11-deoxycortisol, elevated 11-deoxycorticosterone, and low cortisol. Females present at birth with atypical genitalia.

Liddle syndrome (Answer D) is an autosomal dominant disorder due to increased activity of the epithelial sodium channel (ENaC) leading to sodium retention and hypertension. Affected individuals present with hypokalemia, suppressed aldosterone and renin, and metabolic alkalosis.

Educational Objective

Construct the differential diagnosis for primary hyperaldosteronism and diagnose glucocorticoid-remediable hyperaldosteronism in a patient with primary hyperaldosteronism.

Reference(s)

Funder JW, Carey RM, Mantero F, et al. The management of primary aldosteronism: case detection, diagnosis, and treatment: an Endocrine Society clinical practice guideline. *J Clin Endocrinol Metab.* 2016;101(5):1889-1916. PMID: 26934393

Ozdede M. Monogenic hypertension linked to the renin-angiotensin-aldosterone system. *Anatol J Cardiol.* 2024;28(9):417-428. PMID: 38872497

Sarafoglou K, Reiner W, Hindmarsh PC. Congenital adrenal hyperplasia. In: Sarafoglou K, Hoffmann GF, Roth KS, eds. *Pediatric Endocrinology and Inborn Errors of Metabolism.* 2nd edition. McGraw-Hill Education; 2017:533-559.

98 ANSWER: A) Add recombinant FSH

In boys, the onset of puberty, which typically occurs by age 14 years in the absence of pathology, is manifested by increases in the circulating concentrations of the pituitary hormones FSH and LH. Production of FSH and LH is stimulated by pulsatile secretion of the hypothalamic hormone GnRH. Pubertal initiation occurs after an interval of quiescence in GnRH secretion following the mini-puberty of infancy. FSH stimulates Sertoli cells to proliferate, which, in postpubertal boys, leads to both testicular growth and spermatogenesis. LH stimulates Leydig cells to produce testosterone, leading to virilization.

This patient has hypogonadotropic hypogonadism following treatment of craniopharyngioma. This diagnosis is supported by the absence of pubertal development on physical examination at nearly 14 years of age, undetectable gonadotropins on laboratory testing, and the presence of other anterior pituitary hormone deficiencies. The goals of pubertal induction include virilization (ie, secondary sexual characteristics) along with the other benefits of sex steroid exposure such as improved sexual function, bone health, muscle mass and strength, and quality of life. For some individuals, achieving fertility is a goal. Most often, pubertal induction is achieved with testosterone, which provides virilization effects but does not produce fertility or lead to the increases in testicular volume characteristic of physiologic puberty. In contrast, pubertal induction with gonadotropins, which have a relatively limited but growing evidence base, has the capacity to address both virilization and fertility issues and also increase testicular volume.

Current guidelines recommend a discussion of available options with patients and families, taking care to mention the heterogeneity of gonadotropin treatment approaches and the paucity of long-term outcome data, especially with respect to future fertility. At the time of this writing, there is not clear evidence to support a particular approach, and in the United States, pubertal induction with hCG is not currently routine clinical practice. Counseling such patients should also include discussion around available options for preserving future fertility, including possible referral to colleagues in urology or reproductive endocrinology with specific clinical expertise.

This patient and his family elected to start pubertal induction with gonadotropins. Treatment with hCG, which is structurally similar to LH (also a glycoprotein and active at the same receptor), is sufficient to produce increased circulating testosterone and associated virilization. The addition of recombinant FSH (Answer A) is required for stimulation of Sertoli cells to engage in spermatogenesis, which is required for the patient's requested sperm cryopreservation.

Increasing the hCG dosage (Answer D) is not the most appropriate next step because it will not lead to spermatogenesis. Similarly, continuing hCG for a longer duration (Answer C) is not likely to lead to further increases in testicular volume.

Germ cells, production of which requires recombinant FSH, constitute the largest proportion of volume in the mature testis. Some authors advocate for pretreatment with recombinant FSH before combination therapy with recombinant FSH and hCG because this approach more closely recapitulates typical physiologic pubertal progression and may optimize induction of spermatogenesis. However, long-term controlled data are lacking.

Adding testosterone (Answer B) is not necessary as his current testosterone concentration is appropriate for his Tanner stage. Moreover, exogenous testosterone would interfere with the benefits of gonadotropin treatment.

Pausing hCG to assess for spontaneous puberty (Answer E) is not warranted and not worth the adverse effects of discontinuation. The presence of other pituitary hormone deficiencies in this patient following treatment of craniopharyngioma makes recovery extremely unlikely.

Educational Objective

Explain the mechanism of pubertal induction with gonadotropins in males with hypogonadotropic hypogonadism.

Reference(s)

Alexander EC, Faruqi D, Farquhar R, et al. Gonadotropins for pubertal induction in males with hypogonadotropic hypogonadism: systematic review and meta-analysis. *Eur J Endocrinol.* 2024;190(1):S1-S11. PMID: 38128110

Abreu AP, Kaiser UB. Pubertal development and regulation. *Lancet Diabetes Endocrinol.* 2016;4(3):254-64. PMID: 26852256

Nordenstrom A, Ahmed SF, van den Akker E, et al. Pubertal induction and transition to adult sex hormone replacement in patients with congenital pituitary or gonadal reproductive hormone deficiency: an Endo-ERN clinical practice guideline. *Eur J Endocrinol.* 2022;186(6):G9-G49. PMID: 35353710

Rey RA. Recent advancement in the treatment of boys and adolescents with hypogonadism. *Ther Adv Endocrinol Metab.* 2022;13:20420188211065660. PMID: 35035874

Rohayem J, Hauffa BP, Zacharin M, Kliesch S, Zitzmann M, German Adolescent Hypogonadotropic Hypogonadism Study Group. Testicular growth and spermatogenesis: new goals for pubertal hormone replacement in boys with hypogonadotropic hypogonadism? -a multicentre prospective study of hCG/rFSH treatment outcomes during adolescence. *Clin Endocrinol (Oxf).* 2017;86(1):75-87. PMID: 27467188

99 ANSWER: C) Normal testosterone, very low estradiol, normal LH, high FSH

The patient in this vignette has the classic presentation of aromatase deficiency. Aromatase deficiency is a very rare autosomal recessive disorder due to pathogenic variants in the aromatase gene (*CYP19A1*). Aromatase is responsible for the conversion of testosterone to estradiol. Based on rare individuals with either aromatase deficiency or estrogen resistance, it has been discovered that estrogen is the hormone primarily responsible for growth plate fusion. Additionally, estrogen provides feedback to the pituitary to enhance GH production during puberty and is thus instrumental in the pubertal growth spurt in both males and females. As can be seen in this patient's growth chart, individuals with estrogen deficiency have a prolonged growth period with delay (or frank lack) of epiphyseal fusion and an absent pubertal growth spurt. Eunuchoid body proportions may develop, with increased arm span as compared with height.

Estrogen is also very important for increasing bone density. Estrogen deficiency leads to osteopenia and increases fracture risk. Other features seen in aromatase deficiency include abdominal adiposity, early-onset metabolic syndrome, genu valgum, acanthosis nigricans, dyslipidemia, bone pain, oligospermia, increased testicular volume, and scoliosis. Additionally, aromatase has an important role in the placenta, which is produced from fetal tissue, where it protects the mother from exposure to the fetus's androgens. When a fetus has aromatase deficiency, the mother can develop signs of virilization that reverse after the baby is delivered.

The hormonal profile characteristic of aromatase deficiency includes a very low estradiol concentration with a typically normal testosterone concentration (although this is variable), normal LH, and high FSH (Answer C).

Estrogen resistance due to pathogenic variants in the gene encoding the estrogen receptor can have a very similar phenotypic presentation, but from a hormonal perspective, affected persons have a very high estradiol concentration and high LH and FSH concentrations (Answer D). There is no virilization of the mother during pregnancy in patients with estrogen resistance.

Answers A and B represent hypogonadotropic and hypergonadotropic hypogonadism, respectively. While some of the features can overlap, the patient's robust testicular size and other clinical features make both conditions quite unlikely.

Answer E is the typical pattern for androgen insensitivity, which would not present in this fashion.

Educational Objective

Identify the hormonal profile expected in aromatase deficiency.

Reference(s)

Albuquerque EVA, Scalco RC, Jorge AAL. Management of endocrine disease: diagnostic and therapeutic approach of tall stature. *Eur J Endocrinol.* 2017;176(6):R339-R353. PMID: 28274950

Carani C, Qin K, Simoni M, et al. Effect of testosterone and estradiol in a man with aromatase deficiency. *N Engl J Med.* 1997;337(2):91-95. PMID: 9211678

Rochira V, Carani C. Aromatase deficiency in men: a clinical perspective. *Nat Rev Endocrinol.* 2009;5(10):559-568. PMID: 19707181

100 ANSWER: D) Initiate treatment with an estradiol patch, 6.25 mcg daily (one-quarter of 25 mcg patch)

Some girls with Turner syndrome have spontaneous thelarche and/or menarche. About 20% to 40% show some degree of pubertal development, with menarche in approximately 16% to 20% and regular menstrual cycles in 6%. However, 80% or more of girls with Turner syndrome need estrogen replacement therapy to initiate, progress, or maintain pubertal development. As indicated by some observations, an FSH concentration less than 10.0 mIU/mL (<10.0 IU/L) at 12 years or less than 6.7 mIU/mL (<6.7 IU/L) during mid-childhood (6-10 years) could be an indicator of spontaneous puberty and menstruation, but, most likely, treatment will be necessary at some point. Estradiol replacement for most girls should be initiated around 11 years of age. Estrogen depletion can adversely affect bone mineral density, and there is no reason to delay treatment initiation in this child who has signs of premature ovarian insufficiency.

Clinical guidelines recommend the use of low-dosage estradiol (E2) administered by the transdermal route. Incremental dose increases every 6 months can mimic normal puberty until the adult dosing is reached within a 2- to 3-year period. An acceptable starting dosage is 6.25 mcg per day (Answer D). As this child has no breast development at all, an initial dosage of 50 mcg twice weekly (Answer C) would be too high.

Observation without intervention until she is 15 years old (Answer E) is not appropriate in this child who already has signs of ovarian insufficiency.

Bone age (Answer A) can be used to estimate final adult height and help with the decision of whether initiation of estradiol treatment may be appropriate for some girls with Turner syndrome when they are younger than 11 years. Starting puberty induction at a younger age can result in a shorter final height than starting treatment at an older age, but this might be less of a concern in girls with tall predicted height (estimated from bone age). However, this child is already on GH treatment.

Progesterone is usually added after puberty induction or during sex hormone replacement to sustain puberty in girls after breakthrough bleeding or after at least 2 years of estradiol treatment. This girl has never been exposed to estradiol therapy; therefore, adding progesterone now (Answer B) is not necessary. Furthermore, addition of progesterone early in the treatment course can impair breast development.

Educational Objective

Initiate treatment to induce puberty in girls with Turner syndrome and premature ovarian insufficiency.

Reference(s)

Gravholt CH, Andersen NH, Christin-Maitre S, et al. Clinical practice guidelines for the care of girls and women with Turner syndrome. *Eur J Endocrinol.* 2024;190(6):G53-G151. PMID: 38748847

Gravholt CH, Andersen NH, Conway GS, et al, the International Turner Syndrome Consensus Group. Clinical practice guidelines for the care of girls and women with Turner syndrome: proceedings from the 2016 Cincinnati International Turner Syndrome Meeting. *Eur J Endocrinol.* 2017;177(3)G1-G70. PMID: 28705803

Nordenström A, Ahmed SF, van den Akker E, et al. Pubertal induction and transition to adult sex hormone replacement in patients with congenital pituitary or gonadal reproductive hormone deficiency: an Endo-ERN clinical practice guideline. *Eur J Endocrinol.* 2022;186(6):G9-G49. PMID: 35353710

Question-Mapping Index

PEDIATRIC ENDOCRINE SELF-ASSESSMENT PROGRAM 2025-2026

Part III

*This question-mapping index groups question topics according to the 7 umbrella sections of Pediatric ESAP (Adrenal, Bone, Carbohydrate and Lipid Metabolism/Obesity, Growth, Pituitary, Reproductive System, and Thyroid). Relevant **question numbers** follow each topic.*

ADRENAL

BONE

CARBOHYDRATE AND LIPID METABOLISM/OBESITY

GROWTH

PITUITARY

REPRODUCTIVE SYSTEM

THYROID

www.ingramcontent.com/pod-product-compliance
Ingram Content Group UK Ltd.
Pitfield, Milton Keynes, MK11 3LW, UK
UKHW050146040626
12888UKWH00039B/32

9 781936 704644